the best
Low-carb
cookbook

the best
Low-carb
cookbook

from Robert Rose

The Best Low-Carb Cookbook
Text and photographs copyright © 2005 Robert Rose Inc.

For complete cataloguing information, see page 370.

Disclaimer
The recipes in this book have been carefully tested by our kitchen and our tasters. To the best of our knowledge, they are safe and nutritious for ordinary use and users. For those people with food or other allergies, or who have special food requirements or health issues, please read the suggested contents of each recipe carefully and determine whether or not they may create a problem for you. All recipes are used at the risk of the consumer.

We cannot be responsible for any hazards, loss or damage that may occur as a result of any recipe use.

For those with special needs, allergies, requirements or health problems, in the event of any doubt, please contact your medical advisor prior to the use of any recipe.

Cover image: Turkiaki Fiesta (see recipe, page 241)

We acknowledge the financial support of the Government of Canada through the Book Publishing Industry Development Program (BPIDP) for our publishing activities.

Published by Robert Rose Inc.
120 Eglinton Avenue East, Suite 800, Toronto, Ontario, Canada M4P 1E2
Tel: (416) 322-6552; Fax: (416) 322-6936

Printed in Canada

1 2 3 4 5 6 7 8 9 FP 12 11 10 09 08 07 06 05 04

Contents

Introduction

Insulin resistance, pre-diabetes, glycemic index, low-carbohydrate — these are terms for our 21st century. What do these terms mean and, more importantly, what do they mean to us individually?

Over the last 20 years, nutritionists have guided the public to reduce fat intake according to U.S. government guidelines — in other words, 30% or less of the calories we take in should come from fat. But the guidelines did not differentiate among the types of fat. In order to reach this percentage, carbohydrates were added to many recipes. Since that time, despite our current obsession with dieting, we have become fatter, and a large percentage of our population is pre-diabetic, including an epidemic among young children.

The combination of a sedentary lifestyle and poor eating habits helps to explain the current rise of obese and overweight North Americans. A study from the University of California at Berkeley states that sweets, desserts, soft drinks and alcoholic beverages make up 25% of the total calories consumed by Americans. Salty snacks and fruit-flavored drinks make up another 5%.

Insulin resistance affects almost half of all Americans and an even higher percentage of those who are overweight. People with insulin resistance produce higher-than-normal amounts of insulin after eating carbohydrates. This promotes an increase in fat storage. The National Institutes of Health have cited insulin resistance as the "epidemic of the modern era." If you have an apple shape or a beer belly, have food cravings or can't lose weight — even if you don't cheat — there's a good chance that you are insulin resistant or **pre-diabetic**. As always, it is best to check with your doctor for a complete diagnosis.

The **glycemic index** was developed in the 1970s to measure how consumption of different types of foods increases blood sugar level. At that time, researchers found that eating a piece of white bread or a baked potato rapidly increased blood sugar levels. Lower glycemic foods cause blood sugar to rise and fall more slowly, and satisfy hunger longer.

Foods at the high end of the glycemic index should be avoided. These include sugary sodas; baked goods such as donuts and white-flour bagels; root vegetables (French fries, instant potatoes, pumpkin, parsnips), sweets (candies, jams); and snack foods such as corn chips and pretzels. A rule of thumb is to stay away from white foods and go for those that are green and brown. This means lots of green vegetables and limited amounts of brown rice or 100% whole wheat bread or pasta. A caution: read labels carefully. A loaf of bread may say 100% wheat, but you should look for 100% whole wheat. Other baked goods that may look brown are simply colored with caramel coloring. Ask for the nutrition information at a bakery. If they don't have it or won't give it to you, the likelihood is that the product is not made with whole wheat flour.

The theory behind a **low-carbohydrate** lifestyle is that cutting down on carbohydrates — not consuming a big plate of pasta as a main course, for example — prevents us from overstimulating insulin production, preventing peaks and valleys in blood sugar levels. It's important to eat a well-balanced meal three times a day and to have two small snacks during the day to keep a steady, even flow of insulin. What is a well-balanced meal? This is a question many medical people have a hard time answering. Outside of grilling a piece of fish and steaming vegetables, the answer seems to baffle them.

But you won't be in the same boat. The recipes in this book will help you plan delicious and healthful meals. No more diet boredom. With the recipes in this book, you can cut your carbs, but not the flavor or fun. This is a chance for those who have been a slave to their diets, following everything exactly as it is written, to expand their repertoire. Simply decide on the amount of carbohydrates that fits your lifestyle (See "Counting Carbs") and then select from the 500 recipes in this book. Variety will add spice to your meals. There are recipes from all around the world here. You can have Chinese one night, Italian the next and Cajun another evening.

The recipes in this book give you a wide choice of foods to fit every mood and palate. Plan your meals with them, and enjoy a happy and healthy low-carb lifestyle.

Carbohydrates, Fats and Proteins

There are three basic food elements, carbohydrates, fats and protein, all of which provide calories. All foods fit into at least one of these three categories.

CARBOHYDRATES

A carbohydrate is composed of carbon, hydrogen and oxygen. Bread, pasta, rice, corn and root vegetables are all carbohydrates, as are sugar, sweets, popcorn and pretzels. Look for complex carbohydrates such as brown rice or whole wheat pasta. Discard donuts, muffins, English muffins, Danish pastries, cookies, cakes and candies. A warning: there are several low-carb baked products available. Remember that even if a brownie has only 4 net carbs (see below), it still may have 350 calories — and these are empty calories. It's better to have a nourishing snack (see examples on page 12) that will stop your hunger and not simply add extra calories to your daily count.

Net carbs

Many labels say "net carbs," "net impact carbs" or "net effective carbs." What do these terms mean? The formula for net carbs, net impact carbs or net effective carbs is: carbs less fiber and sugar alcohols. This gives a net carb number. While it is correct to deduct fiber, as explained on page 9, it is not widely agreed upon whether deducting sugar alcohols is appropriate.

Sugar alcohols are sugar-free sweeteners such as sorbitol, malititol and mannitol. Sugar alcohols are neither sugar nor alcohol. They are called this because part of their structure chemically resembles sugar and part is similar to alcohols. The manufacturers say they subtract all sugar-alcohol grams from carbohydrate grams because, for the most part, sugar alcohols do not cause a sudden increase in blood glucose levels. However, many food scientists and chemists say we might absorb between 10% and 50%, depending on the sugar alcohol and the person consuming the food. They advise that half of sugar-alcohol grams should be counted, rather than zero. For example, if a low-carb candy bar has 20 g of carbs as sugar alcohol, you should count 10 g, not zero as the label says.

Fiber

Fiber is another story and an important one. What Grandma called roughage, scientists know as fiber. Fiber is an indigestible complex carbohydrate found in plants. Vegetables, seeds, oat bran, dried beans, oatmeal, barley, rye and fruits such as apples, oranges, pears, peaches and grapes are high in fiber. We need fiber in our diet. The recommended fiber intake is at least 25 to 30 g per day. Most of us do not get that amount. Remember, the purpose of a low-carb diet is not to cut out all carbs. It's to eat the types of foods that are slowly digested so that insulin is produced at a slow, even pace. Fiber helps slow digestion. This is why it can be deducted from the total carb count on a label. According to the American Diabetes Association, when you're counting carbs, if the meal has at least 5 g of fiber, you may subtract those grams from the total carb count. For example, if a meal contains 13 g of carbohydrates and 5 g of fiber, then the net count is 8 g of carbohydrates for that meal.

When counting carbohydrate grams, the bottom line is it is okay to subtract grams of fiber. However, subtract only half the grams of sugar alcohols.

FATS

There are "good" fats and "bad" fats. Monounsaturated fats such as canola or olive oil are considered good fats. Saturated fats, those from animal products such as meat or butter, should be eaten in moderation. Trans fats — processed fats made by adding hydrogen to liquid vegetable oil and then adding pressure — should be avoided. Trans fats can be found in cookies, crackers, icing, potato chips, margarine, microwave popcorn and most fried foods. Many manufacturers started including trans fats in their processed foods about 20 years ago to prolong the products' shelf life, but public health experts warn that these kinds of fats clog arteries and cause obesity. Avoid canola, soybean or cottonseed oil labeled "hydrogenated" or "partially hydrogenated." The order of ingredients in processed foods is also important. If hydrogenated fats are listed first, second or third, there are a lot of them in the food.

PROTEINS

Protein helps build many parts of the body, including muscle, bone, skin and blood. It is found in foods such as meat, fish, poultry, eggs, dairy products, beans, nuts and tofu. It is important to include proteins in a balanced, healthful diet.

Counting Carbs

The information out there about diets is very confusing, even statements as basic as "If we take in too many calories and don't expend energy, we gain weight." Can we eat cookies for breakfast, lunch and dinner, up to 1,200 calories worth, and lose weight? Obviously not. It's the type of calories that counts. The question is, what kinds of calories should we eat? A well-balanced, carb-conscious diet should include foods from all three food categories, including monounsaturated fats, lean proteins and complex carbohydrates.

Each recipe in this book has a nutritional analysis to help you choose the meal that best fits your needs. The nutritional analyses list values for calories and six different nutrients: protein, fat, carbohydrates, fiber, sodium and cholesterol. Keep in mind that the nutritional analyses are *per serving*. If the recipe yield gives a range of servings, such as "Serves 4 to 6," the analysis is always based on the larger number. In this example, the values would represent the amount of each nutrient in each of six servings of the recipe.

There are a few different stages to making the transition to a low-carbohydrate diet. First, you'll want to cut way back on carbs to lose weight quickly. Once you've reached your target weight, you'll want to gradually reintroduce the right carbs into your diet. Eventually, you'll get back up to the optimal amount of carbs you need each day to maintain a healthy weight.

The following guidelines tell you how much carbohydrate you should be aiming for over the course of a day. Remember, you need to divide this up into meals. So if you are aiming for, say, 40 g of carbohydrates in a day, you might want to take in 10 g at each of your three main meals, and 5 g for each of your snacks.

QUICK WEIGHT LOSS

To lose weight quickly, most low-carbohydrate proponents suggest an intake of about 30 to 40 g of carbohydrates per day. These meals should include lots of vegetables, at least 2 cups (500 mL) per meal. You should also exercise and drink plenty of water.

ADDING BACK SOME CARBS

Once you've lost weight, start reintroducing carbohydrates into your meals. Try to consume 75 to 85 g per day. These should be complex carbohydrates in measured amounts. Continue to eat plenty of vegetables and add a little fruit.

MAINTAINING YOUR WEIGHT LOSS

Finally, to maintain your weight loss and to achieve a balanced, healthy lifestyle, plan to eat an average of 125 to 135 g of carbohydrates per day on a permanent basis.

Tips for a Low-Carb Kitchen

STOCKING YOUR PANTRY AND REFRIGERATOR

The first step in adopting a low-carbohydrate lifestyle is to go through your pantry and refrigerator. Here are some tips on what to include and what to discard:

- Discard high glycemic foods such as white rice, bread and bagels made from white flour, jams, jellies, raisins, popcorn, crackers, pretzels, sugary syrups, cakes, cookies and candies. Also avoid highly processed or prepared foods.
- Remove processed low-fat foods. "Low-fat" or "no-fat" foods are usually high in carbohydrates. Remember, all foods fit into three categories: carbohydrates, fats and proteins. If a low-fat dressing has little fat and no protein, what's left? Just carbohydrates and chemicals.
- Keep small amounts of flour and sugar available, sugar for visiting friends and flour to lightly coat some foods and to thicken sauces.
- Herbs, seasonings and condiments are important flavor enhancers. Examples of foods that help add flavor to recipes without carbs are paprika, chili powder, curry powder, Chinese five-spice, mustard, horseradish, chili peppers, sesame seeds, capers, anchovies, sun-dried tomatoes, sweet pimentos, dried wild mushrooms, peanut butter, olive oil, canola oil, real oil-and-vinegar salad dressings, low-sodium soya sauce and hot pepper sauce.
- Keep canned tuna, salmon and tomatoes on hand for quick meals.
- Keep lots of fresh vegetables in the refrigerator, along with eggs, lower-fat cheese, cottage cheese, lean proteins (fish, poultry) and fresh herbs. Also stock mayonnaise made with soybean, corn or olive oil.

- Keep lots of frozen vegetables for those meals when you haven't had a chance to buy fresh. Tofu freezes well and adds protein to many dishes. Sausages can also be made into a quick meal.

EXAMPLES OF HEALTHFUL SNACKS
- ¼ cup (50 mL) nuts (almonds, pecans, walnuts, peanuts or a mixture)
- 2 celery stalks with 1 tablespoon (15 mL) chunky peanut butter
- 2 thin slices of lower-fat ham, chicken breast or turkey breast
- 2 ounces (60 g) lower-fat string cheese or other lower-fat cheese
- 1 hard-boiled egg
- edamame (soy beans)

COOKING TIPS
Stir-frying
- When using a wok, make sure it is very hot before adding ingredients. The oil should be smoking.
- To keep the ingredients crisp, let them sit in the wok for a few minutes before tossing. This allows the wok to regain heat that is lost when cold ingredients are added.
- So you don't have to look back at a recipe when stir-frying, place all of the ingredients on a plate or cutting board in the order of use.

Steaming
- If using a steamer, bring the water to a boil before adding the steaming basket with the food.
- Make sure the steaming basket does not touch the water.

Cooking protein
- Protein becomes rubbery when boiled. A hard-cooked egg should be simmered, not boiled. The poaching liquid for seafood or chicken should be brought just to the simmering point.

Sautéing
- When browning meat, add a little at a time. Wait several minutes before adding another piece. This gives the skillet a chance to regain its heat and make a caramelized crust on the meat.

ENTERTAINING

Weekend parties don't have to mean disaster for your low-carb lifestyle. There are many creative, festive dishes in this book that are low in carbohydrates. The "Appetizer" section, for example, has over 80 recipes. You can choose Mediterranean, Asian or Caribbean as your theme. For example, plan an entire party around Mediterranean tapas. Place an array of foods on a buffet table, along with a stack of small plates. Everyone can taste the various dishes and change their plates as they go. It makes for a fun evening and creates movement so that people can meet and talk.

Barbecues are a great way to entertain casually. Use spice rubs and oil-and-vinegar marinades instead of sugary barbecue sauces. Fill the table with an array of colorful foods from the "Side Dishes" section.

Brunch can be fun without the muffins and bagels. Look for the omelet and crustless quiche recipes in the "Vegetarian Meals" section, and add attractive salads from "Soups and Salads."

Most parties seem to end with everyone milling around the kitchen. Select two or three recipes from the soups in "Soups and Salads" and leave large pots on the stove. Let everyone come into the kitchen and help themselves.

Tips for Eating Out

About 60% of our meals are prepared outside the home. They're either eaten out or brought in. In addition, portion sizes have steadily grown over the years. The latest edition of *Joy of Cooking* proves this point. Meals that fed 4 to 6 in the original book now feed 2 to 3. Restaurant portions can often feed two instead of one. When in a restaurant, ask to take some of your meal home. It will make a good snack or lunch the next day.

Have a snack (see page 12) before going out to a cocktail party or dinner. The usual strategy before one of these events is to eat very little for lunch, or no lunch. The result can be disaster. You sit down at the table, and the bread basket is staring at you. It's hard to resist, especially if you've ordered a drink or a glass of wine. (One tip is to ask for the bread to be brought with the main course.) Or, if you're out at a cocktail party, you'll probably grab the first piece of food that comes along, and it's likely to be fried in thick batter or served on bread or crackers. The solution is to eat a well-balanced lunch and have a small snack around 4 p.m.

Alcohol is another issue. The American Diabetes Association recommends a maximum of one glass of wine (that's a 3.5-ounce glass) or one drink per day for women and two glasses of wine or two drinks for men. Watch out for the mixers. Many, such as tonic, have a lot of carbs. Read the labels. If you are on a strict low-carbohydrate diet, alcohol should be avoided.

Here are some tips to help you stick to your diet while you're out at a restaurant:

- Avoid sugary drinks.
- Opt for roasted or grilled meats.
- Make sure to include vegetables with your meal.
- Ask for two vegetables rather than a vegetable and a starch.
- Ask for the salad dressing on the side.
- If you can't finish the meal without dessert, order one for the table and take only a few bites.

FAST FOOD

Many fast-food restaurants now offer healthier meals. Look for restaurants that have good salads and grilled meats. Avoid french fries and potato chips, and go easy on the ketchup. Here are some good choices for a low-carb meal:

- grilled chicken or fish without bread
- a hamburger without the bun
- salads with regular dressing (not lower-fat)
- diet drinks or water

CHINESE

Be careful: most Chinese sauces contain sugar to balance the salt and cornstarch for thickening. Avoid rice or rice dishes, noodles, wonton soup, egg rolls and ribs or chicken in a thick sauce. Instead, look for:

- clear soups with meat and vegetables
- stir-fried dishes with a minimum of sauce

JAPANESE

Sushi has become a world-wide favorite. The problem for those on a low-carb diet is that it always includes white rice, which is usually cooked with a little sugar. Stick to these:

- miso soup
- cooked meats
- vegetables

MEXICAN

This is a difficult category. Most restaurants have tortilla chips and salsa on the table when you sit down to dinner. I suggest having just one or two chips with salsa, then eat salsa with a spoon. Mexican restaurants also feature items such as rice, refried beans and nachos. These should be avoided. Most Mexican entrées, such as enchiladas and fajitas, come wrapped in flour tortillas. It's fine to eat one of these. If you're still hungry after that, take the meat and vegetables out of the tortilla and eat them on their own.

ITALIAN

Italian restaurants are a good choice because they have a wide variety of meats and vegetables. Choose vegetable or cold meat dishes from an antipasto table and avoid pasta, risotto and polenta.

FRENCH

This is another good category. There are many options on French menus, and you can always ask for vegetables rather than a starch with your main course.

EATING ON THE ROAD

It's important to stick with a low-carb lifestyle even when you're traveling. More and more hotel chains and restaurants now cater to low-carb guests, offering low-carb options on their menus. But it's always a good idea to ask for the nutritional information if it is not displayed. It's also best to stick with fresh foods that are not heavily sauced. That way, you don't have to worry that someone in the kitchen isn't following the recipe guidelines.

Appetizers, Dips and Spreads

Continued on next page...

Hot Three-Cheese Dill Artichoke Bake

1	can (14 oz/398 mL) artichoke hearts, drained and halved	1
1/2 cup	shredded part-skim mozzarella cheese (about 2 oz/50 g)	125 mL
1/3 cup	shredded Swiss cheese (about 1 1/2 oz/35 g)	75 mL
1/3 cup	minced fresh dill (or 1 tsp/5 mL dried)	75 mL
1/4 cup	light sour cream	50 mL
3 tbsp	light mayonnaise	45 mL
1 tbsp	freshly squeezed lemon juice	15 mL
1 tsp	minced garlic	5 mL
Pinch	cayenne pepper	Pinch
1 tbsp	grated Parmesan cheese	15 mL

Make Ahead

Prepare up to 1 day in advance. Bake just before serving.

SERVES 6 TO 8
Preheat oven to 350°F (180°C) • Small casserole dish

1. In a food processor, combine artichoke hearts, mozzarella and Swiss cheeses, dill, sour cream, mayonnaise, lemon juice, garlic and cayenne. Process on and off just until combined but still chunky. Place in a small casserole dish. Sprinkle with Parmesan cheese.

2. Bake uncovered 10 minutes. Broil 3 to 5 minutes just until top is slightly browned. Serve warm with crudités.

Tip
- This tastes like the traditional hot artichoke dip loaded with fat and calories, but has less than half the fat.

Nutritional Analysis (Per Serving)
- Calories: 79
- Protein: 5 g
- Fat: 5 g
- Carbohydrates: 6 g
- Fiber: 2 g
- Sodium: 271 mg
- Cholesterol: 10 mg

Artichoke Nuggets

1	bottle (6 oz/170 mL) artichoke hearts, drained	1
1/2 cup	seasoned crouton crumbs (about 1 cup/250 mL croutons)	125 mL
1 tbsp	olive oil	15 mL
1 tbsp	grated Parmesan cheese	15 mL
1	egg, beaten	1
2 tsp	lemon juice	10 mL
1	clove garlic, mashed	1
	Grated Parmesan cheese for coating	

MAKES 12 MEDIUM NUGGETS
Preheat oven to 350°F (180°C) • Baking sheet

1. In a small bowl, mash artichoke hearts. Stir in crouton crumbs, oil, cheese, egg, lemon juice and garlic. Form into small balls. Roll each ball in additional Parmesan cheese (about 1/4 cup/50 mL).

2. Bake on sheet in preheated oven for 10 minutes for small nuggets, 15 minutes for medium.

Tip
- These nuggets freeze well before they are baked. Keep a supply in the freezer and they will be ready to serve at a moment's notice. If frozen, bake for 5 minutes longer than recipe specifies.

Nutritional Analysis (Per Nugget)
- Calories: 45
- Protein: 2 g
- Fat: 2 g
- Carbohydrates: 4 g
- Fiber: 0 g
- Sodium: 194 mg
- Cholesterol: 36 mg

Eggplant, Tomato and Fennel Appetizer

2 tsp	vegetable oil	10 mL
2 tsp	minced garlic	10 mL
1 cup	chopped fennel	250 mL
1 cup	chopped onions	250 mL
1 cup	chopped red bell peppers	250 mL
3 cups	diced unpeeled eggplant	750 mL
2 cups	chopped plum tomatoes	500 mL
¼ cup	sliced green olives	50 mL
1½ tbsp	balsamic vinegar	22 mL
4 tsp	drained capers	20 mL
2 tsp	dried basil	10 mL

Make Ahead

Prepare up to 2 days in advance.

SERVES 6

1. In a nonstick saucepan, heat oil over medium-high heat. Add garlic, fennel, onions and red peppers; cook, stirring occasionally, 4 minutes. Add eggplant; cook 5 minutes longer, stirring occasionally. Stir in tomatoes, olives, vinegar, capers and basil; reduce heat to medium-low and simmer 15 minutes.

2. Transfer to a food processor; pulse on and off until chunky. Chill.

Tip

- For an interesting salad, omit Step 2, then serve chilled on top of green beans.

Nutritional Analysis (Per Serving)
- Calories: 69
- Protein: 2 g
- Fat: 3 g
- Carbohydrates: 11 g
- Fiber: 4 g
- Sodium: 529 mg
- Cholesterol: 0 mg

Eggplant Tapas

1	small eggplant (about ¾ lb/375 g)	1
1	medium green bell pepper	1
1	medium red bell pepper	1
2 tbsp	lemon juice	25 mL
1 tbsp	red wine vinegar	15 mL
1 tsp	olive oil	5 mL
1	clove garlic, minced	1
	Freshly ground black pepper	

Tapas — tasty nibblers served with drinks — originated in Spain, where the practice of meeting friends for appetizers and drinks before dinner is a treasured tradition.

SERVES 6 OR MAKES 2 CUPS (500 ML)
Preheat oven to 400°F (200°C) • Baking sheet

1. Place eggplant and peppers on baking sheet. Bake in preheated oven for about 30 minutes or until tender and peppers are charred. (Note: Peppers may be cooked before eggplant.) Remove skin from peppers and eggplant. Cut eggplant into chunks; cut peppers into thin slices.

2. Combine lemon juice, vinegar, oil, garlic, and pepper to taste. Pour over vegetables and stir. Cover and refrigerate for several hours.

Tip

- You can also cook the eggplant and peppers on the barbecue. Roast until charred, then place in a plastic bag to "sweat" before removing skins.

Nutritional Analysis (Per Serving)
- Calories: 104
- Protein: 0 g
- Fat: 1 g
- Carbohydrates: 4 g
- Fiber: 1 g
- Sodium: 4 mg
- Cholesterol: 0 mg

Palm Hearts Niçoise

1	can (14 oz/398 mL) hearts of palm, drained and rinsed	1
1/4 cup	bottled oil and vinegar dressing	50 mL
2 tbsp	finely chopped parsley	25 mL
2 tbsp	drained capers	25 mL
1	bag (10 oz/300 g) washed salad greens or 4 cups (1 L) torn lettuce, washed and dried	1
1	avocado, cut into 1/4-inch (0.5 cm) wedges (see tip, at right)	1
2	hard-cooked eggs, peeled and cut into quarters	2

SERVES 6

1. Cut hearts of palm into 1/2-inch (1 cm) slices.
2. In a bowl, combine palm hearts, dressing, parsley and capers. Toss to combine. Refrigerate for at least 1 hour or overnight.
3. Arrange salad greens over a deep platter. Top with chilled palm heart mixture, sliced avocado and eggs. Serve immediately.

Tip

- Cut the avocado just before serving; otherwise it will turn brown.

Nutritional Analysis (Per Serving)
- Calories: 82
- Protein: 3.4 g
- Fat: 6.8 g
- Carbohydrates: 3.2 g
- Fiber: 2.2 g
- Sodium: 112 mg
- Cholesterol: 71 mg

Marinated Greek Mushrooms

1 lb	button mushrooms, cleaned	500 g
1/2 cup	chopped fresh coriander	125 mL
1/2 cup	chopped red onions	125 mL
1/3 cup	sliced black olives	75 mL
1/3 cup	balsamic vinegar	75 mL
2 tbsp	water	25 mL
2 tbsp	olive oil	25 mL
1 tbsp	freshly squeezed lemon juice	15 mL
1 tsp	minced garlic	5 mL
1/2 to 3/4 tsp	chili powder or 1/2 tsp (2 mL) minced fresh jalapeño pepper	2 to 4 mL
1/4 tsp	freshly ground black pepper	1 mL
2 oz	feta cheese, crumbled	50 g

Make Ahead

Prepare 1 day in advance. Stir before serving.

SERVES 6 TO 8

1. In a large bowl, stir together mushrooms, coriander, red onions, olives, vinegar, water, olive oil, lemon juice, garlic, chili powder, pepper and feta.
2. Cover and chill 1 hour or overnight, mixing occasionally.

Tips

- The longer the mushrooms marinate, the more flavorful they will be.
- If you can't find small button mushrooms, use larger mushrooms and cut into quarters.
- To make this a vegan dish, just eliminate the cheese.

Nutritional Analysis (Per Serving)
- Calories: 71
- Protein: 2 g
- Fat: 5 g
- Carbohydrates: 5 g
- Fiber: 1 g
- Sodium: 125 mg
- Cholesterol: 6 mg

Brie-Stuffed Mushrooms

16 to 20	medium mushrooms	16 to 20
2 oz	Brie cheese	50 g
1/4 cup	chopped roasted red peppers	50 mL
1/4 cup	chopped green onions	50 mL
3 tbsp	dried bread crumbs	45 mL
1 tsp	minced garlic	5 mL
1/2 tsp	dried basil	2 mL

Make Ahead

Fill mushroom caps up to 1 day in advance. Bake just before serving.

SERVES 4

Preheat oven to 400°F (200°C) • Baking sheet

1. Wipe mushrooms; remove stems and reserve for another use. (See tip, below.) Place on baking sheet.
2. In a small bowl, stir together Brie, red peppers, green onions, bread crumbs, garlic and basil. Divide mixture among mushroom caps, approximately 1 1/2 tsp (7 mL) per cap.
3. Bake 15 minutes, or until mushrooms release their liquid. Serve warm or at room temperature.

Tips

- Don't throw out those mushroom stems — use them in salads or soups, or sauté in a nonstick skillet and serve as a side vegetable dish.
- Roast your own red bell peppers or buy water-packed roasted red peppers.
- Use another soft cheese of your choice to replace the Brie.

Nutritional Analysis (Per Serving)
- Calories: 86
- Protein: 5 g
- Fat: 4 g
- Carbohydrates: 9 g
- Fiber: 1 g
- Sodium: 205 mg
- Cholesterol: 13 mg

Spinach-Stuffed Mushrooms with Walnuts

18	jumbo mushrooms	18
2 tbsp	olive oil	25 mL
2 tbsp	lemon juice, divided	25 mL
2 cups	chopped spinach	500 mL
1	small onion, chopped	1
8 oz	tofu	250 g
1	egg	1
1½ tsp	ground cumin	7 mL
¼ tsp	each salt and black pepper	1 mL
18	walnut halves	18

Serve this simple yet elegant appetizer to your most discriminating guests. Not only is it delicious, it is also easy to make.

SERVES 6

Preheat oven to 375°F (190°C) • 13- by 9-inch (3 L) baking dish

1. Clean mushrooms. Remove stems and chop; set aside. In a skillet over medium heat, heat oil and 1 tbsp (15 mL) of the lemon juice. Add mushroom caps; cover and steam for 2 to 3 minutes, turning once. Drain on paper towels.

2. To pan juices, add chopped mushroom stems, spinach and onion; cook, stirring, for 2 minutes. Drain off excess moisture; cool.

3. In a food processor or blender, purée tofu until smooth. Combine with egg, cumin, salt, pepper, remaining lemon juice and spinach mixture. Spoon into mushroom caps. Place walnut half on top of each. Place in 13- by 9-inch (3 L) baking dish. Bake in preheated oven for 20 to 25 minutes or until heated through. Serve warm.

Tips

- One way to clean mushrooms is to brush them with a soft brush to remove any dirt, then wipe gently with a paper towel.

- In this recipe, tofu is a lower-fat alternative to cream cheese. Since tofu is quite bland on its own (it takes on the flavor of ingredients it is combined with), the spinach and walnuts add both taste and fiber to these appetizing treats.

Nutritional Analysis (Per Serving)
- Calories: 147
- Protein: 7 g
- Fat: 11 g
- Carbohydrates: 7 g
- Fiber: 3 g
- Sodium: 126 mg
- Cholesterol: 36 mg

Madrid Mushrooms

25	button mushrooms (about 1½ inches/4 cm in diameter), wiped with damp paper towels, stems discarded	25
1 tbsp	olive oil	15 mL
¼ tsp	black pepper	1 mL
Pinch	salt	Pinch
3 oz	prosciutto, trimmed of excess fat and finely chopped	75 g
¼ cup	mayonnaise	50 mL
1	small clove garlic, pressed through a garlic press	1
	Watercress (tough stems discarded)	
	Paprika	

Make Ahead

Stuffed mushrooms can be refrigerated, covered, for up to 4 hours before baking. Garlic mayonnaise can be refrigerated, covered, for up to 24 hours.

MAKES 25
Preheat oven to 400°F (200°C) • Baking sheet

1. In a medium bowl, combine mushrooms, olive oil, pepper and salt; toss well.
2. Arrange mushrooms, stem-side up, in a single layer on baking sheet. Divide prosciutto evenly among mushroom caps. Bake in preheated oven for 10 to 15 minutes or until tender and juicy.
3. Meanwhile, in a small bowl, combine mayonnaise and garlic; stir until well combined.
4. When mushrooms are ready, spoon a small dollop of mayonnaise on top of each. Arrange mushrooms on a serving platter; surround with watercress. Sprinkle mushrooms very lightly with paprika. Serve at once.

Tips
- If using very lean prosciutto, you'll need only 2 oz (50 g).
- If you don't have a garlic press, use a knife to mince the garlic very finely.
- Reserve mushroom stems for use in another recipe, such as soup or stock.

Nutritional Analysis (Per Serving)
- Calories: 157
- Protein: 9.3 g
- Fat: 11.0 g
- Carbohydrates: 8.3 g
- Fiber: 2.5 g
- Sodium: 262 mg
- Cholesterol: 13 mg

Antipasto Nibblers

24	stuffed green olives or Kalamata olives	24
8 oz	Fontina cheese, cut into 3/4-inch (2 cm) cubes	250 g
1	small red bell pepper, cut into 1-inch (2.5 cm) squares	1
1	small green bell pepper, cut into 1-inch (2.5 cm) squares	1
1 tbsp	olive oil	15 mL
1 tbsp	balsamic vinegar	15 mL
	Freshly ground black pepper	
2 tbsp	chopped fresh basil leaves or parsley	25 mL

SERVES 6

1. Thread 1 olive, 1 cheese cube, then 1 pepper square on cocktail toothpicks. Arrange in attractive shallow serving dish. Cover and refrigerate until serving time.

2. In a small bowl, whisk together oil and balsamic vinegar; pour over kabobs. Season generously with pepper; sprinkle with basil and serve.

Tip

- This recipe can be varied according to what you have on hand. Thin slices of salami or ham folded in half, cocktail onions and marinated artichoke pieces make for other easy combinations.

Nutritional Analysis (Per Serving)
- Calories: 199
- Protein: 10.3 g
- Fat: 16.1 g
- Carbohydrates: 4.2 g
- Fiber: 1.0 g
- Sodium: 674 mg
- Cholesterol: 44 mg

Roasted Pear with Brie Cheese

1	6-inch (15 cm) round Brie cheese	1
1 tbsp	melted butter or margarine	15 mL
2	ripe pears, peeled and thinly sliced	2
1 tsp	chopped fresh thyme or 1/2 tsp (2 mL) dried thyme	5 mL

Roasted pears put a new twist on baked Brie cheese to make this a favorite cocktail munchy.

SERVES 8

Preheat oven to 425°F (220°C)

1. Remove top rind from cheese and discard.

2. Brush a baking sheet with melted butter. Arrange pear slices on sheet. Roast in preheated oven for 15 minutes. Turn slices and roast for 10 minutes more or until edges are caramelized. Let cool.

3. Top cheese with pears, overlapping slices and refrigerate (for up to 4 hours) until ready to bake.

4. Just before serving, heat cheese and pears in 350°F (180°C) oven for 10 minutes or until cheese is softened. Sprinkle with thyme and serve.

Nutritional Analysis (Per Serving)
- Calories: 237
- Protein: 12.6 g
- Fat: 18.1 g
- Carbohydrates: 6.7 g
- Fiber: 1.1 g
- Sodium: 389 mg
- Cholesterol: 63 mg

Greek Egg Rolls with Spinach and Feta

2 tsp	vegetable oil	10 mL
2 tsp	minced garlic	10 mL
³⁄₄ cup	diced onions	175 mL
1²⁄₃ cup	diced mushrooms	400 mL
1 tsp	dried oregano	5 mL
half	package (10 oz/300 g) frozen chopped spinach, thawed and drained	half
2 oz	feta cheese, crumbled	50 g
10	egg roll wrappers	10

Make Ahead

Prepare early in the day, cover and keep refrigerated until ready to bake.

MAKES 10
Preheat oven to 425°F (220°C) • Baking sheet sprayed with vegetable spray

1. In nonstick skillet, heat oil over medium-high heat. Add garlic, onions, mushrooms and oregano; cook for 5 minutes or until softened. Add spinach and feta; cook, stirring, for 2 minutes or until well mixed and cheese melts.

2. Keeping rest of egg roll wrappers covered with a cloth to prevent drying out, put one wrapper on work surface with a corner pointing towards you. Put 2 tbsp (25 mL) of the filling in the center. Fold the lower corner up over the filling, fold the two side corners in over the filling and roll the bundle away from you. Place on prepared pan and repeat until all wrappers are filled. Bake for 12 to 14 minutes until browned, turning the egg rolls at the halfway point.

Nutritional Analysis (Per Serving)
- Calories: 60
- Protein: 2 g
- Fat: 3 g
- Carbohydrates: 7 g
- Fiber: 1 g
- Sodium: 96 mg
- Cholesterol: 5 mg

Roasted Garlic Sweet Pepper Strips

4	large sweet peppers (combination of green, red and yellow)	4
2 tbsp	olive oil	25 mL
1¹⁄₂ tsp	crushed garlic	7 mL
1 tbsp	grated Parmesan cheese	15 mL

Make Ahead

These peppers can be prepared ahead of time and served cold.

SERVES 4
Preheat oven to 400°F (200°C)

1. On baking sheet, bake whole peppers for 15 to 20 minutes, turning occasionally, or until blistered and blackened. Place in paper bag; seal and let stand for 10 minutes.

2. Peel off charred skin from peppers; cut off tops and bottoms. Remove seeds and ribs; cut into 1 inch (2.5 cm) wide strips and place on serving platter.

3. Mix oil with garlic; brush over peppers. Sprinkle with cheese.

Nutritional Analysis (Per Serving)
- Calories: 95
- Protein: 1 g
- Fat: 7 g
- Carbohydrates: 7 g
- Fiber: 2 g
- Sodium: 26 mg
- Cholesterol: 1 mg

Tomatoes and Arugula with Ricotta and Basil Oil

³/₄ cup	grapeseed oil or olive oil	175 mL
¹/₂ cup	packed fresh basil leaves	125 mL
2	beefsteak tomatoes or 3 hothouse tomatoes	2
8 cups	arugula, washed and dried, tough stems discarded and larger leaves torn into pieces	2 L
12 oz	regular (10%) ricotta cheese	375 g
¹/₂ tsp	black pepper	2 mL
¹/₄ tsp	salt	1 mL

Make Ahead

Basil oil must be refrigerated, covered, for 24 hours before serving.

SERVES 6

1. In a mini-chopper or food processor, combine oil and basil leaves. Process until well combined and basil is finely chopped. Refrigerate, covered, for 24 hours to allow the flavor to develop (do not store basil oil for longer than 24 hours).

2. Thirty minutes before serving, remove basil oil from refrigerator; let stand at room temperature.

3. Just before serving, scoop out tough stem ends from tomatoes with a small sharp knife; slice tomatoes thinly. Divide arugula among 6 dinner plates; arrange a circle of tomato slices on top of each portion. Spoon an equal amount of cheese in center of circle of tomatoes; sprinkle with pepper and salt. Whisk basil oil; drizzle about 2 tbsp (25 mL) over each serving. Serve at once.

Tip

• This salad is best prepared in late summer using fresh local tomatoes. At other times of the year, buy hothouse tomatoes (with stems intact) and let stand at room temperature for 5 to 7 days or until the stems are dry and the tomatoes are fully ripe. Never, ever refrigerate tomatoes or their texture will become woolly.

Nutritional Analysis (Per Serving)
- Calories: 378
- Protein: 8.7 g
- Fat: 35.4 g
- Carbohydrates: 8.0 g
- Fiber: 1.9 g
- Sodium: 161 mg
- Cholesterol: 31 mg

Zucchini Algis

1	tomato	1
1/4 cup	olive oil	50 mL
1/4 tsp	salt	1 mL
1/4 tsp	freshly ground black pepper	1 mL
3 cups	diagonally sliced zucchini	750 mL
1	onion, sliced	1
1 3/4 cups	thickly sliced mushrooms	425 mL
2 to 3	cloves garlic, thinly sliced	2 to 3
2 tbsp	white wine or water	25 mL
	Few sprigs fresh basil and/or dill, chopped	

SERVES 4

1. Blanch tomato in boiling water for 30 seconds. Over a bowl, peel, core and deseed it. Chop tomato into chunks and set aside. Strain any accumulated tomato juices from bowl; add the juices to the tomato.

2. In a large frying pan, heat olive oil on high heat for 30 seconds. Add salt and pepper and stir. Add zucchini and onions. Stir-fry for 3 to 4 minutes, until the zucchini is slightly charred.

3. Add mushroom slices and continue stir-frying (gently, so as not to injure the zucchini) for 2 to 3 minutes. Add garlic and stir-fry for 1 minute. Add reserved tomato and its juice, and stir-fry for 2 to 3 minutes until a sauce begins to form.

4. Remove from heat and stir in wine. You should have a spare but luscious sauce. Transfer to a serving dish and garnish with the basil and/or dill. Serve immediately.

Nutritional Analysis (Per Serving)
- Calories: 176
- Protein: 3.1 g
- Fat: 13.9 g
- Carbohydrates: 10.9 g
- Fiber: 2.8 g
- Sodium: 153 mg
- Cholesterol: 0 mg

Lemon Pesto Pita Pizza

1/2 cup	Lemon Pesto Sauce (see recipe, page 60)	125 mL
2 tbsp	grated Parmesan cheese	25 mL
3	whole-wheat pita breads	3
1/2 cup	chopped red bell pepper	125 mL
1 cup	shredded part-skim mozzarella cheese	250 mL

Here's another way to use Lemon Pesto Sauce and one more reason for keeping a supply on hand in the freezer.

SERVES 12
Preheat oven to 450°F (230°C) • Baking Sheet

1. Combine Lemon Pesto Sauce and Parmesan. Spread over pitas. Sprinkle with red pepper and mozzarella. Bake in preheated oven until cheese melts. Cut into triangles.

Tip

- Whole-wheat pita breads are a nutritious and versatile convenience food. Use them as a base for pizza or a pouch for sandwich fillings, or cut them into triangles and load them with dips.

Nutritional Analysis (Per Serving)
- Calories: 97
- Protein: 5 g
- Fat: 4 g
- Carbohydrates: 10 g
- Fiber: Trace
- Sodium: 216 mg
- Cholesterol: 11 mg

Piquant Marinated Vegetables

2 cups	cauliflower florets	500 mL
2 cups	broccoli florets	500 mL
1 cup	fresh button mushrooms	250 mL
½	red bell pepper, cut into strips	½
1 cup	cut-up green beans	250 mL
8	small white pickling onions	8
1	carrot, cut into rounds	1
	Lettuce leaves	
	Cherry tomatoes, chopped	
	fresh parsley	

MARINADE

1 cup	red wine vinegar	250 mL
1 tsp	dried oregano	5 mL
1 tsp	dried tarragon	5 mL
½ tsp	granulated sugar	2 mL
½ tsp	salt	2 mL
¼ tsp	freshly ground black pepper	1 mL
¼ cup	olive oil	50 mL

SERVES 10

1. In a bowl, combine cauliflower, broccoli, mushrooms, red pepper, green beans, onions and carrot.

2. *Marinade:* In a saucepan, heat vinegar and seasonings; add oil and pour over vegetables. Cool slightly and transfer mixture to a large plastic bag. Refrigerate for 24 hours before serving.

3. Serve in bowl lined with lettuce; garnish with cherry tomatoes and parsley. Provide toothpicks for spearing vegetables.

Tips

- Here's a great way to have a vegetable snack available in the fridge. Cauliflower and broccoli are members of the cruciferous family of vegetables. They contribute antioxidants to our diets, which may help to reduce the incidence of some diseases.

- When purchasing cauliflower or broccoli, take note of the smell. If these vegetables have passed their peak, they will have a strong, unpleasant odor.

- This intriguing combination of vegetables can be served as a first course salad on leaf lettuce, or as a side salad to a meat entrée as well as an appetizer. Make the entire recipe. It improves with time and keeps very well.

Nutritional Analysis (Per Serving)
- Calories: 53
- Protein: 2 g
- Fat: 3 g
- Carbohydrates: 6 g
- Fiber: 3 g
- Sodium: 129 mg
- Cholesterol: 0 mg

Frittata di Menta
(Open-Faced Omelette with Fresh Mint)

3 tbsp	olive oil	45 mL
1	onion, finely chopped	1
1 cup	whole fresh mint leaves, washed and dried thoroughly	250 mL
¼ cup	chopped flat-leaf parsley	50 mL
8	eggs	8
3 tbsp	fresh bread crumbs	45 mL
3 tbsp	grated Pecorino Romano	45 mL
2 tsp	light (10%) cream	10 mL
2 tsp	all-purpose flour	10 mL
½ tsp	salt	2 mL
¼ tsp	freshly ground black pepper	1 mL

Swiss chard or peppery greens like rapini are often used as frittata fillings, as are thin asparagus, artichoke hearts and zucchini flowers.

SERVES 4 TO 6

1. In a large ovenproof skillet, heat 4 tsp (20 mL) of the olive oil over medium heat. Add onion and cook for 6 minutes or until softened. Remove from heat. Stir in mint and parsley. Transfer to a bowl. Wipe skillet clean with paper towel.

2. In another bowl, whisk together eggs, bread crumbs, Pecorino Romano, cream, flour, salt and pepper. Stir in cooled onion-herb mixture.

3. Preheat broiler. Return skillet to medium heat. Add remaining olive oil, swirling to coat surface of skillet. Pour egg mixture into skillet; cook, gently running a narrow metal spatula around the edges to lift cooked egg up and allow uncooked egg to run beneath for 5 minutes or until frittata is set and cooked on the bottom.

4. Place skillet 6 inches (15 cm) beneath broiler. Cook 2 minutes or until top is set and golden brown. Serve immediately or cooled to room temperature, cut into squares or strips.

Nutritional Analysis (Per Serving)
- Calories: 243
- Protein: 12.0 g
- Fat: 17.6 g
- Carbohydrates: 8.4 g
- Fiber: 0.7 g
- Sodium: 409 mg
- Cholesterol: 345 mg

Crab Louis

2	cans (each 4 oz/125 g) crabmeat, drained, or 8 oz (250 g) crabmeat, thawed and drained if frozen	2

LOUIS SAUCE

¾ cup	mayonnaise	175 mL
¼ cup	tomato-based chili sauce	50 mL
2 tbsp	lemon juice	25 mL
1 tbsp	finely chopped red or green onion	15 mL
1 tbsp	finely chopped parsley	15 mL
¼ tsp	Worcestershire sauce	1 mL
	Freshly ground black pepper	

SERVES 4

1. *Louis Sauce:* In a bowl, combine mayonnaise, chili sauce, lemon juice, onion, parsley and Worcestershire sauce. Mix well.

2. Add crab and toss to combine. Season with black pepper to taste.

Variation

- *Even Easier Crab Louis:* Substitute 1 cup (250 mL) prepared Thousand Islands salad dressing for the Louis Sauce. Proceed with Step 2.

Tip

- For a change, add 2 tbsp (25 mL) finely diced green bell pepper along with the onion and add a pinch of cayenne pepper.

Nutritional Analysis (Per Serving)
- Calories: 367
- Protein: 10.8 g
- Fat: 33.5 g
- Carbohydrates: 5.7 g
- Fiber: 0.1 g
- Sodium: 371 mg
- Cholesterol: 68 mg

Crab Celery Sticks

1	can (4.2 oz /120 g) crabmeat, well drained	1
¼ cup	sliced green onions	50 mL
¼ tsp	crushed garlic	1 mL
3 tbsp	chopped fresh dill (or 1 tsp/5 mL dried dillweed)	45 mL
1 tbsp	lemon juice	15 mL
¼ cup	chopped celery	50 mL
¼ cup	chopped sweet red or green pepper	50 mL
2 tbsp	2% yogurt	25 mL
¼ cup	light mayonnaise	50 mL
	Salt and pepper	
24	pieces (2-inch/5 cm) celery stalks	24
	Paprika	

SERVES 4 TO 6 OR MAKES 24 HORS D'OEUVRES

1. In food processor, combine crabmeat, onions, garlic, dill, lemon juice, chopped celery, red pepper, yogurt and mayonnaise. Using on/off motion, process just until combined but still chunky. Season with salt and pepper to taste.

2. Stuff each celery stalk evenly with mixture. Sprinkle with paprika to taste.

Tips

- For a less expensive version, use imitation crab, often called Surimi.

- Serve as a dip with crudités.

Nutritional Analysis (Per Serving)
- Calories: 15
- Protein: 1 g
- Fat: 1 g
- Carbohydrates: 0.6 g
- Fiber: 0 g
- Sodium: 35 mg
- Cholesterol: 5 mg

Steamed Mussels with Julienne Vegetables

3 lb	fresh mussels	1.5 kg
1 tbsp	olive or vegetable oil	15 mL
¼ cup	finely chopped shallots or onions	50 mL
¼ cup	julienned red and green bell peppers	50 mL
¼ cup	minced garlic	50 mL
2	medium tomatoes, diced	2
1 cup	beef stock	250 mL
1 cup	dry white wine (optional)	250 mL
Pinch	saffron (optional)	Pinch

If you enjoy mussels when eating out but have never made them at home, here's your chance to experiment with a fabulous one-pot dish!

SERVES 4

1. Wash mussels, cutting off beards and discarding any that are open.

2. In an 8-cup (2 L) saucepan, heat oil over medium heat; cook shallots, red and green peppers, garlic and tomatoes, stirring, for 2 to 3 minutes. Add mussels, stock and, if using, wine and saffron; increase heat to high. Cover and bring to boil; cook for about 5 minutes or until mussels have opened. Discard any that have not opened. Serve in wide soup plates.

Tips

- To julienne vegetables, cut them into thin strawlike strips about ⅛ inch (3 mm) thick.

- Mussels should be scrubbed and rinsed in several changes of cold water to get rid of the grit. Any beard on the outer shell should be scrubbed off with a hard brush prior to cooking. Discard any with broken shells before you cook. After cooking, toss any that do not open, as they are not safe to eat.

- Mussels, served in this tasty sauce, are a good source of protein with little added fat. They make an ideal appetizer for a special meal.

Nutritional Analysis (Per Serving)
- Calories: 155
- Protein: 14 g
- Fat: 6 g
- Carbohydrates: 12 g
- Fiber: 2 g
- Sodium: 1174 mg
- Cholesterol: 96 mg

Fresh Mussels with Tomato Salsa

24	mussels	24
1/2 cup	water or wine	125 mL
3/4 cup	finely chopped onions	175 mL
1 1/2 tsp	crushed garlic	7 mL
1 cup	coarsely chopped tomato	250 mL
4 tsp	chopped fresh basil (or 1/2 tsp/2 mL dried)	20 mL
2 tbsp	chopped fresh parsley	25 mL
2 tsp	olive oil	10 mL
1/4 tsp	chili powder	1 mL
	Salt and pepper	

Make Ahead

Prepare and refrigerate mixture early in day to allow flavors to blend. Spoon into shells a couple of hours prior to serving and keep chilled.

You can't change the shape you were born with, but you can change your food and activity habits to achieve a healthier weight. Set small goals for eating better and being more active.

SERVES 4 TO 6 OR MAKES 24 HORS D'OEUVRES

1. Scrub mussels under cold running water; remove any beards. Discard any mussels that do not close when tapped.

2. In saucepan, combine mussels, water, 1/4 cup (50 mL) of the onions and 1 tsp (5 mL) of the garlic; cover and steam just until mussels open, approximately 5 minutes. Discard any that do not open. Let cool then remove mussels from shells, reserving half of shell. Place mussels in bowl.

3. In food processor, combine remaining 1/2 cup (125 mL) onions and 1/2 tsp (2 mL) garlic, tomatoes, basil, parsley, oil, chili powder, and salt and pepper to taste; process using on/off motion just until chunky. Do not purée. Add to mussels and stir to mix. Refrigerate until chilled.

4. Divide mussel mixture evenly among reserved shells and arrange on serving plate.

Tips

- Substitute fresh coriander for the parsley for a change.
- This recipe can also be made with fresh clams.
- Serve as a salad over lettuce.

Nutritional Analysis (Per Serving)
- Calories: 18
- Protein: 2 g
- Fat: 0.5 g
- Carbohydrates: 1 g
- Fiber: 0 g
- Sodium: 47 mg
- Cholesterol: 5 mg

Smoked Salmon and Goat Cheese Cucumber Slices

3 oz	smoked salmon, diced	75 g
3 oz	goat cheese	75 g
2 tbsp	2% yogurt	25 mL
1/2 tsp	lemon juice	2 mL
4 tsp	chopped fresh dill (or 1/2 tsp/2 mL dried dillweed)	20 mL
25	slices (1/4-inch/5 mm thick) cucumber	25

Make Ahead

Prepare and refrigerate mixture up to a day before. Place on cucumber slices just before serving.

SERVES 4 TO 6 OR MAKES 25 HORS D'OEUVRES

1. Reserve about 25 bits of salmon for garnish.
2. In bowl or using food processor, combine goat cheese, yogurt, remaining salmon, lemon juice and dill; mix with fork or using on/off motion just until combined but not puréed.
3. Place spoonful of filling on each cucumber slice. Garnish with bit of reserved salmon.

Tips

- Goat cheese, also known as chèvre, comes in a variety of shapes ranging from logs to pyramids and discs. Some are sprinkled with herbs and spices throughout. Use any variety.
- Serve also as a dip or serve on celery sticks or in hollow cherry tomatoes.

Nutritional Analysis (Per Serving)
- Calories: 92
- Protein: 8 g
- Fat: 6 g
- Carbohydrates: 2 g
- Fiber: 0 g
- Sodium: 156 mg
- Cholesterol: 19 mg

Sizzling Shrimp

1 1/2 lbs	raw large shrimp, peeled and deveined, patted dry	750 g
3	cloves garlic, sliced	3
1/4 tsp	salt	1 mL
1/4 tsp	hot pepper flakes	1 mL
1/2 cup	olive oil	125 mL

This messy but delectable first course is perfect for sharing among good friends. Serve straight from the baking dish.

SERVES 6
Preheat oven to 450°F (230°C) • 9-inch (22.5 cm) ovenproof earthenware dish or glass pie plate

1. Spread out shrimp in baking dish; tuck slices of garlic in amongst shrimp. Sprinkle with salt and hot pepper flakes. Drizzle oil evenly over shrimp.
2. Bake in preheated oven for 10 to 12 minutes, stirring once or twice, until shrimp are pink and opaque and oil is bubbling. Serve at once.

Nutritional Analysis (Per Serving)
- Calories: 282
- Protein: 23.1 g
- Fat: 20.0 g
- Carbohydrates: 1.6 g
- Fiber: 0.1 g
- Sodium: 265 mg
- Cholesterol: 172 mg

Shrimp-Stuffed Avocado

8 oz	cooked salad shrimp, thawed and drained if frozen, or 2 cans (each 3¾ oz/106 g) shrimp, rinsed and drained	250 g
1 tbsp	lemon juice	15 mL
½ cup	finely chopped celery	125 mL
2 tbsp	finely chopped green onion (white part only)	25 mL
¼ cup	mayonnaise	50 mL
	Salt and freshly ground black pepper	
2	avocados	2

Depend upon avocados, one of nature's own convenience foods, for ease of preparation and the perfect combination of flavor and texture. This dish makes an elegant starter for any meal, and this quantity also makes a delicious and nutritious light dinner for two. Look for cooked salad shrimp at your supermarket fish counter.

SERVES 4

1. In a bowl, combine shrimp and lemon juice. Toss to combine. Add celery, green onion, mayonnaise and salt and black pepper to taste. Mix well.
2. Cut each avocado in half and remove pits.
3. Place one avocado half on each plate. Fill with shrimp mixture (it will spill over the sides) and serve immediately.

Tips

- Do not halve avocados until just before serving; otherwise the flesh will turn brown. Use the tip of a spoon to remove the pit.
- For an extra zip, add 2 tbsp (25 mL) finely chopped dill along with the celery.

Nutritional Analysis (Per Serving)
- Calories: 415
- Protein: 13.8 g
- Fat: 37.9 g
- Carbohydrates: 8.2 g
- Fiber: 4.6 g
- Sodium: 116 mg
- Cholesterol: 102 mg

Thai-Roasted Shrimp

1 lb	raw large shrimp, in their shells	500 g
	Grated zest of 2 limes	
	Freshly squeezed juice of 2 limes	
2 tbsp	sesame oil	25 mL
2 tbsp	chopped fresh coriander	25 mL
1	clove garlic, minced	1
½ tsp	hot pepper sauce	2 mL
¼ tsp	salt	1 mL
	Lettuce leaves	

Make Ahead

If serving shrimp cold, cook then refrigerate, covered, for up to 24 hours.

MAKES ABOUT 35 SHRIMP

Large shallow nonreactive dish • Baking sheet, lightly oiled

1. Remove shells from shrimp, leaving tails and last segment of shell intact. If necessary, with a small sharp knife, slit backs of shrimp just enough to remove dark vein-like intestinal tract from each. Pat shrimp dry on paper towels.

2. In the nonreactive dish, combine lime zest, lime juice, sesame oil, coriander, garlic, hot pepper sauce and salt. Add shrimp; stir gently. Refrigerate, covered, for 1 hour.

3. Preheat the oven to 400°F (200°C). Remove shrimp from marinade, shaking off any excess. Arrange in a single layer on baking sheet. Bake for 5 to 7 minutes or until shrimp are just pink. Do not overcook. Serve hot or cold on a lettuce-lined platter.

Tips

- These moist, flavorful shrimp can be served hot or cold. Do not marinate longer than 1 hour or the shrimp will become mushy.

- Sesame oil is a vibrantly flavored oil that frequently appears in Asian recipes. It has a strong flavor, so use it sparingly. Look for sesame oil in the Asian food section of your supermarket. It will be labeled as pure sesame oil or as a blend of sesame and soybean oils — either type is fine for this recipe.

- A folded damp cloth placed under your chopping board will keep it in place while you chop.

Nutritional Analysis (Per Serving)
- Calories: 71
- Protein: 11.1 g
- Fat: 2.0 g
- Carbohydrates: 1.9 g
- Fiber: 1.0 g
- Sodium: 101 mg
- Cholesterol: 76 mg

Spicy Fried Shrimp with Maple-Mustard Dip

MAPLE-MUSTARD DIP

¼ cup	mayonnaise	50 mL
1 tbsp	Dijon mustard	15 mL
1 tsp	maple syrup	5 mL
1 tsp	Worcestershire sauce	5 mL

SHRIMP

1 tsp	salt	5 mL
1 tsp	ground coriander	5 mL
½ tsp	cayenne pepper	2 mL
½ tsp	ground cumin	2 mL
1 lb	raw large shrimp, peeled, deveined and patted dry	500 g
2 cups	canola or vegetable oil	500 mL
	Fresh coriander sprigs	

Make Ahead

The dip can be refrigerated, covered, for up to 24 hours.

> *These shrimp take just minutes to make — a good thing because they're really addictive!*

SERVES 4 TO 6
Preheat oven to 200°F (100°C)

1. *Maple-Mustard Dip:* In a small serving bowl, combine mayonnaise, Dijon mustard, maple syrup and Worcestershire sauce; stir well. Refrigerate, covered, until ready to serve.

2. *Shrimp:* In a medium bowl, combine salt, coriander, cayenne and cumin. Add shrimp; toss well to coat evenly.

3. In a large deep skillet or in a Dutch oven, heat oil over medium-high heat. In batches fry shrimp, turning once, for 1 minute or until curled and pink. As each batch is ready, remove with a slotted spoon to a paper-towel-lined plate. Keep warm in preheated oven until all shrimp are cooked.

4. To serve, pile shrimp in a napkin-lined basket. Garnish with sprigs of coriander. Serve at once with dip alongside. Discard any dip that's left over after serving.

Nutritional Analysis (Per Serving)
- Calories: 223
- Protein: 18.7 g
- Fat: 15.0 g
- Carbohydrates: 2.6 g
- Fiber: 0.2 g
- Sodium: 641 mg
- Cholesterol: 144 mg

Shrimp and Snow Pea Tidbits

16	snow peas	16
2 tsp	vegetable oil	10 mL
1 tsp	crushed garlic	5 mL
1 tbsp	chopped fresh parsley	15 mL
16	medium shrimp, peeled, deveined, tail left on	16

Make Ahead

If serving cold, prepare and refrigerate early in day.

SERVES 4 TO 6 OR MAKES 16 HORS D'OEUVRES

1. Steam or microwave snow peas until barely tendercrisp. Rinse with cold water. Drain and set aside.

2. In nonstick skillet, heat oil; sauté garlic, parsley and shrimp just until shrimp turn pink, 3 to 5 minutes.

3. Wrap each snow pea around shrimp; fasten with toothpick. Serve warm or cold.

Nutritional Analysis (Per Serving)
- Calories: 31
- Protein: 3 g
- Fat: 1 g
- Carbohydrates: 1 g
- Fiber: 0 g
- Sodium: 31 mg
- Cholesterol: 26 mg

Shrimp with Pesto and Prosciutto

15	large shrimp, peeled and deveined	15
3 tbsp	pesto (see recipe, below)	45 mL
5	thin slices prosciutto	5

Make Ahead

Shrimp can be prepared, covered and refrigerated up to 4 hours before baking.

This is an elegant appetizer that takes just minutes to prepare. Serve these shrimp hot or warm, as a starter or on toothpicks as finger food. If you wish, you can omit the prosciutto (reduce the cooking time by a minute or so).

MAKES 3 TO 4 SERVINGS

1. Pat shrimp dry and place in a large bowl. Add pesto and toss until shrimp are coated.
2. Cut each prosciutto slice lengthwise into 3 pieces. Wrap each shrimp with prosciutto, tucking in ends.
3. Place shrimp, seam side down, in a single layer on lightly greased oven pan.
4. Bake in preheated 400°F (200°C) toaster oven for 8 minutes, or until shrimp are cooked and pink.

Variation

- **Scallops with Pesto and Prosciutto:** Use 15 large scallops (about 1 lb/500 g) instead of shrimp. Bake for 8 minutes, or until scallops are opaque.

Nutritional Analysis (Per Serving)
- Calories: 298
- Protein: 42.3 g
- Fat: 11.2 g
- Carbohydrates: 4.3 g
- Fiber: 0.5 g
- Sodium: 925 mg
- Cholesterol: 259 mg

Pesto

In a food processor, combine 1 cup (250 mL) packed fresh basil leaves, ¼ cup (50 mL) toasted pine nuts, 2 peeled cloves garlic, ¼ tsp (1 mL) salt and ¼ tsp (1 mL) black pepper. Pulse until finely chopped. With machine running, pour ⅓ cup (75 mL) olive oil through feed tube. Blend in ⅓ cup (75 mL) grated Parmesan cheese, scraping down sides of food processor. Makes about 1 cup (250 mL).

Refrigerate pesto for up to 4 days or freeze for up to 6 weeks. To freeze, spoon pesto into 2 tbsp (25 mL) portions on waxed paper-lined baking sheet. Freeze, then transfer to resealable plastic bags.

Eggplant and Tuna Antipasto Appetizer

1 tbsp	olive oil	15 mL
1½ cups	peeled, chopped eggplant	375 mL
1 cup	sliced mushrooms	250 mL
¾ cup	chopped red peppers	175 mL
½ cup	chopped onions	125 mL
2 tsp	minced garlic	10 mL
1 tsp	dried basil	5 mL
½ tsp	dried oregano	2 mL
½ cup	chicken stock or water	125 mL
½ cup	crushed tomatoes (canned or fresh)	125 mL
⅓ cup	sliced pimiento-stuffed green olives	75 mL
⅓ cup	bottled chili sauce	75 mL
2 tsp	drained capers	10 mL
1	can (6.5 oz/184 g) tuna in water, drained	1

Make Ahead
Prepare up to 2 days before and stir before serving cold or before reheating.

SERVES 8 TO 10

1. Spray a nonstick pan with vegetable spray. Heat oil in pan over medium-high heat; add eggplant, mushrooms, red peppers, onions, garlic, basil and oregano. Cook for 8 minutes, stirring occasionally, or until vegetables are softened.

2. Add stock, tomatoes, olives, chili sauce and capers; simmer uncovered for 6 minutes, stirring occasionally until most of the liquid is absorbed.

3. Transfer to bowl of food processor and add tuna; process for 20 seconds or until combined but still chunky.

Tip
• Chill or serve warm.

Nutritional Analysis (Per Serving)
- Calories: 65
- Protein: 5 g
- Fat: 2 g
- Carbohydrates: 6 g
- Fiber: 2 g
- Sodium: 411 mg
- Cholesterol: 3 mg

Seafood Seviche

¼ lb	scallops, sliced	125 g
¼ lb	squid, sliced	125 g
½ cup	finely chopped red onion	125 mL
½ cup	diced sweet red or yellow pepper	125 mL
½ cup	diced tomato	125 mL
1 tsp	crushed garlic	5 mL
¼ cup	fresh lime or lemon juice	50 mL
2 tbsp	chopped fresh cilantro or parsley	25 mL
1 tbsp	olive oil	15 mL
	Lettuce leaves	

SERVES 4

1. In bowl, combine scallops, squid, onion, red pepper, tomato, garlic, lime juice, cilantro and oil; stir to combine.

2. Cover and refrigerate for 2 hours to marinate, stirring occasionally. Serve over lettuce-lined plates.

Tips
• Cilantro, a wonderful herb, is also called coriander or Chinese parsley. If unavailable, substitute fresh parsley.

• If you prefer, use only scallops or only squid.

Nutritional Analysis (Per Serving)
- Calories: 111
- Protein: 11 g
- Fat: 4 g
- Carbohydrates: 7 g
- Fiber: 1 g
- Sodium: 95 mg
- Cholesterol: 76 mg

Seafood Garlic Antipasto

1 lb	scallops, squid or shrimp, or a combination, cut into pieces	500 g
¾ cup	chopped snow peas	175 mL
¾ cup	chopped red peppers	175 mL
½ cup	diced tomatoes	125 mL
⅓ cup	chopped red onions	75 mL
⅓ cup	minced coriander or dill	75 mL
¼ cup	sliced black olives	50 mL
3 tbsp	lemon juice	45 mL
2 tbsp	olive oil	25 mL
1½ tsp	minced garlic	7 mL
	Pepper to taste	

Make Ahead

Prepare early in the day and keep refrigerated. Mix before serving.

SERVES 6

1. In a nonstick skillet sprayed with vegetable spray, cook the seafood over medium-high heat for 3 minutes, or until just done. Drain excess liquid, if any, and place seafood in serving bowl. Let cool slightly.

2. Add snow peas, red peppers, tomatoes, red onions, coriander and olives; mix well. Whisk together lemon juice, olive oil, garlic; pour over seafood mixture. Add pepper to taste. Chill for 1 hour before serving.

Tip

• If suggested seafood is not used, try a firm white fish such as swordfish, haddock, or monkfish.

Nutritional Analysis (Per Serving)
• Calories: 127   • Protein: 14 g   • Fat: 5 g
• Carbohydrates: 6 g   • Fiber: 1 g   • Sodium: 176 mg
• Cholesterol: 25 mg

Oriental Chicken Wrapped Mushrooms

1 tbsp	rice wine vinegar	15 mL
1 tbsp	vegetable oil	15 mL
2 tbsp	soya sauce	25 mL
1 tsp	crushed garlic	5 mL
2 tbsp	finely chopped onion	25 mL
1 tsp	sesame oil	5 mL
2 tbsp	water	25 mL
2 tbsp	brown sugar	25 mL
½ tsp	sesame seeds (optional)	2 mL
¾ lb	boneless skinless chicken breast	375 g
18	medium mushroom caps (without stems)	18

Make Ahead

Refrigerate chicken in marinade early in day. Wrap chicken around mushroom caps and broil just before serving.

SERVES 4 TO 6 OR MAKES 18 HORS D'OEUVRES
Preheat broiler • Baking sheet sprayed with nonstick vegetable spray

1. In bowl, combine vinegar, oil, soya sauce, garlic, onion, sesame oil, water, sugar, and sesame seeds (if using); mix well.

2. Cut chicken into strips about 3 inches (8 cm) long and 1 inch (2.5 cm) wide to make 18 strips. Add to bowl and marinate for 20 minutes, stirring occasionally.

3. Wrap each chicken strip around mushroom; secure with toothpick. Place on baking sheet. Broil for approximately 5 minutes or until chicken is no longer pink inside. Serve immediately.

Nutritional Analysis (Per Serving)
• Calories: 130   • Protein: 15 g   • Fat: 5 g
• Carbohydrates: 7 g   • Fiber: 0 g   • Sodium: 329 mg
• Cholesterol: 36 mg

Saffron-Scented Chicken Kababs

8	skinless boneless chicken breasts	8
1/2 tsp	saffron threads	2 mL
1/2 cup	plain nonfat yogurt, avoiding as much liquid as possible	125 mL
2 tbsp	minced green chilies, preferably serranos, or to taste	25 mL
1 1/2 tbsp	minced peeled gingerroot	22 mL
1 1/2 tbsp	minced garlic	22 mL
1 1/2 tsp	cumin powder	7 mL
3/4 tsp	cardamom powder	4 mL
1/2 tsp	freshly ground black pepper	2 mL
1 1/2 tsp	salt or to taste	7 mL
3 tbsp	lemon or lime juice	45 mL
2 tbsp	vegetable oil (approx.)	25 mL

Saffron adds a special touch to these succulent, bite-size pieces of chicken. They are delicious cooked on a charcoal grill.

SERVES 8

12 to 16 metal skewers, or 16 to 20 bamboo skewers, soaked in water for 30 minutes

1. Rinse chicken and pat dry. Cut into bite-size pieces.

2. Soak saffron in 2 tbsp (25 mL) hot water for 10 minutes.

3. Stir together yogurt, chilies, ginger, garlic, cumin, cardamom, pepper, salt and lemon juice. Stir in saffron threads with liquid. Pour over chicken and mix thoroughly. Refrigerate for at least 2 hours or for up to 12 hours.

4. *To bake in oven:* Preheat oven to 375°F (190°C). Line a rimmed jelly-roll pan or baking sheet with foil. Arrange chicken pieces on pan, discarding extra marinade. Drizzle oil evenly on top. Bake until no longer pink inside, 10 to 12 minutes. Serve immediately.

5. *To cook on grill:* Preheat barbecue to medium. Thread chicken pieces onto metal skewers, 3 to 4 per skewer. If using bamboo skewers, wrap exposed bamboo with foil to prevent burning. Brush lightly with oil and grill, turning once, until no longer pink inside, 3 to 4 minutes.

Tip

- It is not always necessary to thread kababs in Indian cooking. In this recipe, you can bake them without threading or grill them on skewers.

Nutritional Analysis (Per Serving)

- Calories: 234
- Protein: 42.8 g
- Fat: 5.1 g
- Carbohydrates: 1.9 g
- Fiber: 0.2 g
- Sodium: 474 mg
- Cholesterol: 103 mg

Ham Roulades

1 tbsp	soft margarine	15 mL
1 cup	finely chopped mushrooms	250 mL
¼ cup	chopped green onions	50 mL
4 oz	light cream cheese, softened	125 g
½ cup	chopped fresh parsley	125 mL
2 tsp	Dijon mustard	10 mL
1 tsp	lemon juice	5 mL
Pinch	cayenne pepper	Pinch
6	slices cooked lean ham	6

These roll-ups are tasty and so easy to make that even young children can assist in their assembly. Kids have a natural affinity for cooking, and your encouragement will boost their self-esteem.

MAKES 24

1. In a skillet, melt margarine over medium heat; cook mushrooms and green onions for 3 to 5 minutes or until tender. Cool.

2. In a bowl, blend together cheese, parsley, mustard, lemon juice and cayenne; stir in mushroom mixture. Spread evenly over ham slices and roll up. Wrap in plastic wrap. Refrigerate for at least 2 hours or until chilled. Cut each roll into 4 pieces. Serve speared with frilled toothpick.

Tips

- Try substituting smoked turkey, roast beef or prosciutto for the ham in these tasty nibblers.

- This easily prepared appetizer can be made ahead of time. Serve these rolls as part of a tray of finger foods, along with roasted red peppers and Artichoke Nuggets (see recipe, page 19).

Nutritional Analysis (Per Hors d'oeuvre)
- Calories: 29
- Protein: 2 g
- Fat: 2 g
- Carbohydrates: 1 g
- Fiber: Trace
- Sodium: 444 mg
- Cholesterol: 16 mg

Asparagus Wrapped with Ricotta Cheese and Ham

12	medium asparagus, trimmed	12
4 oz	ricotta cheese	125 g
¼ tsp	crushed garlic	1 mL
1 tbsp	finely chopped green onion or chives	15 mL
	Salt and pepper	
4	thin slices cooked ham (about 4 oz/125 g)	4

Make Ahead

Assemble rolls early in day and refrigerate. Serve cold or hot.

SERVES 4
Preheat oven to 400°F (200°C) • Baking sheet sprayed with nonstick vegetable spray

1. Steam or microwave asparagus just until tender-crisp; drain and let cool. Set aside.

2. In small bowl, combine cheese, garlic, onion, and salt and pepper to taste; mix well.

3. Spread evenly over each slice of ham. Top each with 3 asparagus and roll up. Place on baking sheet and bake for 3 to 4 minutes or until hot.

Nutritional Analysis (Per Serving)
- Calories: 94
- Protein: 10 g
- Fat: 4 g
- Carbohydrates: 4 g
- Fiber: 1 g
- Sodium: 378 mg
- Cholesterol: 23 mg

Mushroom and Prosciutto Antipasto with Walnuts

1 cup	walnut pieces (about 4 oz/125 g)	250 mL
3 cups	sliced button mushrooms (about 6 oz/175 g)	750 mL
¾ cup	shaved Parmesan cheese (about 2 oz/50 g)	175 mL
2 oz	prosciutto, trimmed of excess fat and chopped	50 g
¼ cup	fresh lemon juice	50 mL
2 tbsp	chopped fresh Italian flat-leafed parsley	25 mL
2 tbsp	olive oil	25 mL
¼ tsp	black pepper	1 mL
Pinch	salt (optional)	Pinch

Use the finest-quality, freshest walnuts you can find for this easy salad. It is best served within 2 hours of being made. Although it will taste fine the next day, the mushrooms tend to darken on standing.

SERVES 4 TO 6

1. In a small skillet over medium-high heat, toast walnuts, stirring often, for 3 to 5 minutes or until golden and fragrant. (Watch them carefully; they burn easily.) Remove from heat; let cool completely.

2. In a large serving bowl, stir together walnuts, mushrooms, Parmesan cheese and prosciutto. Sprinkle with lemon juice, parsley, olive oil and pepper; toss well. If desired, add salt and additional pepper. Serve at room temperature.

Tips

- Since nuts go stale and rancid very quickly, it's best to buy them in small sealed packages from a store with a sufficiently fast turnover that you know they're fresh. If you're not going to use them immediately, store them in the freezer. For most recipes, you can use nuts straight from the freezer.

- Use a sharp paring knife or vegetable peeler to shave a piece of fresh Parmesan cheese into thin flakes.

Nutritional Analysis (Per Serving)
- Calories: 296
- Protein: 13.3 g
- Fat: 25.5 g
- Carbohydrates: 7.0 g
- Fiber: 2.5 g
- Sodium: 447 mg
- Cholesterol: 16 mg

Baked Goat Cheese

4 oz	soft goat cheese, at room temperature	125 g
¼ cup	toasted pine nuts	50 mL
1 tbsp	drained green peppercorns	15 mL
12 to 14	small lettuce leaves (radicchio, Belgian endive, or inner leaves of Boston or Romaine lettuce)	12 to 14

SERVES 2 AS AN APPETIZER OR 4 TO 6 AS AN HORS D'OEUVRE

Preheat oven to 400°F (200°C) • Baking sheet

1. In a bowl, combine goat cheese, pine nuts and green peppercorns; mix gently but thoroughly. Form cheese mixture into balls measuring about ¾ inch (2 cm). (You should end up with 12 to 14 balls.) Put them on a plate, cover loosely with waxed paper and refrigerate for at least 45 minutes to harden.

2. Place cheese balls on baking sheet, well spaced apart; bake in preheated oven for 4 to 5 minutes, until cheese is bubbling and has started to spread. Remove from oven.

3. Spread leaves of lettuce on a serving tray. Using a small spatula, remove baked cheese balls and carefully transfer each to the middle of a lettuce leaf. (The leaf acts as a platform for the cheese, and is eaten with it.) Serve immediately.

Nutritional Analysis (Per Serving)
- Calories: 326
- Protein: 18.3 g
- Fat: 25.9 g
- Carbohydrates: 8.2 g
- Fiber: 3.5 g
- Sodium: 301 mg
- Cholesterol: 44 mg

Ricotta and Blue Cheese Appetizers

2 oz	blue cheese	50 g
½ cup	ricotta cheese	125 mL
2 tbsp	2% yogurt	25 mL
2 tbsp	chopped fresh dill (or 1 tsp/5 mL dried dillweed)	25 mL
2	Belgian endives	2

Make Ahead

Prepare dip and refrigerate up to a day before. Spoon onto endive leaves just before serving.

SERVES 4 TO 6 OR MAKES 25 HORS D'OEUVRES

1. In food processor, combine blue cheese, ricotta, yogurt and dill; process until creamy and smooth.

2. Separate Belgian endive leaves. Spoon 2 tsp (10 mL) cheese mixture onto stem end of each.

Tips
- For blue cheese lovers, increase to 3 oz (75 g).
- Instead of endive leaves, fill empty mushroom caps, or serve as a dip with crudités.

Nutritional Analysis (Per Serving)
- Calories: 87
- Protein: 6 g
- Fat: 4 g
- Carbohydrates: 6 g
- Fiber: 3 g
- Sodium: 190 mg
- Cholesterol: 13 mg

Cheddar Pepper Rounds

8 oz	aged Cheddar cheese, shredded	250 g
4 oz	cream cheese	125 g
2 tbsp	brandy or sherry	25 mL
¼ cup	finely chopped fresh parsley	50 mL
1 tbsp	cracked black peppercorns (see tip, at right)	15 m

Here's an updated version of the classic cheese ball, an appetizer that dominated the party scene in the 1950s and 1960s. This recipe may seem to call for a lot of peppercorns, but it's not all that peppery. It just has a lively zip.

SERVES 16

1. In a food processor, combine Cheddar cheese, cream cheese and brandy. Process until mixture is very smooth. Transfer to a bowl; refrigerate for 3 hours or until firm.

2. Divide mixture into two pieces; wrap each in plastic wrap. Roll on a flat surface and shape into a smooth log measuring about 6 inches by 1½ inches (15 by 4 cm).

3. Place parsley and cracked peppercorns on a plate. Unwrap cheese logs and roll in parsley-peppercorn mixture until evenly coated. Wrap again in plastic wrap and refrigerate until firm.

4. To serve, cut each log into ¼-inch (0.5 cm) slices and serve on ½-inch (1 cm) cucumber slices.

Tips

- To crack peppercorns, place in a heavy plastic bag and, on a wooden board, crush using a rolling pin or a heavy skillet.

- Cheese logs can be frozen for up to 1 month. Defrost in the refrigerator for several hours before slicing.

Variation

- **Cheddar Walnut Rounds:** Substitute ⅓ cup (75 mL) finely chopped walnuts or pecans for cracked peppercorns.

Nutritional Analysis (Per Serving)
- Calories: 93
- Protein: 4.3 g
- Fat: 7.3 g
- Carbohydrates: 1.8 g
- Fiber: 0.4 g
- Sodium: 110 mg
- Cholesterol: 23 mg

Tea-Scented Goat Cheese

1	round soft unripened goat cheese (about 4 oz/125 g)	1
2 tbsp	flavored tea (such as fruit tisane, Lapsang Souchong, Genmai Cha, jasmine tea, etc.)	25 mL

SERVES 4

1. Wrap cheese in a single layer of cheesecloth with very little overlap.

2. On a piece of plastic wrap large enough to wrap the cheese, spread 1 tbsp (15 mL) of the tea in a band lengthwise down the middle of the plastic wrap. Place the curved edge of the cheese in the tea at one end of the wrap and tightly roll the cheese in the wrap, making sure that the tea is covering the side of the cheese all the way around. Place the cheese with one of the flat sides up and sprinkle half the remaining tea over the cheese. Close the end tightly. Repeat on the remaining side. You should end up with a piece of cheese that is almost completely covered in tea, tightly wrapped in plastic.

3. Refrigerate for 24 hours. (Keep in mind that the longer the cheese is marinated, the stronger the flavor of the tea.) Remove the plastic wrap and cheesecloth from the cheese and serve.

Nutritional Analysis (Per Serving)
- Calories: 103
- Protein: 6.1 g
- Fat: 8.5 g
- Carbohydrates: 0.7 g
- Fiber: 0 g
- Sodium: 146 mg
- Cholesterol: 22 mg

Swiss Cheese Pâté

½ cup	whipping (35%) cream	125 mL
1	clove garlic	1
1 cup	shredded Swiss cheese	250 mL
¼ tsp	freshly ground nutmeg	1 mL

Mellow Swiss cheese adds "up-market" appeal to a pâté. Sitting for a day or so allows time for flavors to mellow. Serve with sliced apples or pears, or as a dip for crudités.

SERVES 6 TO 8

1. In a small saucepan over medium heat, heat cream and garlic just until cream comes to a boil. Remove from heat and discard garlic.

2. Slowly add cheese, stirring after each addition, until cheese has melted. Stir in nutmeg.

3. Transfer to a small serving bowl. Cover and refrigerate until firm.

4. Remove from refrigerator one hour before serving time. Serve warm or at room temperature.

Nutritional Analysis (Per Serving)
- Calories: 118
- Protein: 4.8 g
- Fat: 10.6 g
- Carbohydrates: 1.2 g
- Fiber: 0 g
- Sodium: 47 mg
- Cholesterol: 37 mg

Mushroom Cheese Pâté

1 lb	button mushrooms or a variety of mixed mushrooms	500 g
2 tbsp	butter or margarine	25 mL
1½ cups	shredded Cheddar cheese	375 mL
1 tbsp	horseradish	15 mL

Make this wonderful pâté anytime you have an abundance of mushrooms on hand. Add a sprinkling of chopped fresh parsley for color.

SERVES 12

1. Coarsely chop mushrooms. Set aside.
2. In a nonstick skillet on high heat, melt butter. Add mushrooms and cook, stirring frequently, for 5 minutes or until mushrooms are softened and liquid has evaporated. Set aside to cool slightly.
3. Place mushrooms in a food processor and process until fairly smooth. Add cheese and process again until smooth. Add horseradish to taste. Transfer to a small bowl. Cover and refrigerate until chilled before serving. Store in a covered container in refrigerator for up to one week or freeze for longer storage.

Nutritional Analysis (Per Serving)
- Calories: 5
- Protein: 0.3 g
- Fat: 0.4 g
- Carbohydrates: 0.1 g
- Fiber: 0 g
- Sodium: 8 mg
- Cholesterol: 1 mg

Leek Mushroom Cheese Pâté

2 tsp	vegetable oil	10 mL
1½ tsp	minced garlic	7 mL
1½ cups	chopped leeks	375 mL
½ cup	finely chopped carrots	125 mL
12 oz	oyster or regular mushrooms, thinly sliced	375 g
2 tbsp	sherry or white wine	25 mL
2 tbsp	chopped fresh dill (or 2 tsp/10 mL dried)	25 mL
1½ tsp	dried oregano	7 mL
¼ tsp	coarsely ground black pepper	1 mL
2 oz	feta cheese, crumbled	50 g
2 oz	light cream cheese	50 g
½ cup	5% ricotta cheese	125 mL
2 tsp	freshly squeezed lemon juice	10 mL
2 tbsp	chopped fresh dill	25 mL

Make Ahead

Prepare up to 2 days in advance.

SERVES 8 TO 10
9- by 5-inch (2 L) loaf pan lined with plastic wrap

1. In a large nonstick frying pan sprayed with vegetable spray, heat oil over medium-high heat. Add garlic, leeks and carrots; cook 3 minutes, stirring occasionally. Stir in mushrooms, sherry, dill, oregano and pepper; cook, stirring occasionally, 8 to 10 minutes or until carrots are tender and liquid is absorbed. Remove from heat.
2. Transfer vegetable mixture to a food processor. Add feta, cream cheese, ricotta and lemon juice; purée until smooth. Spoon into prepared loaf pan. Cover and chill until firm.
3. Invert onto serving platter; sprinkle with chopped dill. Serve with crudités.

Nutritional Analysis (Per Serving)
- Calories: 75
- Protein: 4 g
- Fat: 3 g
- Carbohydrates: 6 g
- Fiber: 1 g
- Sodium: 117 mg
- Cholesterol: 11 mg

Mushroom Sun-Dried Tomato Cheese Pâté

1½ tsp	vegetable oil	7 mL
⅓ cup	chopped onions	75 mL
1 cup	chopped mushrooms	250 mL
⅓ cup	finely chopped red bell peppers	75 mL
1½ cups	5% ricotta cheese	375 mL
½ cup	light cream cheese, softened	125 mL
⅓ cup	light sour cream	75 mL
⅓ cup	chopped softened sun-dried tomatoes (see tip, at right)	75 mL
⅓ cup	chopped fresh dill (or 1½ tsp/7 mL dried)	75 mL
2 tbsp	freshly squeezed lemon juice	25 mL
2 tbsp	grated Parmesan cheese	25 mL
1 tsp	minced garlic	5 mL
¼ tsp	freshly ground black pepper	1 mL

Make Ahead

Prepare up to 2 days in advance.

SERVES 8 TO 10

9- by 5-inch (2 L) loaf pan lined with plastic wrap

1. In a nonstick frying pan, heat oil over medium-high heat. Add onions; cook 4 minutes or until softened. Stir in mushrooms and red peppers; cook 4 minutes longer or until vegetables are tender. Remove from heat.

2. In a large bowl, combine ricotta, cream cheese, sour cream, sun-dried tomatoes, dill, lemon juice, Parmesan, garlic and pepper until well mixed. Stir in cooked vegetables. Pour into prepared loaf pan; refrigerate at least 1 hour. Invert onto a serving platter; peel off plastic wrap.

Tips

- Instead of a loaf pan, you can also pour this into a decorative serving dish.

- To soften sun-dried tomatoes, cover with boiling water and let soak 15 minutes; drain and chop.

- Try wild mushrooms, if available. Oyster mushrooms are a good choice.

Nutritional Analysis (Per Serving)
- Calories: 121
- Protein: 8 g
- Fat: 8 g
- Carbohydrates: 6 g
- Fiber 1 g
- Sodium: 212 mg
- Cholesterol: 25 mg

Sardine Lover's Pâté

1	can (3.75 oz/106 g) sardines, drained	1
¼ cup	light sour cream	50 mL
½ tsp	lemon zest	2 mL
1 tbsp	freshly squeezed lemon juice	15 mL

Even non-sardine lovers will enjoy vegetables dipped in this tangy lemon sardine pâté.

SERVES 2

1. In a food processor, combine sardines, sour cream, lemon zest and juice. Pulse with on/off motion until mixture is almost smooth.

2. Store in a covered container in refrigerator for up to one week or freeze for longer storage.

Nutritional Analysis (Per Serving)
- Calories: 148
- Protein: 13.9 g
- Fat: 7.8 g
- Carbohydrates: 1.6 g
- Fiber: 0 g
- Sodium: 280 mg
- Cholesterol: 87 mg

Double Salmon and Dill Pâté

1 cup	5% ricotta cheese	250 mL
1	can (7.5 oz /213 g) salmon, drained and skin removed	1
¼ cup	chopped green onions (about 2 medium)	50 mL
3 tbsp	chopped fresh dill (or 1 tsp/5 mL dried dillweed)	45 mL
2 tbsp	lemon juice	25 mL
4 oz	smoked salmon, cut into thin shreds	125 g

Make Ahead

Prepare up to a day ahead and keep refrigerated.

SERVES 8

1. Place ricotta, canned salmon, green onions, dill and lemon juice in bowl of food processor; process for 20 seconds or until smooth.
2. Transfer mixture to serving bowl and fold in shredded smoked salmon. Serve with crudités.

Tips

- Leaving in the bones from the canned salmon increases the calcium content.
- Leftover cooked salmon can also be used instead of canned.

Nutritional Analysis (Per Serving)
- Calories: 91
- Protein: 10 g
- Fat: 4 g
- Carbohydrates: 1 g
- Fiber: 0 g
- Sodium: 237 mg
- Cholesterol: 18 mg

Do-Ahead Herb Dip

1 cup	creamed cottage cheese	250 mL
½ cup	plain yogurt or sour cream	125 mL
½ cup	light mayonnaise	125 mL
⅓ cup	finely chopped fresh parsley	75 mL
2 tbsp	finely chopped fresh chives or minced green onions	25 mL
1 tbsp	chopped fresh dill	15 mL
1½ tsp	Dijon mustard	7 mL
1 tsp	red wine vinegar or lemon juice	5 mL
	Hot pepper sauce	

This creamy dip relies on lower-fat dairy products and zesty herbs, so it clocks in with a lot less fat and calories than you might imagine. Make it at least a day ahead to let flavors develop. Serve with fresh veggies.

SERVES 4

1. In a food processor, purée cottage cheese, yogurt and mayonnaise until very smooth and creamy.
2. Transfer to a bowl; stir in parsley, chives, dill, mustard, vinegar and hot pepper sauce to taste. Cover and refrigerate.

Tips

- Other fresh herbs, including basil, can be added according to what you have in the fridge or growing in your garden. If you're fond of fresh dill, increase the amount to 2 tbsp (25 mL).
- Store in a covered container in the fridge for up to one week.

Nutritional Analysis (Per Serving)
- Calories: 179
- Protein: 9.1 g
- Fat: 12.7 g
- Carbohydrates: 6.6 g
- Fiber: 0.3 g
- Sodium: 507 mg
- Cholesterol: 19 mg

Cottage Cheese Herb Dip

1 cup	lower-fat cottage cheese	250 mL
1/2 cup	lower-fat plain yogurt	125 mL
1	green onion, chopped	1
1/2 tsp	garlic powder	2 mL
1/2 tsp	celery seed	2 mL
1/4 tsp	dry mustard	1 mL
1/4 tsp	Worcestershire sauce	1 mL
Pinch	black pepper	Pinch
Dash	hot pepper sauce	Dash

This dip will enhance any lazy summer afternoon. For best results, prepare ahead of time and refrigerate.

MAKES 1 1/2 CUPS (375 ML)

1. In a food processor or blender, cream cottage cheese and yogurt until very smooth. Stir in onion and seasonings. Chill overnight.

Tips

- Serve this with Creamy Salmon Quiche (see recipe, page 149), raw vegetables and fresh fruit.

- To keep the calories low, serve with crudités, such as broccoli, cauliflower, green or red bell peppers, zucchini and carrot sticks.

Nutritional Analysis (Per Serving)
- Calories: 11
- Protein: 1 g
- Fat: 0 g
- Carbohydrates: 1 g
- Fiber: 0 g
- Sodium: 263 mg
- Cholesterol: 8 mg

Chunky Artichoke Dip

1	can (19 oz/398 mL) artichoke hearts, drained	1
1/4 cup	5% ricotta cheese	50 mL
1/4 cup	light sour cream or 2% yogurt	50 mL
1/4 cup	chopped fresh parsley	50 mL
1/4 cup	chopped green onions, about 2 medium	50 mL
3 tbsp	light mayonnaise	45 mL
3 tbsp	grated Parmesan cheese	45 mL
1 tsp	minced garlic	5 mL

Make Ahead

Prepare up to a day in advance; stir before serving.

SERVES 8

1. Put artichoke hearts, ricotta, sour cream, parsley, green onions, mayonnaise, Parmesan and garlic in food processor; process until slightly chunky.

Tips

- Serve with crudités.

- Serve either at room temperature or chilled.

Nutritional Analysis (Per Serving)
- Calories: 56
- Protein: 3 g
- Fat: 3 g
- Carbohydrates: 5 g
- Fiber: 0 g
- Sodium: 198 mg
- Cholesterol: 6 mg

Artichoke and Blue Cheese Dip

¾ cup	drained canned artichokes	175 mL
¼ cup	chopped green onions	50 mL
½ tsp	crushed garlic	2 mL
2 oz	blue cheese	50 g
1 tbsp	chopped fresh parsley	15 mL
¼ cup	2% yogurt	50 mL
	Salt and pepper	

Make Ahead

Make and refrigerate up to a day before. Stir just before serving.

SERVES 4 TO 6 OR MAKES 1¼ CUPS (300 ML)

1. In food processor, combine artichokes, onions, garlic, cheese, parsley, yogurt, and salt and pepper to taste; process until smooth. Transfer to serving bowl.

Tips

- If a more subtle flavor is desired, cut back on the blue cheese, using only 1½ oz (40 g).
- Other strong cheeses, such as grated Parmesan or Swiss, can replace the blue cheese.

Nutritional Analysis (Per Serving)
- Calories: 53
- Protein: 3 g
- Fat: 3 g
- Carbohydrates: 4 g
- Fiber: 1 g
- Sodium: 160 mg
- Cholesterol: 7 mg

Tofu and Chickpea Garlic Dip

1 cup	canned chickpeas, rinsed and drained	250 mL
8 oz	soft (silken) tofu, drained	250 g
2 tbsp	tahini	25 mL
2 tbsp	freshly squeezed lemon juice	25 mL
1 tsp	minced garlic	5 mL
¼ cup	chopped fresh dill (or 1 tsp/5 mL dried)	50 mL
¼ cup	chopped green onions	50 mL
¼ cup	chopped green olives	50 mL
¼ cup	chopped red bell peppers	50 mL
¼ tsp	freshly ground black pepper	1 mL

Make Ahead

Prepare up to 1 day in advance. Mix before serving.

SERVES 6 TO 8

1. In a food processor, combine chickpeas, tofu, tahini, lemon juice and garlic; purée. Stir in dill, green onions, olives, red peppers and pepper.
2. Chill. Serve with crudités.

Tips

- Tofu combined with beans, such as the chickpeas used here, gives the dip a butter-like texture.
- Be sure to buy soft (silken) tofu to ensure a creamy dip. Firm or pressed tofu will result in a granular texture.
- Tahini is a sesame paste found in the international section of grocery stores. If you can't find it, try using smooth peanut butter instead.

Nutritional Analysis (Per Serving)
- Calories: 86
- Protein: 5 g
- Fat: 4 g
- Carbohydrates: 8 g
- Fiber: 2 g
- Sodium: 153 mg
- Cholesterol: 0 mg

Creamy Sun-Dried Tomato Dip

4 oz	dry-packed sun-dried tomatoes	125 g
¾ cup	5% ricotta cheese	175 mL
½ cup	chopped fresh parsley	125 mL
⅓ cup	vegetable stock or water	75 mL
3 tbsp	chopped black olives	45 mL
2 tbsp	olive oil	25 mL
2 tbsp	toasted pine nuts	25 mL
2 tbsp	grated Parmesan cheese	25 mL
1 tsp	minced garlic	5 mL

Make Ahead

Prepare up to 3 days in advance.

SERVES 8 OR MAKES 1¾ CUPS (425 ML)

1. In a small bowl, pour boiling water to cover over sun-dried tomatoes. Let stand 15 minutes. Drain and chop.

2. In a food processor combine sun-dried tomatoes, ricotta, parsley, stock, olives, olive oil, pine nuts, Parmesan and garlic; process until well combined but still chunky.

Tips

- To toast pine nuts, bake in 350°F (180°C) oven 8 to 10 minutes or until golden and fragrant. Or, in a nonstick skillet over high heat, toast until browned, about 2 to 3 minutes.

- Avoid sun-dried tomatoes packed in oil; these have a lot of extra calories and fat.

- Great as a dip for crudités.

Nutritional Analysis (Per Serving)
- Calories: 113
- Protein: 7 g
- Fat: 6 g
- Carbohydrates: 10 g
- Fiber: 3 g
- Sodium: 413 mg
- Cholesterol: 7 mg

Spinach and Ricotta Dip

Half	package (10 oz/284 g) fresh spinach	Half
½ cup	2% yogurt	125 mL
¾ cup	ricotta cheese	175 mL
½ tsp	crushed garlic	2 mL
2 tbsp	chopped fresh parsley	25 mL
2 tbsp	grated Parmesan cheese	25 mL
	Salt and pepper	

Make Ahead

Prepare and refrigerate up to a day before. Stir just before serving.

SERVES 4 TO 6 OR MAKES 1½ CUPS (375 ML)

1. Rinse spinach and shake off excess water. With just the water clinging to leaves, cook until wilted; drain and squeeze out excess moisture.

2. In food processor, combine spinach, yogurt, ricotta, garlic, parsley, Parmesan cheese, and salt and pepper to taste; process just until still chunky. Do not purée.

Tips

- You can cook half a package (150 g) frozen spinach instead of the fresh, then continue with recipe.

- Serve in a decorative bowl with vegetable sticks.

Nutritional Analysis (Per Serving)
- Calories: 20
- Protein: 1 g
- Fat: 1 g
- Carbohydrates: 1 g
- Fiber: 0 g
- Sodium: 23 mg
- Cholesterol: 4 mg

Creamy Spinach Dip

1	package (10 oz/300 g) fresh or frozen spinach	1
1 cup	crumbed feta cheese (about 4 oz/125 g)	250 mL
1/3 cup	chopped green onions	75 mL
1/4 cup	chopped fresh dill	50 mL
1	clove garlic, minced	1
1 tsp	grated lemon zest	5 mL
1 1/2 cups	sour cream (regular or light)	375 mL
1/2 cup	light mayonnaise	125 mL

SERVES 6

1. Remove tough stem ends from fresh spinach; wash in cold water. Place spinach with moisture clinging to leaves in a large saucepan. Cook over high heat, stirring, until just wilted. (If using frozen spinach, see tip, page 54.) Place spinach in a colander to drain. Squeeze out moisture by hand; wrap in a clean, dry towel and squeeze out excess moisture.

2. In a food processor, combine spinach, feta, green onions, dill, garlic and lemon zest. Process until very finely chopped.

3. Add sour cream and mayonnaise; process, using on-off turns, just until combined. Transfer to a serving bowl, cover and refrigerate until ready to serve. Serve with vegetable dippers.

Nutritional Analysis (Per Serving)
- Calories: 248
- Protein: 6.4 g
- Fat: 22.2 g
- Carbohydrates: 6.4 g
- Fiber: 1.3 g
- Sodium: 489 mg
- Cholesterol: 49 mg

Roasted Red Pepper Dip

8 oz	feta cheese	250 g
2	roasted red peppers	2

Serve this tasty dip with crudités for an elegant appetizer. Great on its own, it also makes a flavorful addition to a tasting platter.

MAKES ABOUT 1 3/4 CUPS (425 ML)

1. In a food processor, combine cheese and peppers and process until smooth.

Tips

- Make this with creamy feta cheese (about 26% M.F.) as the lower-fat versions tend to produce a drier dip. If your results seem dry, add 1 tsp (5 mL) or so of olive oil and give the mix a final pulse.

- For a zestier version of this dip, add hot pepper sauce to taste before processing.

Nutritional Analysis (Per Serving)
- Calories: 170
- Protein: 8.7 g
- Fat: 12.2 g
- Carbohydrates: 7.1 g
- Fiber: 1.5 g
- Sodium: 636 mg
- Cholesterol: 51 mg

Warm Spinach and Cheese Dip

1	package (10 oz/300 g) fresh or frozen chopped spinach	1
8 oz	cream cheese, softened	250 g
1 cup	mild or medium salsa	250 mL
2	green onions, finely chopped	2
1	clove garlic, minced	1
1/2 tsp	dried oregano leaves	2 mL
1/2 tsp	ground cumin	2 mL
1/2 cup	shredded Monterey Jack or Cheddar cheese	125 mL
1/2 cup	milk (approx.)	125 mL
	Salt	
	Hot pepper sauce	

When you've got the gang coming over, serve this warm dip and watch it disappear. I like to accompany it with white or blue corn tortilla chips.

SERVES 6

1. Remove tough stem ends from fresh spinach; wash in cold water. Place spinach with moisture clinging to leaves in a large saucepan. Cook over high heat, stirring, until just wilted. (If using frozen spinach, see tip, at right.) Place spinach in a colander to drain. Squeeze out moisture by hand; wrap in a clean, dry towel and squeeze out excess moisture.

2. In a medium saucepan, combine spinach, cream cheese, salsa, green onions, garlic, oregano and cumin. Cook over medium heat, stirring, for 2 to 3 minutes or until smooth and piping hot.

3. Stir in cheese and milk; cook for 2 minutes or until cheese melts. Add more milk to thin dip, if desired. Season with salt and hot pepper sauce to taste. Spoon into serving dish.

Microwave Method

1. In an 8-cup (2 L) casserole dish, combine spinach, cream cheese, salsa, onions, garlic, oregano and cumin; cover and microwave at Medium for 4 minutes, stirring once. Add cheese and milk; cover and microwave at Medium-High, stirring once, for 2 to 3 minutes, or until cheese is melted. Season with salt and hot pepper sauce to taste.

Tips

- If you want a hot version, use 2 fresh or pickled jalapeño peppers. Or for a mild version, use 1 can (4 oz/113 g) green chilies, drained and chopped.

- To defrost spinach, remove packaging and place in a 4-cup (1 L) casserole dish. Cover and microwave at High, stirring once, for 6 to 8 minutes or until defrosted and hot. Place in a sieve and press out excess moisture.

Nutritional Analysis (Per Serving)
- Calories: 205
- Protein: 7.7 g
- Fat: 17.1 g
- Carbohydrates: 6.8 g
- Fiber: 2.0 g
- Sodium: 442 mg
- Cholesterol: 53 mg

Quick Roasted Red Pepper Dip

3	roasted red bell peppers, skins and seeds removed	3
¾ cup	feta cheese, drained and crumbled (about 6 oz/175 g)	175 mL
½ tsp	minced garlic	2 mL
¼ tsp	hot pepper flakes	1 mL

SERVES 6 OR MAKES 1½ CUPS (375 ML)

1. In a food processor or blender, purée peppers, feta cheese, garlic and hot pepper flakes. Chill before serving.

Tips

- Roasted red peppers are flavorful and offer key nutrients. No wonder they often appear as an ingredient in recipes. You can roast them yourself and freeze them for later use or purchase them already prepared in a jar.
- Red peppers are high in vitamin C, vitamin A and antioxidants. To increase fiber, serve this delicious dip with raw vegetables.

Nutritional Analysis (Per ¼ cup/50 mL Serving)
- Calories: 58
- Protein: 3 g
- Fat: 3 g
- Carbohydrates: 5 g
- Fiber: 1 g
- Sodium: 211 mg
- Cholesterol: 17 mg

5-Minute Crab Dip

8 oz	cream cheese	250 g
1	can (6 oz/170 mL) crab meat, drained, liquid reserved	1
¼ cup	finely chopped green onions	50 mL
2 tsp	fresh lemon juice	10 mL
½ tsp	Worcestershire sauce	2 mL
¼ tsp	paprika	1 mL
	Hot pepper sauce	

With a can of crab meat in the pantry and cream cheese in the fridge, you're all set to make a quick dip in 5 minutes flat. You can make it in the microwave or just as easily on the stovetop over medium heat.

SERVES 3

1. Place cream cheese in a medium-size microwave-safe bowl; microwave at Medium for 2 minutes or until softened. Stir until smooth.
2. Stir in crab, green onions, 2 tbsp (25 mL) reserved crab liquid, lemon juice, Worcestershire sauce, paprika and hot pepper sauce to taste. Microwave at Medium-High for 2 minutes or until piping hot. Serve warm.

Variation

- **5-Minute Clam Dip:** Substitute 1 can (5 oz/142 g) drained clams for the crab. Stir in 1 minced garlic clove, if desired.

Tip

- Serve with crisp vegetable dippers.

Nutritional Analysis (Per Serving)
- Calories: 318
- Protein: 16.1 g
- Fat: 27.0 g
- Carbohydrates: 3.0 g
- Fiber: 0.3 g
- Sodium: 406 mg
- Cholesterol: 127 mg

Melizzano Despina (Eggplant Dip #1)

1	medium eggplant (about 1 lb/500 g)	1
1 tsp	vegetable oil	5 mL
1	onion	1
2 tbsp	lemon juice	25 mL
¼ cup	olive oil	50 mL
	Few sprigs fresh parsley, chopped	
	Salt and pepper to taste	

SERVES 4
Preheat oven to 450°F (230°C)

1. Brush eggplant lightly with vegetable oil. Using a fork, pierce the skin lightly at 1-inch (2.5-cm) intervals. Place on a baking sheet and bake for 1 hour, or until eggplant is very soft and the skin is dark brown and caved in.

2. Transfer eggplant to a working surface. Cut off 1 inch (2 cm) at the stem end and discard (this part never quite cooks through). Peel the eggplant by picking at an edge from the cut end, then pulling upward. The skin should come off easily in strips.

3. Cut the eggplant lengthwise and place each half with the interior facing you. With a spoon scoop out the tongues of seed-pods, leaving as much of the flesh as possible. To remove the additional seed-pods hiding inside, cut each piece of eggplant in half and repeat the deseeding procedure. Once deseeded, let cleaned eggplant flesh sit to shed some of its excess water.

4. Transfer drained eggplant flesh to a bowl. Using a wooden spoon, mash and then whip the pulp until smooth and very soft. Coarsely grate onion directly into the eggplant (the onion juice that results is very important to this dip). Add lemon juice and whip with a wooden spoon until perfectly integrated. Keep beating and add olive oil in a very thin stream; the result should be a frothy, light colored emulsion. Season to taste with salt and pepper. Transfer to a serving bowl and garnish with chopped parsley.

Tip

- This dip can be served immediately or it can wait, covered and unrefrigerated, for up to 2 hours. If refrigerated, let it come back to room temperature and give it a couple of stirs before serving.

Nutritional Analysis (Per Serving)
- Calories: 166
- Protein: 1 g
- Fat: 15 g
- Carbohydrates: 9 g
- Fiber: 0 g
- Sodium: 4 mg
- Cholesterol: 0 mg

Melizzano Lambrino (Eggplant Dip #2)

1	medium eggplant (about 1 lb/500 g)	1
1 tsp	vegetable oil	5 mL
½ cup	chopped onion	125 mL
¼ cup	chopped fresh parsley, packed down	50 mL
1 tbsp	freshly squeezed lemon juice	15 mL
1 tsp	red wine vinegar	5 mL
1 tsp	Dijon mustard	5 mL
½ tsp	dried basil leaves	2 mL
½ tsp	dried oregano leaves	2 mL
2	cloves garlic, roughly chopped	2
¼ cup	olive oil	50 mL
	Salt and freshly ground black pepper to taste	
¼ cup	whole black olives (about 8)	50 mL

SERVES 4
Preheat oven to 450°F (230°C)

1. Brush eggplant lightly with vegetable oil. Using a fork, pierce the skin lightly at 1-inch (2.5 cm) intervals. Place on a baking sheet and bake for 1 hour, or until eggplant is very soft and the skin is dark brown and caved in.

2. Transfer eggplant to a working surface. Cut off 1 inch (2.5 cm) at the stem end and discard (this part never quite cooks through). Peel the eggplant by picking at an edge from the cut end, then pulling upward. The skin should come off easily in strips.

3. Cut the eggplant lengthwise and place each half with the interior facing you. With a spoon scoop out the tongues of seed-pods, leaving as much of the flesh as possible. To remove the additional seed-pods hiding inside, cut each piece of eggplant in half and repeat the deseeding procedure. Once deseeded, let cleaned eggplant sit to shed some of its excess water.

Nutritional Analysis (Per Serving)
- Calories: 190
- Protein: 1.9 g
- Fat: 15.9 g
- Carbohydrates: 12.2 g
- Fiber: 4.2 g
- Sodium: 97 mg
- Cholesterol: 0 mg

Hot Salsa Cheese Dip

2 cups	mild or medium salsa	500 mL
1 lb	Monterey Jack cheese, cubed	500 g
1	avocado, peeled and diced	1
2 tbsp	chopped fresh cilantro	25 mL

This delicious appetizer is great served as a dip with endive spears.

SERVES 12
Preheat oven to 350°F (180°C) • 9-inch (2.5 L) square or (23 cm) round baking dish

1. Spread salsa in bottom of baking dish. Top with cheese cubes.

2. Bake in preheated oven for 25 minutes or until cheese melts and salsa is heated. Remove from oven. Top with avocado and cilantro. Serve warm.

Nutritional Analysis (Per Serving)
- Calories: 179
- Protein: 9.7 g
- Fat: 14.0 g
- Carbohydrates: 4.0 g
- Fiber: 1.4 g
- Sodium: 392 mg
- Cholesterol: 34 mg

Spicy Mexican Dip

1 cup	canned refried beans	250 mL
1/3 cup	minced red onion	75 mL
1/3 cup	finely diced sweet red pepper	75 mL
3/4 tsp	crushed garlic	4 mL
2 tsp	chili powder	10 mL
2 tbsp	chopped fresh parsley	25 mL
2 tbsp	2% yogurt	25 mL
2 tsp	lemon juice	10 mL
3 tbsp	crushed bran cereal*	45 mL
	Parsley sprigs	

* Use a wheat bran breakfast cereal

Make Ahead

Make and refrigerate up to a day before. Stir before garnishing.

SERVES 6 TO 8 OR MAKES 2 CUPS (500 ML)

1. In bowl, combine beans, onion, red pepper, garlic, chili powder, parsley, yogurt, lemon juice and cereal; stir until blended. Place in serving bowl and garnish with parsley sprigs.

Nutritional Analysis (Per Serving)
- Calories: 11
- Protein: 0.6 g
- Fat: 0 g
- Carbohydrates: 2 g
- Fiber: 0.5 g
- Sodium: 37 mg
- Cholesterol: 0 mg

Avocado Tomato Salsa

2 cups	finely chopped plum tomatoes	500 mL
1/2 cup	finely chopped ripe but firm avocado (about 1/2 avocado)	125 mL
1/3 cup	chopped fresh coriander	75 mL
1/4 cup	chopped green onions (about 2 medium)	50 mL
1 tbsp	olive oil	15 mL
1 tbsp	lime or lemon juice	15 mL
1 tsp	minced garlic	5 mL
1/8 tsp	chili powder	1 mL

Make Ahead

Prepare up to 4 hours ahead; stir before serving.

SERVES 8

1. In serving bowl, combine tomatoes, avocado, coriander, green onions, olive oil, lime juice, garlic and chili powder; let marinate 1 hour before serving.

Tip

- For an authentic, intense flavor, use 1/2 tsp (2 mL) finely diced chili pepper, or more chili powder.

Nutritional Analysis (Per Serving)
- Calories: 53
- Protein: 1 g
- Fat: 4 g
- Carbohydrates: 4 g
- Fiber: 1 g
- Sodium: 8 mg
- Cholesterol: 0 mg

Pico de Gallo (Mexican Hot Sauce)

1	medium tomato, cut into ¼-inch (0.5 cm) cubes	1
¼ cup	finely diced red onions	50 mL
2	jalapeño peppers, finely diced (with or without seeds, depending on desired hotness)	2
½ tsp	salt	2 mL
1 tbsp	lime juice	15 mL
1 tbsp	vegetable oil	15 mL
	Few sprigs fresh coriander, chopped	

MAKES ABOUT I CUP (250 ML)

1. In bowl combine tomato, onions, jalapeño, salt and lime juice. Stir to mix well. Add oil and stir again.
2. Transfer to a serving bowl and scatter chopped coriander on top. Let rest for about 1 hour, covered and unrefrigerated, for best flavor. Serve alongside main courses and appetizers.

Tips

- This delicious, versatile and explosive sauce requires no cooking, and can live in the fridge nicely for 2 to 3 days, though it is best about an hour after it's freshly made. The hotness of the sauce can be regulated by modifying the amount of jalapeño pepper seeds used.
- When working with hot peppers, be sure to wear gloves; otherwise, wash hands thoroughly.

Nutritional Analysis (Per Serving)
- Calories: 44
- Protein: 1 g
- Fat: 4 g
- Carbohydrates: 3 g
- Fiber: 1 g
- Sodium: 365 mg
- Cholesterol: 0 mg

Pesto Sauce

½ cup	well-packed chopped fresh parsley	125 mL
½ cup	well-packed chopped fresh basil	125 mL
¼ cup	water or chicken stock	50 mL
1 tbsp	toasted pine nuts	15 mL
2 tbsp	grated Parmesan cheese	25 mL
3 tbsp	olive oil	45 mL
¾ tsp	crushed garlic	4 mL

Make Ahead

Refrigerate for up to a week or freeze for up to 6 weeks.

MAKES ¾ CUP (I75 ML)

1. In food processor, combine parsley, basil, water, pine nuts, Parmesan, oil and garlic; process until smooth.

Tips

- You can be creative with pesto sauces by substituting different leaves such as spinach or coriander, or using a combination of different leaves.
- Serve over cooked fish or chicken.

Nutritional Analysis (Per I tbsp/I5 mL Serving)
- Calories: 39
- Protein: 1 g
- Fat: 4 g
- Carbohydrates: 1 g
- Fiber: 0.3 g
- Sodium: 17 mg
- Cholesterol: 1 mg

Creamy Pesto Dip

1 cup	well-packed basil leaves	250 mL
2 tbsp	toasted pine nuts	25 mL
2 tbsp	grated Parmesan cheese	25 mL
2 tbsp	olive oil	25 mL
2 tsp	lemon juice	10 mL
1 tsp	minced garlic	5 mL
$\frac{1}{2}$ cup	5% ricotta cheese	125 mL
$\frac{1}{4}$ cup	light sour cream	50 mL

Make Ahead

Prepare early in the day and keep covered and refrigerated.

SERVES 6 TO 8

1. Put basil, pine nuts, Parmesan, olive oil, lemon juice and garlic in food processor; process until finely chopped, scraping sides of bowl down once. Add ricotta and sour cream and process until smooth. Serve with crudités.

Tips

• To toast pine nuts, put in nonstick skillet over medium-high heat for 3 minutes, stirring occasionally. Or put them on a baking sheet and toast in a 400°F (200°C) oven for 5 minutes. Whichever method you choose, watch carefully — nuts burn quickly.

• If basil is not available, use parsley or spinach leaves.

Nutritional Analysis (Per Serving)
- Calories: 67
- Protein: 4 g
- Fat: 5 g
- Carbohydrates: 2 g
- Fiber: 0 g
- Sodium: 53 mg
- Cholesterol: 8 mg

Lemon Pesto Sauce

1 cup	packed fresh basil leaves (see tip, at right)	250 mL
1	clove garlic	1
1 tbsp	olive oil	15 mL
1 tbsp	almonds or pine nuts	15 mL
4 tsp	lemon juice	20 mL
1 tsp	grated lemon zest	5 mL

Keep a supply of this sauce in the freezer, as it is used in other recipes in this book.

MAKES $\frac{1}{3}$ CUP (75 ML)

1. In a food processor or blender, combine basil, garlic, oil, almonds, lemon juice and zest. Blend until coarsely chopped. Chill or freeze, as desired.

Tips

• When fresh basil is not available, replace with 1 cup (250 mL) fresh parsley leaves and 2 tbsp (25 mL) dried basil.

• Basil contributes to healthy eating because it is a flavor enhancer, which reduces the need for fat and salt.

Nutritional Analysis (Per 1 tbsp/15 mL Serving)
- Calories: 40
- Protein: 1 g
- Fat: 4 g
- Carbohydrates: 2 g
- Fiber: Trace
- Sodium: 2 mg
- Cholesterol: 0 mg

Lemon Pesto Dip

¾ cup	lower-fat plain yogurt	175 mL
¼ cup	Lemon Pesto Sauce (see recipe, page 60)	50 mL
	Raw vegetables	

> *With a supply of Lemon Pesto Sauce in the freezer, you can make this tasty dip in less than 5 minutes.*

MAKES I CUP (250 ML)

1. In a bowl, combine yogurt and Lemon Pesto Sauce. Serve with raw vegetables.

Tip

- Served with raw vegetables, this dip is a lower-fat choice for an appetizer. It can make boosting your vegetable intake easier.

Nutritional Analysis (Per I tbsp/15 mL Serving)
- Calories: 17
- Protein: 1 g
- Fat: 1 g
- Carbohydrates: 1 g
- Fiber: 0 g
- Sodium: 71 mg
- Cholesterol: 2 mg

Fazool

1 cup	white beans	250 mL
1	medium onion, chopped	1
3 tbsp	chopped ginger root	45 mL
¾ tsp	salt	4 mL
3 tbsp	olive oil	45 mL
2 tbsp	balsamic vinegar	25 mL
¼ tsp	hot pepper sauce	1 mL
Pinch	black pepper	Pinch

MAKES 2¼ CUPS (550 ML)

1. Cover beans with water; let soak overnight. Drain and rinse.

2. In a large saucepan, combine beans, onion, ginger, ½ tsp (2 mL) of the salt and enough water to cover; bring to boil. Reduce heat and simmer, uncovered, until beans are tender, 35 to 40 minutes. Drain well.

3. In a food processor, purée beans with oil, vinegar, hot pepper sauce, remaining salt and pepper. Chill.

Tips

- The ginger root, balsamic vinegar and hot pepper sauce in this recipe add loads of flavor without fat.

- Because this tasty spread is lower in fat, it is a healthy alternative to higher-fat spreads.

Nutritional Analysis (Per I tbsp/15 mL Serving)
- Calories: 30
- Protein: 1 g
- Fat: 1 g
- Carbohydrates: 4 g
- Fiber: 1 g
- Sodium: 354 mg
- Cholesterol: 0 mg

Hummus (Chickpea Pâté)

¼ cup	water	50 mL
1 cup	drained canned chickpeas	250 mL
¾ tsp	crushed garlic	4 mL
2 tbsp	lemon juice	25 mL
4 tsp	olive oil	20 mL
¼ cup	tahini	50 mL
1 tbsp	chopped fresh parsley	15 mL

Make Ahead

Prepare dip up to a day before. Stir just before serving and garnish with parsley.

SERVES 4 TO 6 OR MAKES I CUP (250 ML)

1. In food processor, combine water, chickpeas, garlic, lemon juice, oil and tahini; process until creamy and smooth.
2. Transfer to serving dish; sprinkle with parsley.

Tips

- Tahini is a Middle Eastern condiment found in the specialty section of some supermarkets. If unavailable, use peanut butter.
- Surround the dip with fresh vegetable sticks.

Nutritional Analysis (Per Serving)
- Calories: 134
- Protein: 4 g
- Fat: 9 g
- Carbohydrates: 10 g
- Fiber: 2 g
- Sodium: 80 mg
- Cholesterol: 0 mg

Hummus with Tahini

1	can (19 oz/540 mL) chickpeas, drained	1
2	green onions	2
2 to 4	large cloves garlic	2 to 4
¼ cup	each lemon juice and tahini (see tip, at right)	50 mL
½ tsp	each ground cumin and salt	2 mL
	Freshly ground black pepper to taste	
½ cup	lower-fat plain yogurt	125 mL
	Chopped onion, tomato, parsley	

This version of the Middle Eastern dip uses yogurt to replace much of the traditional olive oil. Serve hummus as a dip with vegetable crudités.

MAKES 2¾ CUPS (675 ML)

1. In a food processor or blender, purée chickpeas, green onions, garlic, lemon juice, tahini and seasonings until smooth. Mix in yogurt. Garnish with onion, tomato and parsley. Chill or serve at room temperature.

Tips

- Tahini, a sesame seed paste, is widely available in health food stores. If you cannot find tahini, substitute toasted sesame seeds and process with chickpeas.
- Chickpeas, also known as garbanzo beans, are a great source of plant protein.

Nutritional Analysis (Per I tbsp/I5 mL Serving)
- Calories: 55
- Protein: 3 g
- Fat: 1 g
- Carbohydrates: 8 g
- Fiber: 2 g
- Sodium: 24 mg
- Cholesterol: 0 mg

Sautéed Vegetable Feta Cheese Spread

½ cup	chopped carrots	125 mL
2 tsp	vegetable oil	10 mL
2 tsp	minced garlic	10 mL
¾ cup	chopped red bell peppers	175 mL
¾ cup	chopped leeks	175 mL
½ cup	chopped onions	125 mL
¼ cup	sliced black olives	50 mL
2 tbsp	light sour cream	25 mL
2 tbsp	light mayonnaise	25 mL
1 tbsp	freshly squeezed lemon juice	15 mL
½ tsp	dried oregano	2 mL
2 oz	feta cheese, crumbled	50 g

Make Ahead

Prepare up to 2 days in advance.

SERVES 6 TO 8

1. Boil or steam carrots just until tender, about 5 minutes. Drain, and set aside.

2. In a saucepan heat oil over medium-low heat. Add garlic, red peppers, leeks, onions and carrots; cook, stirring occasionally, for 5 minutes or until tender. Cool.

3. In a food processor combine cooled vegetables, black olives, sour cream, mayonnaise, lemon juice, oregano and feta. Process to desired consistency. Serve with crudités.

Tips

- Pulse food processor on and off for a chunky texture.

- Try goat cheese instead of feta.

- For an attractive-looking spread, line a decorative mold with plastic wrap and unmold after chilled.

Nutritional Analysis (Per Serving)
- Calories: 72
- Protein: 2 g
- Fat: 4 g
- Carbohydrates: 8 g
- Fiber: 1 g
- Sodium: 134 mg
- Cholesterol: 6 mg

Mediterranean Eggplant Spread

2	medium eggplants	2
2 cups	lower-fat plain yogurt	500 mL
2 tbsp	lemon juice	25 mL
1	clove garlic, minced	1
1 tbsp	red wine vinegar	15 mL
1 tbsp	olive oil	15 mL
½ tsp	crumbled dried oregano	2 mL
½ tsp	salt	2 mL
2	medium tomatoes, seeded and diced	2
½ cup	diced celery	125 mL

Make this creamy spread when eggplants and tomatoes are in season for maximum flavor and minimum cost.

MAKES 5 CUPS (1.25 L)
Preheat oven to 375°F (190°C) • Baking sheet, greased

1. Cut eggplants in half lengthwise. Place on greased baking sheet, cut side down; cut 2 or 3 slits in skin. Cover with foil; bake in preheated oven for 35 to 45 minutes or until tender. Cool. Remove stalk, peel and seeds; finely chop eggplants.

2. In a bowl, combine eggplants, yogurt, lemon juice, garlic, vinegar, oil, oregano, salt, tomatoes and celery, mixing well. Cover and chill for at least 30 minutes.

Nutritional Analysis (Per 3 tbsp/45 mL Serving)
- Calories: 21
- Protein: 1 g
- Fat: 1 g
- Carbohydrates: 3 g
- Fiber: Trace
- Sodium: 164 mg
- Cholesterol: 1 mg

Avocado, Tomato and Chili Guacamole

Half	avocado, peeled	Half
3/4 tsp	crushed garlic	4 mL
2 tbsp	chopped green onions	25 mL
1 tbsp	lemon juice	15 mL
1/4 cup	finely diced sweet red pepper	50 mL
1/2 cup	chopped tomato	125 mL
Pinch	chili powder	Pinch

Make Ahead

Make early in day and squeeze more lemon juice over top to prevent discoloration. Refrigerate. Stir just before serving.

SERVES 4 TO 6 OR MAKES 3/4 CUP (175 ML)

1. In bowl, combine avocado, garlic, onions, lemon juice, red pepper, tomato and chili powder; mash with fork, mixing well.

Tips

- Adjust the chili powder to your taste.
- Serve with crudités.

Nutritional Analysis (Per Serving)
- Calories: 35
- Protein: 1 g
- Fat: 3 g
- Carbohydrates: 3 g
- Fiber: 1 g
- Sodium: 5 mg
- Cholesterol: 0 mg

Brandied Cheese Spread

1/2 cup	butter or margarine, softened	125 mL
3 cups	shredded old Cheddar cheese	750 mL
2 tbsp	brandy (see variation, at right)	25 mL
1 tbsp	sesame seeds	15 mL

SERVES 12

1. In a food processor, combine butter, cheese, brandy and sesame seeds. Pulse with on/off motion until smooth.

2. Transfer to a small bowl. Cover and refrigerate before serving. Store in a covered container in refrigerator for up to one week or freeze for longer storage.

3. Return to room temperature for easy spreading.

Variation

- Dry sherry or port is a pleasant change from brandy.

Tip

- It's best to let this spread rest for a few days before serving so the flavors can mellow.

Nutritional Analysis (Per Serving)
- Calories: 158
- Protein: 7.3 g
- Fat: 13.6 g
- Carbohydrates: 0.4 g
- Fiber: 0 g
- Sodium: 215 mg
- Cholesterol: 40 mg

Sun-Dried Tomato Cheese Spread

1	package (8 oz/250 g) cream cheese, softened	1
½ cup	butter or margarine, softened	125 mL
½ cup	freshly grated Parmesan cheese	125 mL
½ cup	chopped oil-packed sun-dried tomatoes, drained	125 mL

Wonderful flavorful things happen when you combine cream cheese with sun-dried tomatoes. Use as a dip with crudités.

SERVES 8

1. In a food processor or bowl using an electric mixer, beat cheese and butter until smooth. Stir in Parmesan cheese and tomatoes.

2. Transfer to a small bowl. Cover and refrigerate before serving. Return to room temperature for easy spreading.

3. Store in a covered container in refrigerator for up to one week or freeze for longer storage.

Nutritional Analysis (Per Serving)
- Calories: 239
- Protein: 4.7 g
- Fat: 23.9 g
- Carbohydrates: 2.6 g
- Fiber: 0.4 g
- Sodium: 312 mg
- Cholesterol: 66 mg

Red Pepper and Feta Spread

1	red bell pepper	1
2 cups	crumbled feta cheese (about 8 oz/250 g)	500 mL
¼ tsp	hot pepper flakes	1 mL
	Fresh oregano or thyme sprigs or chopped fresh parsley	

Make Ahead

The spread can be refrigerated, covered, for up to 3 days.

Serve this spread on short lengths of celery.

SERVES 6

Preheat broiler • Baking sheet

1. Place red pepper on baking sheet. Broil, turning often, for 20 to 30 minutes or until skin is blackened and blistered. (Alternatively, cook pepper on barbecue over medium heat, turning often, for 15 to 20 minutes or until skin is blackened and blistered.) Transfer pepper to a plate; cover with a bowl and let stand for 10 minutes. Remove skin, seeds, stalk and any membrane from pepper; set aside until cool.

2. In a food processor, combine roasted pepper, feta cheese and hot pepper flakes; process until fairly smooth. Spoon into a serving bowl. Garnish with oregano, thyme or parsley.

Nutritional Analysis (Per Serving)
- Calories: 139
- Protein: 7.3 g
- Fat: 10.7 g
- Carbohydrates: 3.7 g
- Fiber: 0.5 g
- Sodium: 559 mg
- Cholesterol: 45 mg

Salsa, Crab and Cheese Spread

1	8-oz (250 g) package cream cheese, softened	1
1	6-oz (170 g) can crabmeat or tuna, drained and broken up	1
1 cup	tomato salsa	250 mL
1 cup	grated Cheddar cheese	250 mL
2 tbsp	chopped fresh parsley or cilantro	25 mL

Make Ahead

The spread can be assembled, covered and refrigerated up to 8 hours before baking.

MAKES 6 TO 8 SERVINGS

1. Spread cheese over bottom of a shallow 8-inch (20 cm) round or square ovenproof serving dish. Top with crabmeat. Spread with salsa and sprinkle with Cheddar.
2. Bake in preheated 325°F (160°C) toaster oven for 15 to 18 minutes, or until cheese melts and spread is hot.
3. Sprinkle with parsley. Let stand for 10 minutes before serving.

Tip

- For a lighter version of this spread, use light cream cheese, and for a very rich and creamy version, use chèvre (goat cheese). You can also use ¾ cup (175 mL) diced cooked chicken or turkey or 1 cup (250 mL) drained and rinsed cooked black beans in place of the crab. Serve in the baking dish with a small spoon for spreading on fresh vegetables.

Nutritional Analysis (Per Serving)
- Calories: 210
- Protein: 11.4 g
- Fat: 17.0 g
- Carbohydrates: 3.4 g
- Fiber: 0.6 g
- Sodium: 429 mg
- Cholesterol: 71 mg

Oriental Crab Spread

⅓ cup	light cream cheese	75 mL
1 tbsp	soy sauce	15 mL
1 tsp	granulated sugar	5 mL
Pinch	white pepper	Pinch
1	can (4.2 oz/120 g) crabmeat, drained	1
½ cup	finely chopped water chestnuts	125 mL
⅓ cup	finely chopped red bell pepper	75 mL
1	green onion, thinly sliced	1
2 tbsp	lower-fat plain yogurt	25 mL

Spread on cucumber slices or celery sticks, this mixture is delicious.

MAKES 1¾ CUPS (425 ML)

1. In a bowl, combine first 4 ingredients. Stir in remaining ingredients. Cover and refrigerate until chilled.

Tips

- Try using sodium-reduced soy sauce. Generally, soy sauce labeled "light" has a reduced sodium content, but check the label to be certain.
- Increase fiber by serving this spread with an assortment of fresh vegetables.

Nutritional Analysis (Per 1 tbsp/15 mL Serving)
- Calories: 15
- Protein: 1 g
- Fat: 1 g
- Carbohydrates: 1 g
- Fiber: 0 g
- Sodium: 270 mg
- Cholesterol: 39 mg

Rosy Shrimp Spread

4 oz	light cream cheese, softened	125 g
1/4 cup	light sour cream or plain yogurt	50 mL
2 tbsp	prepared chili sauce	25 mL
1 tsp	prepared horseradish	5 mL
	Hot pepper sauce, to taste	
1	can (4 oz/113 g) small shrimp rinsed and drained	1
1 tbsp	minced green onion tops or chives	15 mL

Make Ahead

Spread can be prepared up to 2 days ahead, covered and refrigerated.

MAKES 1 1/4 CUPS (300 ML)

1. In a bowl, beat cream cheese until smooth. Stir in sour cream, chili sauce, horseradish and hot pepper sauce.
2. Fold in shrimp and green onions. Transfer to serving dish; cover and refrigerate until serving time.

Tips

- Microwave cold cream cheese at Medium for 1 minute to soften.
- Serve with crudités.
- Instead of shrimp, try using 1 can (6 oz/170 g) crab.

Nutritional Analysis (Per 2 tbsp/25 mL Serving)
- Calories: 48
- Protein: 4 g
- Fat: 3 g
- Carbohydrates: 2 g
- Fiber: 0 g
- Sodium: 127 mg
- Cholesterol: 27 mg

Tuna and White Bean Spread

1 cup	canned, cooked white kidney beans, drained	250 mL
1	can (6.5 oz/184 g) tuna in water, drained	1
1 1/2 tsp	minced garlic	7 mL
2 tbsp	lemon juice	25 mL
2 tbsp	light mayonnaise	25 mL
1/4 cup	5% ricotta cheese	50 mL
3 tbsp	minced red onions	45 mL
1/4 cup	minced fresh dill (or 1 tsp/5 mL dried)	50 mL
1 tbsp	grated Parmesan cheese	15 mL
1/4 cup	diced red pepper	50 mL

Make Ahead

Prepare up to a day ahead; keep covered and refrigerated. Stir before using.

SERVES 8

1. Place beans, tuna, garlic, lemon juice, mayonnaise and ricotta in food processor; pulse on and off until combined but still chunky. Place in serving bowl.
2. Stir onions, dill, Parmesan and red pepper into bean mixture.

Tip

- White navy pea beans can also be used. If you cook your own dry beans, 1/2 cup (125 mL) dry yields approximately 1 1/2 cups (375 mL) of cooked beans.

Nutritional Analysis (Per Serving)
- Calories: 73
- Protein: 8 g
- Fat: 2 g
- Carbohydrates: 7 g
- Fiber: 2 g
- Sodium: 188 mg
- Cholesterol: 6 mg

Tunnato Spread

¾ cup	mayonnaise (see tip, at right)	175 mL
1	can (6 oz/170 g) tuna, preferably Italian, packed in olive oil, drained	1
20	parsley leaves	20
	Crudités	

Don't be fooled by the simplicity of this recipe: it is a mouth-watering combination. Amazingly versatile, this ambrosial mixture excels as a dip. Make it the centerpiece of a tasting platter, surrounded by celery sticks and cucumber slices or tender leaves of Belgian endive. It also performs well as a sauce for plated appetizers or salade composé (for which the ingredients are arranged on a plate rather than tossed together).

SERVES 4

1. In a food processor, combine mayonnaise, tuna and parsley. Process until smooth.
2. Transfer to a small bowl and serve surrounded by crudités for dipping. If not using immediately, cover and refrigerate for up to 3 days.

Variations

- **Tunnato-Stuffed Eggs (Serves 6 to 8):** Hard-cook 4 eggs. Let cool and peel. Cut in half lengthwise. Pop out the yolks and mash with ¼ cup (50 mL) Tunnato Spread. Mound the mixture back into the whites. Dust with 1 tsp (5 mL) paprika, if desired. If you prefer a plated appetizer, simply cut the peeled cooked eggs in half, arrange them on a platter and spoon the sauce over top.

- **Asparagus with Tunnato (Serves 4):** Arrange 1 can or jar (16 oz/330 g approx.) white asparagus, drained, on a small platter or serving plate. Top with ¼ cup (50 mL) Tunnato Spread. Use fresh green asparagus in season, if desired. You can also turn this into a salad by spreading a layer of salad greens over a large platter. Arrange the asparagus over the greens and top with Tunnato Spread.

Tips

- Don't confuse real mayonnaise with "mayonnaise-type" salad dressings, which are similar in appearance. Mayonnaise is a combination of egg yolks, vinegar or lemon juice, olive oil and seasonings. Imitators will contain additional ingredients, such as sugar, flour or milk. Make sure the label says mayonnaise and check the ingredients.

- For added flavor, add 1 to 2 tbsp (15 to 25 mL) drained capers and/or 1 to 2 tbsp (15 to 25 mL) finely chopped green onions.

Nutritional Analysis (Per Serving)
- Calories: 384
- Protein: 12.6 g
- Fat: 3.6 g
- Carbohydrates: 0.5 g
- Fiber: 0.3 g
- Sodium: 154 mg
- Cholesterol: 8 mg

Tapenade

1	can (6 oz/170 g) tuna, preferably Italian, packed in olive oil, drained	1
4	anchovies	4
2 tbsp	drained capers	25 mL
1 tbsp	lemon juice	15 mL
1 tsp	minced garlic	5 mL
10	pitted black olives	10
¼ cup	olive oil	50 mL

SERVES 3

1. In a food processor, combine tuna, anchovies, capers, lemon juice, garlic and olives. Process until ingredients are combined but still chunky. Add olive oil and pulse until blended. Spoon into a bowl, cover tightly and refrigerate until ready to use.

Variation

- *Tapenade-Stuffed Eggs:* Hard-cook eggs. Let cool and peel. Cut in half lengthwise. Pop out the yolks and add 1 tsp (5 mL) tapenade per yolk. Mash together and use this mixture to fill the whites. Dust with paprika, if desired.

Nutritional Analysis (Per Serving)
- Calories: 305
- Protein: 28.0 g
- Fat: 37.3 g
- Carbohydrates: 2.4 g
- Fiber: 0.8 g
- Sodium: 397 mg
- Cholesterol: 23 mg

Smoked Salmon and Red Caviar Mousse

8 oz	smoked salmon	250 g
½ to ¾ cup	whipping (35%) cream (see tip, at right)	125 to 175 mL
1 tbsp	lemon juice	15 mL
2 tbsp	red lumpfish roe	25 mL
	Freshly ground black pepper	

This is so easy to prepare, yet elegant enough to start the most sophisticated meal.

SERVES 8

1. In a food processor, combine smoked salmon, cream and lemon juice. Process until smooth. Fold in lumpfish roe. Season with black pepper to taste. Spoon into a serving bowl. Refrigerate until ready to serve.

Tip

- The quantity of cream required depends upon the kind of smoked salmon you are using. You may need more cream if using wild salmon, which is likely to have a heavier texture than the farmed variety. The mousse mixture should be light enough to fold in the red caviar without appearing to crush the delicate roe.

Nutritional Analysis (Per Serving)
- Calories: 118
- Protein: 8.6 g
- Fat: 8.8 g
- Carbohydrates: 0.8 g
- Fiber: 0 g
- Sodium: 229 mg
- Cholesterol: 53 mg

Smoked Salmon Mousse

1/3 cup	dry white wine or water	75 mL
1	package (1/4 oz/7 g) unflavored gelatin	1
1	can (7 1/2 oz/213 g) sockeye salmon, drained, skin removed	1
1 cup	sour cream	250 mL
1/2 tsp	grated lemon zest	2 mL
1 tbsp	fresh lemon juice	15 mL
1/4 tsp	salt	1 mL
	Hot pepper sauce to taste	
4 oz	smoked salmon, finely chopped	125 g
2 tbsp	minced green onions	25 mL
2 tbsp	finely chopped fresh dill	25 mL
1/2 cup	whipping (35%) cream, whipped	125 mL
	Dill sprigs and lemon zest for garnish	

> *This recipe delivers a wonderful smoked salmon flavor, but uses relatively little of that costly ingredient.*

SERVES 6

1. Place wine in a small bowl; sprinkle gelatin over. Let stand 5 minutes to soften. Microwave at Medium for 1 minute or until dissolved.
2. In a food processor, combine canned salmon, sour cream, lemon zest and juice, salt and hot pepper sauce; process until smooth. Add gelatin mixture; process until combined.
3. Transfer mixture to a bowl. Stir in smoked salmon, green onions and dill; fold in whipped cream.
4. Spoon mixture into a serving dish. Cover loosely with plastic wrap (it should not touch surface of the mousse); refrigerate for 4 hours or overnight. Garnish top with dill sprigs and lemon zest.

Tips

- Use canned sockeye salmon (instead of the pink variety) for its superior color and flavor.
- The mousse can be prepared up to four days ahead for easy entertaining.
- To get more juice out of a lemon, roll on counter top or microwave at High for 20 seconds before squeezing.

Nutritional Analysis (Per Serving)
- Calories: 224
- Protein: 12.9 g
- Fat: 17.2 g
- Carbohydrates: 2.3 g
- Fiber: 0.1 g
- Sodium: 287 mg
- Cholesterol: 65 mg

Soups and Salads

Continued on next page...

Babsi's Broccoli Soup

2 cups	chopped broccoli (stems and florets)	500 mL
2 cups	chicken broth	500 mL
1 cup	buttermilk	250 mL
1/2 tsp	dried basil	2 mL
1/2 tsp	dried tarragon	2 mL
	Salt and black pepper to taste	
	Small broccoli florets, lower-fat plain yogurt, chives, shredded Cheddar cheese	

Not only is this soup delicious and nutritious, it is quick and easy to make. It looks elegant when garnished and can be served all year round.

SERVES 6 OR MAKES 3 CUPS (750 ML)

1. In a saucepan over medium-high heat, cook broccoli in chicken broth for 10 minutes or until tender. Refrigerate in broth until chilled.

2. In a food processor or blender, purée chilled mixture, buttermilk and seasonings until smooth. Taste and adjust seasonings. Reheat just to serving temperature, or chill and serve as cold soup. Serve garnished with broccoli, yogurt, chives and Cheddar cheese.

Tip

- This is a great way to use leftover broccoli and a delicious way to add a serving of vegetables to your daily plan. Serve this soup with Creamy Salmon Quiche (see recipe, page 149) and a tossed green salad. Finish with a seasonal dessert. Your meal will be abundant in folic acid, vitamins A and C, and calcium.

Nutritional Analysis (Per Serving)
- Calories: 73
- Protein: 7 g
- Fat: 2 g
- Carbohydrates: 7 g
- Fiber: 2 g
- Sodium: 241 mg
- Cholesterol: 2 mg

Chilled Cucumber Soup

2	English cucumbers, peeled and coarsely chopped	2
2 cups	plain yogurt or light sour cream	500 mL
2 tbsp	chopped fresh dill	25 mL
1 tsp	freshly squeezed lemon juice	5 mL
6	ice cubes	6
	Salt and white pepper	

Flavors really improve when this refreshing soup is made a day ahead. The recipe makes more than you may want, but it can be easily halved. It keeps refrigerated for several days. It was adapted from an Ontario Greenhouse Growers booklet.

MAKES 6 CUPS (1.5 L), ABOUT 5 SERVINGS

1. In a food processor or blender, purée cucumber, yogurt, dill, lemon juice and ice cubes until very smooth.

2. Transfer to a covered container. Refrigerate for 2 hours or until well chilled. Season with salt and pepper to taste.

Nutritional Analysis (Per Serving)
- Calories: 72
- Protein: 6.3 g
- Fat: 0.4 g
- Carbohydrates: 11.2 g
- Fiber: 0.7 g
- Sodium: 78 mg
- Cholesterol: 2 mg

Curried Fiddlehead Soup

1 lb	fresh or frozen fiddleheads	500 g
2 cups	each chicken broth and 1% milk	500 mL
2 tsp	each margarine and curry powder	10 mL
¼ cup	gin (optional)	50 mL

Fiddleheads, the young shoots of the ostrich fern, are a springtime delicacy. If you have access to a supply, freeze a batch and enjoy this soup year-round.

SERVES 5

1. In a large saucepan, cook fiddleheads in chicken broth for 15 to 20 minutes; don't overcook or they will go brown. Remove fiddleheads with slotted spoon and purée in food processor; return to broth. Stir in milk; simmer until hot.

2. In a small skillet, heat margarine over low heat; stir in curry powder and cook, stirring, for 2 to 3 minutes. Add to soup. Stir in gin, if desired.

Tip

- Fiddleheads contain vitamin C, which helps the body absorb iron. Serve this elegant soup followed by Flank Steak Stir-Fry (see recipe, page 247).

Nutritional Analysis (Per Serving)
- Calories: 91
- Protein: 8 g
- Fat: 4 g
- Carbohydrates: 9 g
- Fiber: Trace
- Sodium: 295 mg
- Cholesterol: 4 mg

Spanish Garlic Soup

10	cloves garlic, peeled and sliced	10
3 tbsp	olive oil	45 mL
5 cups	beef stock	1.25 L
1 cup	dry sherry	250 mL
	Salt and freshly ground black pepper	

This soup is reminiscent of the classic French onion soup, but because the stock is clear, it is lighter. The garlic flavor is distinct, but not harsh. Serve this soup with grated Parmesan cheese.

MAKES 6 CUPS (1.5 L), ABOUT 5 SERVINGS

1. In a large saucepan over medium heat, sauté garlic in oil for 1 minute or until golden (but not browned).

2. Add stock and sherry. Bring to a boil. Reduce heat, cover and cook slowly for 30 minutes. Season with salt and pepper to taste. Strain garlic and discard.

Nutritional Analysis (Per Serving)
- Calories: 209
- Protein: 3.1 g
- Fat: 10.2 g
- Carbohydrates: 10.7 g
- Fiber: 0.3 g
- Sodium: 718 mg
- Cholesterol: 0 mg

Gazpacho

4 cups	tomato juice	1 L
1/3 cup	red wine vinegar	75 mL
1	each green bell pepper and English cucumber, finely chopped	1
2	medium tomatoes, diced	2
1	small onion, chopped	1
2	cloves garlic, crushed	2
2 tbsp	chopped chives	25 mL
1/4 tsp	paprika	1 mL

This soup, Spanish in origin, produces maximum impact with minimal effort.

SERVES 6 OR MAKES 7 CUPS (1.75 L)

1. In a large bowl, mix together ingredients. Chill for 3 hours.

Tips

- Prepare with a food processor or blender, if desired.
- If you like spice, add finely chopped chili pepper.
- This versatile soup adds pizzazz to any meal. It has minimal fat and is a tasty way to increase vitamin C intake.

Nutritional Analysis (Per Serving)
- Calories: 52
- Protein: 2 g
- Fat: 0 g
- Carbohydrates: 12 g
- Fiber: 1 g
- Sodium: 19 mg
- Cholesterol: 0 mg

Gazpacho with Baby Shrimp

2 1/2 cups	tomato juice	625 mL
4 tsp	red wine vinegar	20 mL
1 tsp	crushed garlic	5 mL
1 cup	diced sweet green pepper	250 mL
1 cup	diced sweet red or yellow pepper	250 mL
1 1/4 cups	diced tomatoes	300 mL
1 cup	diced cucumber	250 mL
1 cup	chopped green onions	250 mL
1 cup	diced celery	250 mL
1/4 cup	chopped fresh parsley (or 1 tbsp/15 mL dried)	50 mL
2 tbsp	chopped fresh basil (or 2 tsp/10 mL dried)	25 mL
1 tbsp	lemon juice	15 mL
2 oz	cooked baby shrimp	50 g
Dash	Tabasco	Dash
	Pepper	
	Chopped fresh chives	

SERVES 4 TO 6

1. In large bowl, combine tomato juice, vinegar and garlic.
2. Mix together green and red peppers, tomatoes, cucumber, green onions and celery; add half to bowl. Place remaining half in food processor; purée until smooth. Add to bowl.
3. Add parsley, basil, lemon juice, shrimp, Tabasco, and pepper to taste; stir gently to combine well. Refrigerate until chilled. To serve, garnish each bowl with sprinkle of chives.

Tips

- Shrimp can be replaced with crabmeat or imitation seafood.
- Serve with a spoonful of yogurt on each serving.

Nutritional Analysis (Per Serving)
- Calories: 58
- Protein: 4 g
- Fat: 0.5 g
- Carbohydrates: 11 g
- Fiber: 3 g
- Sodium: 413 mg
- Cholesterol: 18 mg

Oriental Mushroom Soup

5 cups	chicken broth	1.25 L
4 tsp	finely chopped gingerroot	20 mL
½ lb	sliced mushrooms (shiitake, oyster, portobello or a combination), about 2 cups (500 mL)	250 g
2 tbsp	sodium-reduced soy sauce	25 mL
1 tsp	sesame oil	5 mL
8 oz	firm tofu, cut into small cubes	250 g
1	green onion, thinly sliced	1

For an elegant touch, cut the tofu into stars with cookie cutters.

SERVES 6

1. In a saucepan, combine broth, ginger root and mushrooms; bring to a boil. Reduce heat and simmer, uncovered, for 15 minutes. Stir in soy sauce and sesame oil.
2. Place tofu and green onion in individual soup bowls or tureen. Add soup and serve.

Tips

- Be sure to use firm tofu in this soup. Otherwise, it won't retain its shape.
- Sesame oil is available in large supermarkets and specialty food shops. All you need is a teaspoon (5 mL) to enhance the flavor of this soup.

Nutritional Analysis (Per Serving)
- Calories: 107
- Protein: 11 g
- Fat: 5 g
- Carbohydrates: 5 g
- Fiber: 2 g
- Sodium: 657 mg
- Cholesterol: 0 mg

Tomato Bisque

3 cups	chicken or vegetable stock	750 mL
½ cup	finely chopped onion	125 mL
1	can (19 oz/398 mL) tomatoes	1
⅓ cup	red wine or stock	75 mL
	Salt and freshly ground black pepper	

MAKES 6 CUPS (1.5 L), ABOUT 5 SERVINGS

1. In a large saucepan over high heat, bring stock and onions to a boil. Add tomatoes and wine. Reduce heat, cover and cook slowly for 25 minutes.
2. Remove from heat. Cool slightly before puréeing half of soup in a food processor or blender until almost smooth. Repeat with remaining soup. Return to saucepan.
3. Reheat to serving temperature or refrigerate for up to 2 days and then reheat. Season with salt and pepper to taste.

Nutritional Analysis (Per Serving)
- Calories: 45
- Protein: 2.2 g
- Fat: 0.1 g
- Carbohydrates: 6.9 g
- Fiber: 1.92 g
- Sodium: 353 mg
- Cholesterol: 0 mg

Tomato Basil Soup

3 cups	chicken stock	750 mL
3	cloves garlic, minced	3
1	can (28 oz/798 mL) diced tomatoes	1
1 cup	fresh basil leaves, thinly sliced	250 mL
	Salt and freshly ground black pepper	

This very quick version of the classic tomato soup is just right for a refreshingly light supper. Serve it hot in winter or cold in summer. Look to the fresh tomato variation above for even more flavor when tomatoes are in season.

MAKES 6 CUPS (1.5 L), ABOUT 5 SERVINGS

1. In a large saucepan over high heat, bring stock, garlic and tomatoes to a boil. Reduce heat. Cover and cook slowly for 20 minutes.
2. Remove from heat. Cool slightly before puréeing half of soup in a food processor or blender until smooth. Repeat with remaining soup.
3. Return to saucepan. Add basil and reheat to serving temperature. Season with salt and pepper to taste.

Variation

- **Fresh Tomato Basil Soup:** Replace canned tomatoes with 6 large peeled and diced tomatoes. Add $1/4$ cup (50 mL) tomato paste during the cooking and follow method using all ingredients.

Nutritional Analysis (Per Serving)
- Calories: 43
- Protein: 2.6 g
- Fat: 0.2 g
- Carbohydrates: 8.3 g
- Fiber: 1.5 g
- Sodium: 356 mg
- Cholesterol: 0 mg

Curried Zucchini Sweet Potato Soup

2 tsp	vegetable oil	10 mL
1 tsp	minced garlic	5 mL
1 tsp	curry powder	5 mL
1 cup	chopped onions	250 mL
4 cups	chopped zucchini	1 L
2 1/2 cups	chicken stock	625 mL
1 1/2 cups	peeled, chopped sweet potato	375 mL

Make Ahead

Make early in the day and gently reheat, adding more stock if necessary.

SERVES 6

1. In large nonstick saucepan sprayed with vegetable spray, heat oil over medium heat. Add garlic, curry powder, onions and zucchini; cook for 4 minutes or until vegetables are slightly softened.
2. Add stock and potatoes; bring to a boil, cover and reduce heat to low. Cook for 20 minutes or until potato is tender. Transfer to food processor or blender and purée.

Tip

- Yellow or green zucchini is fine to use.

Nutritional Analysis (Per Serving)
- Calories: 85
- Protein: 2 g
- Fat: 3 g
- Carbohydrates: 3 g
- Fiber: 3 g
- Sodium: 473 mg
- Cholesterol: 0 g

Fish and Vegetable Chowder

1	large onion, chopped	1
1	clove garlic, minced	1
2 tbsp	butter or margarine	25 mL
1 cup	green bell pepper strips (or green and red bell peppers mixed)	250 mL
1 cup	cauliflower florets	250 mL
1 cup	broccoli florets	250 mL
1 cup	chopped tomato	250 mL
$\frac{1}{2}$ cup	chopped celery	125 mL
1 tbsp	chopped fresh parsley	15 mL
1 lb	cod fillets, cut into chunks	500 g
$2\frac{1}{2}$ cups	hot chicken broth	625 mL
1 tsp	salt	5 mL
$\frac{1}{4}$ tsp	dried thyme	1 mL
$\frac{1}{4}$ tsp	dried basil	1 mL
$\frac{1}{4}$ tsp	freshly ground black pepper	1 mL

This hearty and flavorful soup is the perfect match for cod, if you are lucky enough to find it. If not, use any firm white fish, such as turbot, halibut or haddock.

SERVES 6 OR MAKES 6 CUPS (1.5 L)

1. In a large saucepan over medium heat, cook onion and garlic in butter for 3 minutes. Add pepper strips, cauliflower, broccoli, tomato, celery and parsley; cook for 2 minutes. Add fish; cover and cook for 2 minutes. Add chicken broth and seasonings and simmer for about 5 minutes or until fish flakes with a fork and vegetables are tender-crisp.

Tips

- This is a great pantry soup, as you can use canned tomatoes and frozen pepper strips if desired.
- Although canned or frozen vegetables usually provide essentially the same nutrients as fresh, canned vegetables may have added salt, making them higher in sodium. If using canned tomatoes, you may need to adjust the seasoning accordingly.

Nutritional Analysis (Per Serving)
- Calories: 191
- Protein: 23 g
- Fat: 8 g
- Carbohydrates: 7 g
- Fiber: 2 g
- Sodium: 726 mg
- Cholesterol: 42 mg

Chinese Scallop and Shrimp Broth with Snow Peas

4 cups	chicken stock	1 L
$1\frac{1}{2}$ tsp	minced fresh gingerroot	7 mL
2 cups	chopped snow peas	500 mL
2 oz	scallops, diced	50 g
2 oz	shrimp, diced	50 g
1 tbsp	soya sauce	15 mL
1	green onion, chopped	1

SERVES 4 TO 6

1. In medium saucepan, bring chicken stock and ginger to boil. Add snow peas, scallops, shrimp and soya sauce.

2. Reduce heat and simmer for 2 to 3 minutes or just until scallops are opaque and shrimp are pink. Serve sprinkled with green onion.

Nutritional Analysis (Per Serving)
- Calories: 68
- Protein: 9 g
- Fat: 1 g
- Carbohydrates: 4 g
- Fiber: 1 g
- Sodium 735: mg
- Cholesterol: 21 mg

Curried Tomato and Shellfish Broth

6	scallops, thinly sliced	6
8	prawns, peeled and deveined	8
	Salt and freshly ground white pepper to taste	
2 tsp	vegetable oil	10 mL
1	small onion, sliced	1
1 tbsp	curry powder, preferably madras	15 mL
5 cups	chicken stock	1.25 L
4	small tomatoes, seeded and quartered	4
12	clams, scrubbed	12
2 cups	thinly sliced mustard greens or sui choy (Napa cabbage)	500 mL
	Salt and pepper to taste	

Mustard greens, which are available in Chinese markets, give this broth an interesting bite. The combination of tomatoes and curry provides a fabulous complement to the seafood.

SERVES 4 TO 6

1. Season seafood with salt and pepper; set aside.

2. In a large saucepan or soup pot, heat oil over medium heat for 30 seconds. Add onion and curry powder; sauté for 1 minute. Add chicken stock; bring to a boil. Add tomatoes and cook for 3 minutes. Add clams; cook until they open, about 2 to 5 minutes, depending on size. Skim off any impurities that rise to the top.

3. Add scallops, prawns and mustard greens or cabbage; bring to a boil. Remove from heat. Season to taste with salt and pepper. Cover and allow to steep for 2 minutes. Serve immediately.

Nutritional Analysis (Per Serving)
- Calories: 167
- Protein: 21.4 g
- Fat: 3.3 g
- Carbohydrates: 12.8 g
- Fiber: 2.2 g
- Sodium: 734 mg
- Cholesterol: 60 mg

Shrimp Broth with Coriander

1 lb	raw large shrimp, shelled and deveined, shells reserved	500 g
8 cups	chicken stock or fish stock	2 L
¼ cup	chopped green onions	50 mL
1	clove garlic, peeled but left whole	1
1	1-inch (2.5 cm) piece ginger root, thinly sliced	1
2	2-inch (5 cm) strips lemon zest	2
1 tsp	whole black peppercorns	5 mL
2 or 3	large sprigs fresh coriander	2 or 3
⅓ cup	chopped fresh coriander	75 mL

Make Ahead

Shrimp can be shelled, chopped and refrigerated, covered, for up to 24 hours.

Stock can be boiled with flavorings, then strained and refrigerated, covered, for up to 24 hours.

Dinner guests always seem to enjoy the drama of having something cooked at the table. In this simple but exquisite recipe, chopped shrimp cook almost instantly when boiling stock is poured over them. (Of course, if such theatrics are not to your taste, you can always add the stock in the kitchen and carry the finished soup to the table.)

SERVES 6

1. Cut shrimp crosswise into ¼-inch (5 mm) pieces; refrigerate, covered, until ready to serve.

2. In a large saucepan over high heat, combine shrimp shells, stock, green onions, garlic, ginger, lemon zest, peppercorns and coriander sprigs; bring to a boil. Reduce heat to low; simmer gently, covered, for 1 hour. Strain stock through a fine sieve into a 3-cup (750 mL) pitcher; discard flavorings.

3. When ready to serve, warm a 10-cup (2.5 L) soup tureen or serving bowl. Pour stock into a large saucepan; bring to a full rolling boil over high heat. Place shrimp and chopped coriander in soup tureen. At the table, pour boiling stock into soup tureen; stir once or twice. When shrimp are pink and firm, ladle soup into warm soup bowls. Serve at once.

Nutritional Analysis (Per Serving)
- Calories: 116
- Protein: 18.7 g
- Fat: 2.1 g
- Carbohydrates: 5.3 g
- Fiber: 2.2 g
- Sodium: 875 mg
- Cholesterol: 115 mg

Hot and Sour Chicken Soup

6	dried Chinese mushrooms	6
5 cups	chicken broth	1.25 L
2 cups	shredded cooked chicken (7 oz/200 g)	500 mL
1 tbsp	finely chopped gingerroot	15 mL
1	chili pepper, chopped (or ½ tsp/2 mL crushed chili flakes)	1
1 cup	diced firm tofu	250 mL
2 tbsp	white wine vinegar	25 mL
1 tbsp	sodium-reduced soy sauce	15 mL
1 tbsp	dry sherry	15 mL
1 tbsp	cornstarch	15 mL
1 tbsp	cold water	15 mL
3	egg whites, lightly beaten	3
2	shallots, thinly sliced (optional)	2

Impress friends and family with your own version of this Chinese classic.

SERVES 6

1. Cover Chinese mushrooms with hot water and soak for 10 minutes. Drain, discard stems and slice caps.

2. In a large saucepan, bring broth to a boil; add mushrooms, chicken, ginger root and chili pepper. Reduce heat and simmer, covered, for 5 minutes. Add tofu, vinegar, soy sauce and sherry; simmer for 2 minutes.

3. Stir cornstarch with water until smooth; gradually stir into soup and simmer for 2 to 3 minutes or until thickened slightly. Remove from heat; immediately swirl egg whites through soup. Garnish with shallots, if desired.

Tips

- Use thin green or red chilies or Thai finger chilies in this recipe rather than jalapeño chilies. If using a fresh chili pepper, wash your hands thoroughly after chopping.

- The tofu, chicken and egg whites in this soup combine to make a good source of protein.

Nutritional Analysis (Per Serving)
- Calories: 145
- Protein: 18 g
- Fat: 5 g
- Carbohydrates: 6 g
- Fiber: 1 g
- Sodium: 591 mg
- Cholesterol: 21 mg

Summer Artichoke Salad

6	baby artichokes, cooked or 14-oz (398 mL) can artichoke hearts, rinsed and drained	6
1/2	red bell pepper, cut into thin strips	1/2
1/4 cup	thinly sliced red onion	50 mL
1	1-inch (2.5 cm) piece English cucumber, thinly sliced	1
5	black olives, pitted and halved	5
1	ripe large tomato, cut into 1/2-inch (1 cm) wedges	1
12	seedless grapes, halved	12
1 tsp	drained capers	5 mL
1	clove garlic, pressed	1
2 tbsp	extra virgin olive oil	25 mL
1 tbsp	white wine vinegar	15 mL
1 tbsp	freshly squeezed lemon juice	15 mL
1/4 tsp	salt	1 mL
1/8 tsp	freshly ground black pepper	0.5 mL
	Few sprigs fresh parsley, chopped	

SERVES 4

1. Cut artichokes in half and put in a salad bowl. Add red pepper, onions, cucumber, olives, tomato, grapes and capers. Toss gently to mix.

2. In a small bowl, whisk together garlic, olive oil, vinegar, lemon juice, salt and pepper until slightly emulsified. Drizzle over the salad and toss gently to dress all the pieces, but without breaking up the artichokes too much. Garnish with parsley, and serve within 1 hour (cover if it has to wait, but do not refrigerate).

Nutritional Analysis (Per Serving)
- Calories: 141
- Protein: 1.7 g
- Fat: 1.0 g
- Carbohydrates: 12.3 g
- Fiber: 2.3 g
- Sodium: 353 mg
- Cholesterol: 0 mg

Lettuce and Avocado Salad

8 cups	lettuce (any variety), washed, dried and torn into bite-size pieces	2 L
4	green onions, chopped	4
1 tsp	drained capers	5 mL
	Few sprigs fresh coriander, roughly chopped	
2	ripe avocados	2
1/4 tsp	salt	1 mL
1/4 tsp	freshly ground black pepper	1 mL
2 tbsp	white wine vinegar	25 mL
4 oz	feta cheese, crumbled in large chunks	125 g
2 tbsp	extra virgin olive oil	25 mL

SERVES 4

1. In a salad bowl, toss together lettuce, green onions, capers and coriander. Peel and slice (or scoop) avocado and add to lettuce. Immediately add salt and pepper; sprinkle vinegar all over the avocado (to avoid discoloration). Toss well to combine.

2. Add feta crumbles and drizzle olive oil over everything. Toss well, getting as much as possible of the feta back on top. Serve within 10 to 15 minutes.

Nutritional Analysis (Per Serving)
- Calories: 309
- Protein: 7.9 g
- Fat: 28.0 g
- Carbohydrates: 11.3 g
- Fiber: 6.6 g
- Sodium: 504 mg
- Cholesterol: 25 mg

Asian Caesar Salad

DRESSING

4 tbsp	light mayonnaise	60 mL
2 tbsp	oyster sauce	25 mL
1 tbsp	minced garlic	15 mL
1 tbsp	lemon juice	15 mL
1 tbsp	rice vinegar	15 mL
1 tbsp	chopped cilantro	15 mL
	Salt and pepper to taste	

SALAD

1	head romaine lettuce, washed	1
1	red or yellow bell pepper, seeded and cut into 1/2-inch (1 cm) dice	1
1 cup	diced seedless cucumbers	250 mL
1	green onion, thinly sliced	1
	Sesame seeds for garnish	
	Freshly ground black pepper to taste	

This is a simple and delicious rendition of an all-time favorite. The oyster sauce stands in for traditional anchovies and complements the garlic.

SERVES 4

1. In a small bowl, combine mayonnaise, oyster sauce, garlic, lemon juice, vinegar and cilantro. Season with salt and pepper; whisk until well mixed.

2. Remove root end from lettuce and wash leaves well under cold water. Tear lettuce into pieces, approximately 2 inches (5 cm) square and dry in a salad spinner or by wrapping in a clean, dry kitchen cloth. Refrigerate at least 15 minutes.

3. In a large salad bowl, combine lettuce, red or yellow bell pepper, cucumbers and green onion. Top with dressing; toss. Serve on individual salad plates with a generous sprinkling of sesame seeds and a grind of fresh pepper.

Tip

- You can easily transform this into a main course by adding slices of grilled vegetables, smoked salmon, cooked chicken, beef or seafood.

Nutritional Analysis (Per Serving)
- Calories: 90
- Protein: 2.6 g
- Fat: 5.4 g
- Carbohydrates: 9.7 g
- Fiber: 3.2 g
- Sodium: 256 mg
- Cholesterol: 5 mg

Cabbage and Carrot Slaw

2 cups	thinly sliced cabbage	500 mL
1 cup	small carrot strips	250 mL
2 tbsp	cider vinegar	25 mL
1 tbsp	extra virgin olive oil	15 mL
	Salt and freshly ground black pepper	

This traditional coleslaw is an especially great salad to make for a potluck — it travels well because it does not contain any mayonnaise.

SERVES 4

1. In a salad bowl, combine cabbage and carrots.

2. Add vinegar and oil and toss to combine. Season lightly with salt and pepper. Cover and refrigerate for at least one hour before serving.

Nutritional Analysis (Per Serving)
- Calories: 53
- Protein: 0.8 g
- Fat: 3.5 g
- Carbohydrates: 5.4 g
- Fiber: 1.7 g
- Sodium: 17 mg
- Cholesterol: 0 mg

Oriental Coleslaw

¾ cup	chopped snow peas	175 mL
3 cups	shredded green cabbage	750 mL
3 cups	shredded red cabbage	750 mL
1 cup	sliced water chestnuts	250 mL
1 cup	sliced red peppers	250 mL
¾ cup	canned mandarin oranges, drained	175 mL
2	medium green onions, chopped	2

DRESSING

3 tbsp	brown sugar	45 mL
2 tbsp	rice wine vinegar	25 mL
2 tbsp	vegetable oil	25 mL
1 tbsp	soya sauce	15 mL
1 tbsp	sesame oil	15 mL
1 tsp	minced garlic	5 mL
1 tsp	minced gingerroot	5 mL

Make Ahead

Prepare salad and dressing early in the day. Best if tossed just before serving.

SERVES 8 TO 10

1. In saucepan of boiling water or microwave, blanch snow peas just until tender-crisp, approximately 1 to 2 minutes; refresh in cold water and drain. Place in serving bowl with shredded cabbage, water chestnuts, red peppers, mandarin oranges and green onions; toss well to combine.
2. In small bowl whisk together brown sugar, vinegar, vegetable oil, soya sauce, sesame oil, garlic and ginger; pour over salad and toss well.

Tips

- Other vegetables, such as green beans or broccoli, can replace snow peas.
- This is a great variation on the usual coleslaw.

Nutritional Analysis (Per Serving)
- Calories: 81
- Protein: 1 g
- Fat: 4 g
- Carbohydrates: 12 g
- Fiber: 2 g
- Sodium: 116 mg
- Cholesterol: 0 mg

Coleslaw for a Crowd

8 cups	chopped green savoy cabbage	2 L
2 cups	chopped red apples (crisp or tart)	500 mL
1½ cups	grated carrots	375 mL
1½ cups	chopped celery	375 mL
1 cup	chopped green bell peppers	250 mL
½ cup	chopped green onions	125 mL
⅔ cup	light mayonnaise	150 mL
1 tsp	granulated sugar	5 mL
½ tsp	salt	2 mL

Make Ahead

Once made, the salad keeps well in the refrigerator for about 3 days.

SERVES 16 OR MAKES 12 CUPS (3 L)

1. In a very large bowl, combine cabbage, apples, carrots, celery, green peppers and green onions.
2. In a small bowl or measuring cup, blend together mayonnaise, sugar and salt. Add to cabbage mixture; toss to blend well. Chill for 2 hours or overnight. (Don't worry if salad appears to need more dressing; after chilling, the mixture becomes creamier as the vegetables give off some juice.)

Nutritional Analysis (Per Serving)
- Calories: 58
- Protein: 1 g
- Fat: 3 g
- Carbohydrates: 7 g
- Fiber: 2 g
- Sodium: 60 mg
- Cholesterol: 6 mg

Baby Corn, Broccoli and Cauliflower Salad in a Creamy Citrus Dressing

SALAD

2 cups	broccoli florets	500 mL
2 cups	cauliflower florets	500 mL
2 cups	chopped baby corn cobs	500 mL
2 cups	chopped red bell peppers	500 mL
1 cup	chopped water chestnuts	250 mL
¾ cup	chopped green onions	175 mL

DRESSING

⅓ cup	chopped fresh coriander	75 mL
3 tbsp	olive oil	45 mL
3 tbsp	light sour cream	45 mL
2 tbsp	freshly squeezed lemon juice	25 mL
2 tbsp	freshly squeezed lime juice	25 mL
2 tbsp	light mayonnaise	25 mL
2 tsp	honey	10 mL
1½ tsp	minced garlic	7 mL
1 to 2 tsp	minced fresh jalapeño peppers	5 to 10 mL

Make Ahead

Prepare salad up to 1 day in advance. The salad will marinate.

SERVES 6 TO 8

1. Boil or steam broccoli and cauliflower 5 minutes or until tender-crisp. Rinse under cold water and drain. Put in a serving bowl.

2. Stir baby corn, red peppers, water chestnuts and green onions into broccoli-cauliflower mixture.

3. Make the dressing: In a small bowl, whisk together coriander, olive oil, sour cream, lemon juice, lime juice, mayonnaise, honey, garlic and jalapeño peppers. Pour over salad; toss to coat. Chill and serve.

Tips

- For the best flavor, be sure to use fresh citrus juices. Bottled juice concentrates tend to be more acidic.

- 1 tsp (5 mL) chili powder can replace jalapeño peppers.

- Replace coriander with fresh dill or basil.

Nutritional Analysis (Per Serving)
- Calories: 102
- Protein: 3 g
- Fat: 6 g
- Carbohydrates: 11 g
- Fiber: 2 g
- Sodium: 460 mg
- Cholesterol: 0 mg

Cool Cucumber Salad

3 cups	thinly sliced English cucumber unpeeled, about 1 large	750 mL
½ tsp	salt	2 mL
½ cup	yogurt cheese (see technique, at right)	125 mL
½ tsp	lemon juice	2 mL
¼ tsp	minced garlic	1 mL
¼ tsp	ground ginger	1 mL

This creamy salad is a perfect palate cooler to serve with any spicy meat or poultry dish.

SERVES 6 OR MAKES 3 CUPS (750 ML)

1. Place cucumber slices in a large colander; sprinkle with salt. Let stand for 10 to 15 minutes over a large bowl (or in the sink) to drain. Rinse well under cold water. Pat dry and transfer to a bowl. Set aside.

2. In a separate bowl, blend together yogurt cheese, lemon juice, garlic and ginger. Add mixture to cucumber; toss gently. Chill before serving.

Nutritional Analysis (Per ½ cup/125 mL Serving)
- Calories: 27
- Protein: 2 g
- Fat: 1 g
- Carbohydrates: 3 g
- Fiber: 0 g
- Sodium: 227 mg
- Cholesterol: 1 mg

To make 1 cup (250 mL) yogurt cheese

Use 2 cups (500 mL) lower-fat plain yogurt (Balkan-style, not stirred, made without gelatin). Line a sieve with a double thickness of paper towel or cheesecloth. Pour yogurt into the sieve and place over a bowl. Cover well with plastic wrap and refrigerate for at least 2 hours. Discard liquid and keep solids in an airtight container in the refrigerator for up to 1 week.

If you want to drain the yogurt overnight, use 3 cups (750 mL) yogurt to get 1 cup (250 mL) yogurt cheese. The longer you drain the yogurt, the more tart it becomes.

Cucumbers in Sour Cream

1	cucumber, peeled and sliced	1
¼ cup	sour cream	50 mL
	Salt and freshly ground black pepper	
	Finely chopped dill (optional)	

This combination is particularly good when cucumbers are in season and at their peak of sweetness.

SERVES 2

1. In a serving bowl, combine cucumber and sour cream. Toss well. Season with salt and black pepper to taste. Garnish with dill, if using.

Nutritional Analysis (Per Serving)
- Calories: 37
- Protein: 0.8 g
- Fat: 2.7 g
- Carbohydrates: 2.8 g
- Fiber: 0.5 g
- Sodium: 8 mg
- Cholesterol: 5 mg

Raita Cucumber Salad

1	medium English cucumber, thinly sliced	1
1	large tomato, diced	1
1	medium onion, thinly sliced	1
2½ cups	lower-fat plain yogurt	625 mL
1 tbsp	chopped fresh parsley	15 mL
¾ tsp	ground cumin	4 mL
½ tsp	each ground coriander and salt	2 mL
½ tsp	each grated lemon zest and orange zest	2 mL
¼ tsp	hot pepper sauce	1 mL
Pinch	each paprika and black pepper	Pinch

This refreshing salad cools the palate and goes especially well with spicy ethnic dishes such as curries.

SERVES 8

1. In a bowl, combine vegetables. Whisk remaining ingredients together and toss with vegetables. Cover and chill thoroughly.

Tips

- If you prefer a salad with milder flavor, omit the hot pepper sauce.
- The quantity of lower-fat yogurt in this soothing salad will boost your calcium intake.

Nutritional Analysis (Per Serving)
- Calories: 66
- Protein: 5 g
- Fat: 1 g
- Carbohydrates: 9 g
- Fiber: 1 g
- Sodium: 61 mg
- Cholesterol: 2 mg

Asian Cucumber Salad

2 tbsp	rice vinegar (see tip, at right)	25 mL
1 tbsp	soy sauce	15 mL
1 tbsp	vegetable oil	15 mL
1	cucumber, peeled and sliced	1
	Salt and freshly ground black pepper	

This simple salad makes a delicious addition to any meal.

SERVES 2

1. In a serving bowl, combine vinegar, soy sauce and oil. Add cucumber and toss to combine. Season with salt and black pepper to taste. Serve.

Tip

- Made from fermented rice, this Asian vinegar, which is milder than traditional North American vinegars, is now widely available in supermarkets. Keep a bottle on hand to add its unique flavor to Asian-inspired dishes.

Nutritional Analysis (Per Serving)
- Calories: 272
- Protein: 29.1 g
- Fat: 14.3 g
- Carbohydrates: 7.5 g
- Fiber: 2.6 g
- Sodium: 333 mg
- Cholesterol: 100 mg

Escarole Salad with Olives and Anchovies

8 cups	washed, dried and torn escarole	2 L
⅔ cup	olive oil	150 mL
¼ cup	red wine vinegar	50 mL
1	clove garlic, minced	1
½ tsp	black pepper	2 mL
½ cup	chopped fresh parsley	125 mL
1	can (2 oz/50 g) anchovies, drained and coarsely chopped	1
½ cup	pitted black olives	125 mL
½ cup	pitted green olives	125 mL

Make Ahead

Escarole can be washed, dried and torn, then wrapped loosely in paper towels and refrigerated in a sealed plastic bag for up to 2 days. The dressing can be refrigerated for up to 1 week. Let stand at room temperature for 30 minutes, then shake well before using.

SERVES 6

1. Place escarole in a large salad bowl; refrigerate, covered, until ready to serve.
2. In a small jar with a lid, combine olive oil, vinegar, garlic and pepper; shake until well mixed.
3. Just before serving, add dressing and parsley to escarole; toss well. Scatter anchovies, black olives and green olives over top. Serve at once.

Tips

- Always store cans of anchovies, whether opened or not, in the refrigerator. Once opened, pat the anchovies dry with paper towels. Leftovers can be frozen, wrapped in plastic wrap, for up to 1 month.

- If you prefer, omit the anchovies — but their robust flavor adds an interesting dimension to this salad.

Nutritional Analysis (Per Serving)

- Calories: 256
- Protein: 4.3 g
- Fat: 26.0 g
- Carbohydrates: 3.3 g
- Fiber: 0.3 g
- Sodium: 464 mg
- Cholesterol: 8 mg

Eggplant with Mint

1	large eggplant (about 1½ lbs/750 g)	1
1 tsp	vegetable oil	5 mL
¼ cup	olive oil	50 mL
2 tbsp	freshly squeezed lemon juice	25 mL
2 tbsp	chopped fresh mint or 1 tbsp (15 mL) dried	25 mL
3	cloves garlic, minced	3
1	fresh chili, finely chopped (with or without seeds, depending on desired hotness)	
	Salt to taste	
1	small tomato, cut into wedges	1
¼ cup	black olives (about 8)	50 mL

SERVES 4

Preheat oven to 450°F (230°C)

1. Brush eggplant lightly with vegetable oil. Using a fork, pierce the skin lightly at 1-inch (2.5 cm) intervals. Place on an oven pan and bake for 1 hour.

2. Meanwhile prepare the dressing: In a small bowl combine the olive oil, lemon juice, mint, garlic and chili (with seeds, if desired); mix well and set aside.

3. Transfer eggplant to a work surface. Cut off 1 inch (2.5 cm) at the stem end and discard (this part never quite cooks through). Peel the eggplant by picking at an edge from the cut end, then pulling upward. The skin should come off easily in strips.

4. Cut the eggplant lengthwise and place each half with the interior facing you. With a spoon scoop out the tongues of seed-pods, leaving as much of the flesh as possible. To remove the additional seed-pods hiding inside, cut each piece of eggplant in half and repeat the deseeding procedure. Once deseeded, cut the eggplant flesh into strips 2 inches (5 cm) long and 1 inch (2.5 cm) wide. Transfer the strips to a serving bowl.

5. Whisk the reserved dressing and add salt to taste. Add to the eggplant. Fold gently to dress all the pieces, then garnish with tomato wedges and black olives. Serve right away, or let wait covered and unrefrigerated for up to 2 hours.

Tip

• When working with hot peppers, be sure to wear gloves; otherwise, wash hands thoroughly afterwards.

Nutritional Analysis (Per Serving)

• Calories: 189   • Protein: 2.1 g   • Fat: 15.9 g
• Carbohydrates: 11.9 g   • Fiber: 4.3 g   • Sodium: 82 mg
• Cholesterol: 0 mg

Jellied Gazpacho Salad

1 tbsp	unflavored gelatin (1 package)	15 mL
1¼ cups	vegetable juice cocktail, divided	300 mL
1 tsp	beef bouillon powder	5 mL
2 tbsp	cider vinegar or vinegar	25 mL
1 tsp	Worcestershire sauce	5 mL
Dash	hot pepper sauce	Dash
1	medium tomato, peeled	1
½	large green bell pepper	½
½	large cucumber, peeled and seeded	½
1	small onion	1
1	small clove garlic	1
1	small celery stalk with leaves	1
	Celery leaves	

A new twist on the classic soup — all the zesty flavors of gazpacho prepared as a jellied salad. Loaded with crunch but light on fat, this will fit the bill whenever you are looking for a cool salad.

SERVES 6

6-cup (1.5 L) mold

1. In a medium saucepan, sprinkle gelatin over ¼ cup (50 mL) of the vegetable juice. Stir over low heat for 3 minutes or until gelatin is completely dissolved. Stir in beef bouillon, ¾ cup (175 mL) of the remaining vegetable juice, vinegar, Worcestershire sauce and hot pepper sauce. Refrigerate, stirring occasionally, until mixture is consistency of unbeaten egg whites, about 30 minutes.

2. In a food processor or blender, purée half the tomato, the green pepper, cucumber, onion and garlic with remaining vegetable juice until smooth. Coarsely chop remaining tomato and celery. Stir purée and chopped vegetables into gelatin mixture. Pour into a rinsed 6-cup (1.5 L) mold. Cover and refrigerate until firm, at least 3 hours.

3. To serve, unmold gazpacho onto serving plate. Garnish with celery leaves.

Nutritional Analysis (Per Serving)
- Calories: 31
- Protein: 2 g
- Fat: 0 g
- Carbohydrates: 6 g
- Fiber: 1 g
- Sodium: 83 mg
- Cholesterol: 0 mg

Greek Salad

2	large tomatoes	2
1	medium cucumber	1
1	medium red onion	1
1	sweet red or green pepper	1
3 oz	feta cheese, crumbled	75 g
¼ cup	black olives, sliced	50 mL
DRESSING		
3 tbsp	lemon juice	45 mL
4 tsp	red wine vinegar	20 mL
1 tsp	crushed garlic	5 mL
2 tsp	dried oregano (or 2 tbsp/ 25 mL chopped fresh)	10 mL
3 tbsp	vegetable oil	45 mL
	Salt and pepper	

SERVES 6

1. Cut tomatoes, cucumber, onion and red pepper into large chunks. Place in large salad bowl. Add cheese and olives.

2. *Dressing:* In small bowl, combine lemon juice, vinegar, garlic and oregano; whisk in oil. Season with salt and pepper to taste. Pour over salad and gently mix well.

Nutritional Analysis (Per Serving)
- Calories: 136
- Protein: 3 g
- Fat: 10 g
- Carbohydrates: 8 g
- Fiber: 1 g
- Sodium: 216 mg
- Cholesterol: 12 mg

Fast and Easy Greek Salad

2 cups	diced tomatoes	500 mL
2 cups	diced cucumbers	500 mL
1 cup	cubed feta cheese (about 8 oz/250 g)	250 mL
1/2 cup	thinly sliced onions	125 mL
1/4 cup	sliced black olives (optional)	50 mL
2 tbsp	white wine vinegar	25 mL
2 tbsp	olive oil	25 mL
1/2 tsp	minced garlic	2 mL
1/2 tsp	dried basil	2 mL
1/2 tsp	dried oregano	2 mL
	Black pepper to taste	

Here's a simple salad that's sure to please. It's especially good when tomatoes are in season.

SERVES 4 OR MAKES 6 CUPS (1.5 L)

1. In a large bowl, combine tomatoes, cucumbers, cheese, onions and, if using, olives. Set aside.
2. In a small bowl or measuring cup, whisk together vinegar, oil, garlic, basil, oregano and pepper. Add to tomato mixture; toss gently to combine. Chill before serving.

Tips

- If desired, substitute 1 tbsp (15 mL) chopped fresh basil for the dried.
- This salad is higher in fat, so it is best served with lower-fat dishes. If you don't have time to make the dressing, use a bottled oil-and-vinegar-type dressing. Choose a dressing that contains less than 3 g of fat per 1 tbsp (15 mL) to help cut the fat.

Nutritional Analysis (Per Serving)
- Calories: 177
- Protein: 6 g
- Fat: 14 g
- Carbohydrates: 9 g
- Fiber: 2 g
- Sodium: 471 mg
- Cholesterol: 34 mg

Greek Winter Salad

1	head romaine lettuce, cut into 1/4-inch (0.5 cm) strips	1
4 or 5	green onions, green part only, cut into 1/4-inch (0.5 cm) pieces	4 or 5
	Few sprigs fresh dill, chopped	
1/4 cup	olive oil	50 mL
1 tbsp	red wine vinegar	15 mL
	Salt and freshly ground black pepper to taste	
4 oz	feta cheese, crumbled in large chunks	125 g
Pinch	dried oregano leaves	Pinch
1/2 cup	whole black olives, preferably Calamata (about 16)	125 mL

SERVES 4 TO 6

1. In a wide salad bowl, lay out lettuce strips; sprinkle with green onions and dill. Toss lightly to combine.
2. In a small bowl, whisk together olive oil and vinegar until emulsified. Season to taste with salt and pepper. Pour over the lettuce and toss well.
3. Crumble feta over the salad and sprinkle with oregano. Garnish with black olives and serve immediately.

Nutritional Analysis (Per Serving)
- Calories: 185
- Protein: 4.6 g
- Fat: 17.3 g
- Carbohydrates: 4.4 g
- Fiber: 1.8 g
- Sodium: 382 mg
- Cholesterol: 20 mg

Green and Yellow Salad

8 oz	fresh green beans, trimmed	250 g
8 oz	fresh yellow beans, trimmed	250 g
1 tbsp	lime juice	15 mL
1	ripe avocado	1
	Salt and freshly ground black pepper to taste	
3 tbsp	olive oil	45 mL
3	green onions, finely chopped	3
4 oz	feta cheese, crumbled into large chunks	125 g
	Few sprigs fresh coriander, roughly chopped	

SERVES 4 TO 6

1. Boil green and yellow beans over high heat for 5 to 7 minutes. Drain and immediately refresh in a bowl of ice-cold water. Drain, and put in a wide salad bowl.

2. Put lime juice in a bowl. Peel avocado and cut into slices (or scoop out with a small spoon), and add to the lime juice. Fold avocado into the juice until well coated. Scatter avocado slices (or scoops) decoratively over the beans, along with any leftover lime juice. Season to taste with salt and pepper.

3. Drizzle olive oil over salad, and garnish with chopped green onions. Distribute feta over the salad, and top with a scattering of the chopped coriander. The salad can wait up to 1 hour, covered and unrefrigerated.

Nutritional Analysis (Per Serving)
- Calories: 223
- Protein: 5.7 g
- Fat: 19.1 g
- Carbohydrates: 10.3 g
- Fiber: 4.8 g
- Sodium: 264 mg
- Cholesterol: 20 mg

Heart to Heart Salad

3 tbsp	extra-virgin olive oil	45 mL
1 tbsp	lemon juice	15 mL
1 tbsp	finely diced red or green onion	15 mL
1/2 tsp	crushed dried thyme	2 mL
1	can (14 oz/398 mL) artichoke hearts, drained and quartered	1
1 tbsp	shredded Gruyère or grated Sbrinz cheese	15 mL
1 tbsp	finely chopped fresh parsley	15 mL

SERVES 4

1. In a bowl, combine first 4 ingredients. Add artichokes and stir to coat. Cover and chill thoroughly.

2. To serve, sprinkle with cheese and parsley.

Tip

- Mixing your own salad dressings allows you to control the amount and type of oil used and is less expensive than using store-bought dressings.

Although it takes only minutes to make this salad, for best results marinate overnight.

Nutritional Analysis (Per Serving)
- Calories: 84
- Protein: 3 g
- Fat: 6 g
- Carbohydrates: 7 g
- Fiber: 3 g
- Sodium: 295 mg
- Cholesterol: 8 mg

Green Bean and Plum Tomato Salad

1 lb	young green beans, trimmed	500 g
8	small plum tomatoes (about 1 lb/500 g)	8
2	green onions, sliced	2
DRESSING		
¼ cup	olive oil	50 mL
4 tsp	red wine vinegar	20 mL
1 tbsp	grainy mustard	15 mL
1	clove garlic, minced	1
½ tsp	granulated sugar	2 mL
¼ tsp	salt	1 mL
¼ tsp	freshly ground black pepper	1 mL
¼ cup	chopped fresh parsley	50 mL

SERVES 6

1. In a medium saucepan of boiling salted water, cook beans for 3 to 5 minutes or until just tender-crisp. Drain and rinse under cold water to chill; drain well. Pat dry with paper towels or wrap in a clean, dry towel.

2. Cut plum tomatoes in half lengthwise; using a small spoon, scoop out centers. Cut each piece again in half lengthwise; place in a bowl. Just before serving, combine beans, tomatoes and green onions in a serving bowl.

3. *Dressing:* In a small bowl, whisk together oil, vinegar, mustard, garlic, sugar, salt and pepper. Stir in parsley. Pour dressing over salad and toss well.

Tips

- Use the terrific mustardy dressing with other favorite vegetable salad mixtures and crisp greens.

- When preparing this dish ahead, keep the blanched green beans, tomatoes and dressing separate and toss them just before serving to prevent the salad from getting soggy.

Nutritional Analysis (Per Serving)
- Calories: 131
- Protein: 2.7 g
- Fat: 9.4 g
- Carbohydrates: 11.5 g
- Fiber: 4.3 g
- Sodium: 138 mg
- Cholesterol: 0 mg

Minted Green Salad

6 cups	mixed greens	1.5 L
¼ cup	coarsely chopped mint	50 mL
2 tbsp	extra virgin olive oil	25 mL
	Juice and zest of 1 lemon	
	Salt and freshly ground black pepper	

SERVES 6

1. In a large salad bowl, combine mixed greens and mint.

2. In a small bowl, whisk together oil, lemon juice and zest, salt and pepper. Toss dressing with greens at serving time.

Nutritional Analysis (Per Serving)
- Calories: 49
- Protein: 0.9 g
- Fat: 4.6 g
- Carbohydrates: 1.6 g
- Fiber: 1.0 g
- Sodium: 4 mg
- Cholesterol: 0 mg

Sautéed Mushrooms on Wilted Greens

1 lb	lettuce (one type or mixture of several types), washed, dried and torn into bite-size pieces	500 g
6 tbsp	olive oil	90 mL
½ tsp	salt	2 mL
½ tsp	freshly ground black pepper	2 mL
¾ cup	thinly sliced red onion	175 mL
4 cups	thickly sliced portobello mushrooms	1 L
6	cloves garlic, finely chopped	6
2 tbsp	freshly squeezed lemon juice	25 mL
2 tbsp	white wine	25 mL
1	medium tomato, cut into wedges	1
¼	red bell pepper, cut into thin half-rounds	¼
1 tbsp	grated lemon zest	15 mL
	Few sprigs fresh parsley, roughly chopped	

SERVES 8

1. Place lettuce in a large salad bowl.
2. In a large frying pan, heat olive oil over high heat. Add salt and pepper and stir. Add sliced red onions and stir-fry for 1 minute. Add mushrooms and stir-fry actively, for 4 to 5 minutes, until they are shiny and beginning to char slightly. Add garlic and stir-fry for 1 minute. Add lemon juice and let come to a sizzle, about 30 seconds. Add wine and stir-fry for 1 to 2 minutes, until a syrupy sauce has formed.
3. Transfer the contents of the frying pan with all its juices, evenly over the lettuce. Use a fork to arrange the mushrooms decoratively. Garnish with tomato wedges, red pepper crescents and lemon zest. Top with some chopped parsley, and serve immediately. Toss gently at table, leaving most of the mushrooms on top.

Variation

- If desired, use 1 lb (500 g) whole oyster mushrooms, trimmed, instead of the portobello mushroom strips.

Tips

- Ordinary mushrooms will work in a pinch, but the luxurious texture and flavor of oyster or portobello mushrooms justifies the extra cost.
- This recipe can be easily halved for smaller gatherings.

Nutritional Analysis (Per Serving)
- Calories: 132
- Protein: 3.3 g
- Fat: 10.5 g
- Carbohydrates: 7.7 g
- Fiber: 2.8 g
- Sodium: 155 mg
- Cholesterol: 0 mg

Roasted Portobello Mushroom and Fennel Salad

MUSHROOMS AND FENNEL

1/3 cup	olive oil	75 mL
4	cloves garlic, minced	4
2 tsp	chopped fresh tarragon, or 3/4 tsp (4 mL) dried	10 mL
1/2 tsp	salt	2 mL
1/4 tsp	black pepper	1 mL
6	portobello mushrooms (about 1 1/2 lbs/750 g total), stems removed	6
1	large bulb fennel (about 1 1/2 lbs/750 g), trimmed and cut in 12 wedges	1

BALSAMIC VINAIGRETTE

2 tbsp	balsamic vinegar	25 mL
1 tbsp	lemon juice	15 mL
1 tsp	Dijon mustard	5 mL
2 tbsp	olive oil	25 mL
1/4 tsp	salt	1 mL
1/4 tsp	black pepper	1 mL

SALAD

6 cups	arugula or baby spinach	1.5 L
1/2 cup	toasted pine nuts (see tip, at right)	125 mL

Make Ahead

Prepare dressing, cover and refrigerate for up to two days.

MAKES 6 SERVINGS

1. In a small bowl, whisk together olive oil, garlic, tarragon, salt and pepper.
2. Arrange mushrooms, round side up, on a parchment-lined baking sheet. Brush with half the oil mixture.
3. In a large bowl, toss fennel wedges with remaining oil mixture. Place on another parchment-lined baking sheet.
4. Convection roast mushrooms and fennel in a preheated 400°F (200°C) oven — mushrooms for 12 minutes, fennel for 18 to 20 minutes, or until tender. Cool both slightly. Cut each mushroom diagonally into 4 slices.

Tip

- To toast nuts and seeds, place in a small baking dish. Convection bake in a preheated 300°F (150°C) oven for 5 to 10 minutes, or until golden.

Nutritional Analysis (Per Serving)
- Calories: 267
- Protein: 8.0 g
- Fat: 23.0 g
- Carbohydrates: 11.7 g
- Fiber: 3.7 g
- Sodium: 326 mg
- Cholesterol: 0 mg

Warm Shiitake Mushroom Salad

DRESSING

2 tbsp	toasted pine nuts	25 mL
1 tbsp	finely chopped basil	15 mL
1	clove garlic, chopped	1
2 tbsp	olive oil	25 mL
4 tbsp	vegetable oil	60 mL
2 tbsp	white wine vinegar	25 mL
	Salt and pepper to taste	

SALAD

2 tbsp	olive oil	25 mL
3	large shallots, thinly sliced	3
1 tbsp	finely chopped basil	15 mL
1	clove garlic, chopped	1
8 oz	shiitake mushrooms, stems removed and thinly sliced (about 3 cups/750 mL)	250 g
1/8 cup	toasted pine nuts	25 mL
1 tbsp	fresh lemon juice	15 mL
6 cups	mixed greens (radicchio, arugula and/or endive greens), washed	1.5 L

SERVES 6

1. *Dressing:* In a blender or food processor, blend together all dressing ingredients. Season to taste.

2. *Salad:* In a frying pan, heat olive oil over medium heat. Add shallots and sauté for about 5 minutes. Add basil, garlic and shiitake mushrooms; fry another 2 minutes. Remove from heat and let cool briefly.

3. Add dressing, toasted pine nuts and lemon juice to mushroom mixture; mix thoroughly. Season to taste.

4. Arrange the mixed greens on individual plates and top with equal portions of the mushroom mixture. Serve immediately.

Nutritional Analysis (Per Serving)
- Calories: 164
- Protein: 2.9 g
- Fat: 15.9 g
- Carbohydrates: 4.3 g
- Fiber: 1.4 g
- Sodium: 5 mg
- Cholesterol: 0 mg

Roasted Red Pepper Salad

6	roasted red bell peppers (see tip, at right), each cut into 6 strips	6
1 tbsp	balsamic or red wine vinegar	15 mL
2 tsp	olive oil	10 mL
2 tbsp	chopped fresh basil (optional)	25 mL
	Freshly ground black pepper	

Keep roasted red peppers in your freezer, and you can make this salad any time.

SERVES 6

1. Arrange peppers in the bottom of a serving dish.

2. In a bowl, whisk together vinegar and olive oil; drizzle over peppers. Sprinkle with basil, if using. Season with pepper to taste. Chill for 1 hour.

Tip
- To roast peppers, heat barbecue or broiler; place peppers on grill or broiling pan and cook until skins turn black. Keep turning peppers until skins are blistered and black.

Nutritional Analysis (Per Serving)
- Calories: 48
- Protein: 1 g
- Fat: 2 g
- Carbohydrates: 8 g
- Fiber: 2 g
- Sodium: 3 mg
- Cholesterol: 0 mg

Sweet Pepper Salad with Red Pepper Dressing

2 cups	chopped sweet red, green or yellow pepper	500 mL
1 cup	chopped cucumber	250 mL
1 cup	cherry tomatoes, cut into quarters	250 mL
½ cup	chopped red onion	125 mL
½ cup	chopped celery	125 mL

DRESSING

2 tbsp	diced red onion	25 mL
¼ cup	diced sweet red pepper	50 mL
1 tbsp	lemon juice	15 mL
2 tsp	red wine vinegar	10 mL
1 tbsp	water	15 mL
2 tbsp	olive oil	25 mL
½ tsp	crushed garlic	2 mL
½ tsp	Dijon mustard	2 mL
2 tbsp	chopped fresh parsley	25 mL
	Salt and pepper	

SERVES 4

1. In salad bowl, combine red pepper, cucumber, tomatoes, onion and celery.
2. *Dressing:* In food processor, combine onion, red pepper, lemon juice, vinegar, water, oil, garlic, mustard, parsley, and salt and pepper to taste; process until combined. Pour over salad and toss to combine.

Tip

- Double the recipe for red pepper dressing and save half to serve as a wonderful side sauce for fish or chicken.

Nutritional Analysis (Per Serving)
- Calories: 102
- Protein: 1 g
- Fat: 7 g
- Carbohydrates: 10 g
- Fiber: 2 g
- Sodium: 37 mg
- Cholesterol: 0 mg

Spinach Salad with Creamy Garlic Dressing

1	slice whole-wheat bread	1
10 cups	spinach leaves	2.5 L
1½ cups	sliced mushrooms	375 mL
¼ cup	alfalfa sprouts	50 mL
2 tbsp	grated Parmesan cheese	25 mL

DRESSING

½ cup	lower-fat plain yogurt	125 mL
¼ cup	chopped fresh parsley	50 mL
2 tbsp	light mayonnaise	25 mL
1	large clove garlic, minced	1
Pinch	each salt and black pepper	Pinch

Homemade whole-wheat croutons and yogurt dressing create a light version of this popular salad.

SERVES 6

Preheat oven to 350°F (180°C)

1. Cut bread into cubes; toast in preheated oven for 5 minutes or until crisp and brown.
2. Tear spinach into bite-size pieces. In a large salad bowl, combine toasted bread cubes, spinach, mushrooms, alfalfa sprouts and Parmesan cheese.
3. *Dressing:* Combine yogurt, parsley, mayonnaise, garlic, salt and pepper. Pour dressing over vegetables; toss until well coated.

Tip

- For variety, try adding ½ cup (125 mL) chopped red or green bell pepper, tomatoes, red onion, apple or mandarin orange segments to the salad.

Nutritional Analysis (Per Serving)
- Calories: 74
- Protein: 5 g
- Fat: 3 g
- Carbohydrates: 9 g
- Fiber: 3 g
- Sodium: 199 mg
- Cholesterol: 2 mg

Warm Spinach and Mushroom Salad

DRESSING

3 tbsp	balsamic vinegar	45 mL
4 tsp	olive oil	20 mL
1 tsp	minced garlic	5 mL

SALAD

6 cups	washed, dried and torn spinach leaves	1.5 L
1/2 cup	chopped, softened sun-dried tomatoes (see tip, at right)	125 mL
1/4 cup	toasted chopped walnuts	50 mL
2 tsp	vegetable oil	10 mL
1 tsp	minced garlic	5 mL
2 cups	sliced oyster mushrooms	500 mL
3/4 cup	sliced red onions	175 mL

Make Ahead

Prepare dressing and sauté mushroom mixture early in the day. Do not mix with salad. When ready to serve, reheat mushroom mixture and toss with dressing and salad.

SERVES 4 TO 6

1. In a small bowl, whisk together vinegar, olive oil and garlic. Set aside.
2. Put spinach, sun-dried tomatoes and walnuts in a large serving bowl.
3. In a large nonstick frying pan, heat oil over high heat. Add garlic, mushrooms and red onions; cook 6 minutes, or until mushrooms are browned and any excess liquid is absorbed. Quickly add hot vegetables and dressing to spinach and toss. Serve immediately.

Tips

- To soften sun-dried tomatoes, cover with boiling water and let soak for 15 minutes. Drain and chop.
- Try this recipe with different mushrooms — such as cremini or, for a decadent evening, shiitake or chanterelles.
- Common mushrooms will also work well with this recipe.

Nutritional Analysis (Per Serving)
- Calories: 108
- Protein: 4 g
- Fat: 8 g
- Carbohydrates: 9 g
- Fiber: 3 g
- Sodium: 143 mg
- Cholesterol: 0 mg

The Perfect Tomato Salad

3	large tomatoes, halved	3
1/2 cup	crumbled feta cheese	125 mL
1/4 cup	chopped black olives	50 mL
2 tbsp	extra virgin olive oil	25 mL
	Salt and freshly ground black pepper	

Its ingredients are traditional — black olives, feta cheese and olive oil — but this is definitely not your usual Greek salad. It's a delightful change!

SERVES 6

1. Scoop pulp from center of tomato halves. Reserve pulp. Place halves upside-down on paper towel to drain.
2. In a small bowl, combine half of tomato pulp, cheese, olives, oil, salt and pepper. Chill for 1 hour. At serving time, spoon tomato mixture into tomato halves and serve.

Nutritional Analysis (Per Serving)
- Calories: 93
- Protein: 2.6 g
- Fat: 7.7 g
- Carbohydrates: 4.2 g
- Fiber: 1.2 g
- Sodium: 169 mg
- Cholesterol: 11 mg

Tomato, Avocado and Snow Pea Salad with Blue Cheese Dressing

4 oz	snow peas, cut in half	125 g
	Lettuce leaves	
Half	medium red or sweet onion, sliced	Half
Half	avocado, sliced thinly	Half
1	large tomato, sliced	1

DRESSING

1/4 cup	crumbled blue cheese	50 mL
1/3 cup	2% yogurt	75 mL
1/4 tsp	crushed garlic	1 mL
	Salt and pepper	

Make Ahead

Prepare and refrigerate dressing up to a day before. Prepare salad just prior to serving.

SERVES 4

1. Steam or microwave snow peas just until tender-crisp. Drain and rinse with cold water; drain well and pat dry.

2. Line serving platter with lettuce leaves. Decoratively arrange onion, avocado, tomato and snow peas over lettuce.

3. *Dressing:* In food processor, combine blue cheese, yogurt and garlic; process until just combined. Season with salt and pepper to taste. Drizzle over salad.

Tips

- Since avocado discolors quickly when sliced, assemble the salad just before serving.
- Puréeing dressing gives it a smooth, thin texture. Processing on and off allows pieces of blue cheese to remain.

Nutritional Analysis (Per Serving)
- Calories: 105
- Protein: 5 g
- Fat: 6 g
- Carbohydrates: 8 g
- Fiber: 2 g
- Sodium: 140 mg
- Cholesterol: 7 mg

Basil Marinated Tomatoes

4	medium tomatoes, sliced	4
1/4 cup	chopped fresh parsley	50 mL
3 tbsp	olive oil	45 mL
1 tbsp	each white and red wine vinegar	15 mL
1 tbsp	chopped fresh basil	15 mL
3/4 tsp	granulated sugar	4 mL
1/4 tsp	each salt and black pepper	1 mL

Mouthwatering when tomatoes are at their peak, this is a great addition to summer meals.

SERVES 8

1. Arrange tomatoes on plate. Sprinkle with parsley.

2. Whisk together remaining ingredients and pour over tomatoes. Cover and refrigerate for 1 hour.

Variation

- Add sliced fresh mozzarella or crumbled blue cheese, such as Roquefort or Gorgonzola.

Nutritional Analysis (Per Serving)
- Calories: 81
- Protein: 1 g
- Fat: / g
- Carbohydrates: 5 g
- Fiber: 1 g
- Sodium: 77 mg
- Cholesterol: 0 mg

Over-the-Top Tomato Salad

2 tbsp	coarsely chopped sun-dried tomatoes	25 mL
	Boiling water	
2 tbsp	olive oil	25 mL
1 tbsp	chopped red onion	15 mL
1 tbsp	balsamic vinegar	15 mL
1/4 tsp	granulated sugar	1 mL
1/4 tsp	salt	1 mL
1/4 tsp	black pepper	1 mL
3	beefsteak tomatoes (each about 8 oz/250 g)	3
1/4 cup	small fresh basil or oregano leaves	50 mL

Make Ahead

The dressing can be refrigerated, covered, for up to 1 week. Let stand at room temperature for 30 minutes, then whisk well before using.

In this attractive salad, fresh tomatoes are drizzled with a vibrant sun-dried tomato dressing.

SERVES 6

1. In a small heatproof bowl, combine sun-dried tomatoes with enough boiling water to cover them; set aside for 20 minutes. Drain tomatoes well, reserving water.

2. In a blender or mini-chopper, combine sun-dried tomatoes, 2 tbsp (25 mL) reserved soaking water (use tap water if using oil-packed sun-dried tomatoes), oil, onion, vinegar, sugar, salt and pepper. Blend until finely minced and well combined. (Dressing will be quite thick.)

3. With a small knife, cut out coarse stem ends from beefsteak tomatoes. Cut tomatoes into thin slices; arrange on a serving platter. Just before serving, whisk dressing to combine; spoon evenly over tomatoes. Serve sprinkled with basil leaves.

Tips

- If you use sun-dried tomatoes packed in oil, there's no need to soak them, and you can use their oil in place of the olive oil.

- The easiest way to chop sun-dried tomatoes is to snip them into small pieces with sharp kitchen scissors.

- Wrap leftover red onion tightly in plastic wrap and refrigerate for up to 1 week.

Nutritional Analysis (Per Serving)
- Calories: 72
- Protein: 1.3 g
- Fat: 5.1 g
- Carbohydrates: 6.6 g
- Fiber: 1.8 g
- Sodium: 110 mg
- Cholesterol: 0 mg

Vegetable Salad with Feta Dressing

SALAD

2 cups	chopped celery	500 mL
2 cups	chopped English cucumbers	500 mL
2 cups	chopped red bell peppers	500 mL
2 cups	chopped plum tomatoes	500 mL
1 cup	chopped red onions	250 mL
1/3 cup	sliced black olives	75 mL

DRESSING

2 oz	feta cheese, crumbled	50 g
1/3 cup	light sour cream	75 mL
2 tbsp	2% plain yogurt	25 mL
1 tbsp	freshly squeezed lemon juice	15 mL
1 1/2 tsp	minced garlic	7 mL
1 1/4 tsp	dried oregano	6 mL

Make Ahead

Prepare salad and dressing early in the day. Toss just before serving.

SERVES 4 TO 6

1. In a serving bowl, combine celery, cucumbers, red peppers, tomatoes, red onions and olives.
2. *Make the dressing:* In a food processor or blender, combine feta, sour cream, yogurt, lemon juice, garlic and oregano; process until smooth.
3. Pour dressing over salad; toss to coat.

Tip

- Try goat cheese instead of feta for a change.

Nutritional Analysis (Per Serving)
- Calories: 86
- Protein: 4 g
- Fat: 3 g
- Carbohydrates: 13 g
- Fiber: 3 g
- Sodium: 213 mg
- Cholesterol: 9 mg

Goat Cheese and Sun-Dried Tomato Salad

1/2 tsp	crushed garlic	2 mL
1 tsp	Dijon mustard	5 mL
1 tbsp	red wine vinegar	15 mL
2 tbsp	olive oil	25 mL
1 tbsp	lemon juice	15 mL
2 tbsp	water	25 mL
4 cups	torn lettuce (Boston, radicchio or romaine)	1 L
1 tbsp	pine nuts, toasted	15 mL
2 oz	goat cheese, crumbled	50 g
1/4 cup	sun-dried tomatoes, cut into pieces	50 mL

Make Ahead

Combine dressing ingredients up to a day before. Pour over salad just before serving.

SERVES 4

1. In small bowl, combine garlic, mustard, vinegar, oil, lemon juice and water until well mixed.
2. Place lettuce in serving bowl; sprinkle with nuts, goat cheese and tomatoes. Pour dressing over top and toss gently.

Tips

- Toast nuts in skillet on top of stove for 2 minutes until lightly browned.
- Soften sun-dried tomatoes by placing in boiling water for 10 minutes; then cut.
- If goat cheese is unavailable, substitute feta cheese.

Nutritional Analysis (Per Serving)
- Calories: 149
- Protein: 4 g
- Fat: 11 g
- Carbohydrates: 9 g
- Fiber: 2 g
- Sodium: 193 mg
- Cholesterol: 12 mg

Marinated Vegetable Salad

1/2 cup	broccoli florets	125 mL
1/2 cup	cauliflower florets	125 mL
1/2 cup	sliced carrots	125 mL
1/2 cup	chopped green bell pepper	125 mL
1/2 cup	diagonally sliced celery	125 mL
1/2 cup	coarsely chopped English cucumber	125 mL
1/4 cup	diced red or Spanish onion	50 mL
1	small tomato, cut into wedges	1

DRESSING

3 tbsp	vinegar	45 mL
1 tbsp	olive oil	15 mL
2 tsp	granulated sugar	10 mL
1 1/2 tsp	dried oregano or tarragon	7 mL
Pinch	black pepper	Pinch

Here is a great winter salad to help you get your servings of vegetables. Make this salad more colorful and vary the flavor by using a variety of colored peppers and other vegetables such as snow peas or fennel, if available.

SERVES 4

1. In a large saucepan of boiling water, blanch broccoli, cauliflower and carrots. Drain and plunge into ice water; drain again and place in medium bowl. Add green pepper, celery, cucumber and onion.

2. *Dressing:* In a small bowl or measuring cup, mix together vinegar, oil, sugar, oregano and pepper; pour over vegetables. Marinate at room temperature for 2 to 3 hours, stirring occasionally to ensure vegetables are well coated. Serve garnished with tomato wedges.

Tips

- Use specialty vinegars, such as tarragon, wine, champagne or balsamic, to spice up the flavor of this or any salad. Try using white wine vinegar flavored with tarragon instead of the vinegar and tarragon in this recipe.

- Blanching enhances the colors of vegetables while maintaining their raw texture. To blanch vegetables, drop them into boiling water. Return to a boil and cook for 2 minutes. Drain and plunge into ice water.

Nutritional Analysis (Per Serving)
- Calories: 69
- Protein: 1 g
- Fat: 4 g
- Carbohydrates: 9 g
- Fiber: 2 g
- Sodium: 27 mg
- Cholesterol: 0 mg

Grilled Vegetable Salad

1	medium zucchini	1
1	medium sweet red pepper	1
Half	large red onion	Half
12	small mushrooms	12
3 cups	mixed lettuce leaves (Boston, romaine, radicchio)	750 mL

DRESSING

2 tbsp	lemon juice	25 mL
2 tbsp	water	25 mL
1 tbsp	brown sugar	15 mL
4 tsp	balsamic vinegar	20 mL
1 tsp	crushed garlic	5 mL
2 tbsp	olive oil	25 mL
	Salt and pepper	

SERVES 4

1. Cut zucchini, red pepper and onion into 2-inch (5 cm) chunks. Alternately thread along with mushrooms onto barbecue skewers.

2. *Dressing:* In small bowl, combine lemon juice, water, sugar, vinegar and garlic; gradually whisk in oil. Season with salt and pepper to taste. Pour into dish large enough to hold skewers.

3. Add skewers to dressing; marinate for 20 minutes, turning often.

4. Grill vegetables until tender, basting with dressing and rotating often, approximately 15 minutes.

5. Remove vegetables from skewers and place on lettuce-lined serving platter. Pour any remaining dressing over vegetables.

Nutritional Analysis (Per Serving)
- Calories: 107
- Protein: 2 g
- Fat: 7 g
- Carbohydrates: 10 g
- Fiber: 2 g
- Sodium: 8 mg
- Cholesterol: 0 mg

Warm Salad with Shallots

8 cups	lettuce, washed, dried and torn to bite-size pieces	2 L
Half	red bell pepper, cut into thin strips	Half
2 oz	bocconcini or fresh mozzarella (optional) cut into 1/2-inch (1 cm) cubes	50 g
1/4 cup	olive oil	50 mL
1/2 tsp	salt	2 mL
1/4 tsp	freshly ground black pepper	1 mL
1/2 cup	thinly sliced shallots	125 mL
2	cloves garlic, thinly sliced	2
2 tbsp	balsamic vinegar	25 mL
12	cherry tomatoes	12

SERVES 4

1. In a salad bowl, toss together lettuce, red pepper and cheese (if using); set aside.

2. In a small frying pan, heat oil with salt and pepper over high heat for 1 minute. Add shallots; stir-fry for 3 minutes or until well softened and beginning to brown. Add garlic; stir-fry for 1 minute. Add vinegar; cook, stirring, until it bubbles. Add tomatoes; cook, stirring often, for 1 minute or until glistening and hot to the touch.

3. Immediately scrape all the contents of the pan onto the lettuce. Toss until well combined. (You will notice a slight wilting of the lettuce.)

Nutritional Analysis (Per Serving)
- Calories: 203
- Protein: 6.6 g
- Fat: 16.2 g
- Carbohydrates: 10.5 g
- Fiber: 3.6 g
- Sodium: 371 mg
- Cholesterol: 8 mg

Tomato Mozzarella Salad

VINAIGRETTE

¼ cup	vegetable or olive oil	50 mL
2 tbsp	vinegar	25 mL
1 tbsp	chopped fresh parsley	15 mL
2 tsp	Dijon mustard	10 mL
1 tsp	granulated sugar	5 mL
2	cloves garlic, minced	2
½ tsp	dried basil	2 mL
½ tsp	black pepper	2 mL
¼ tsp	salt	1 mL
2 tbsp	water	25 mL

SALAD

3	large tomatoes, preferably beefsteak	3
16	romaine or Boston lettuce leaves	16
½ cup	cubed part-skim mozzarella cheese	125 mL
6	green onions, sliced	6

SERVES 8

1. *Vinaigrette:* In a jar with tight-fitting lid, whisk together oil, vinegar, parsley, mustard, sugar, garlic, basil, pepper, salt and water; chill. Shake before using.

2. *Salad:* Cut tomatoes in half; cut each half crosswise into slices. Arrange 2 lettuce leaves on each of 8 salad plates. Arrange tomato slices on lettuce; sprinkle with cheese and green onion.

3. At serving time, pour vinaigrette over each salad.

Tip

- When tomatoes are in season, there's no better way to enjoy them than in this simple but delicious salad with an Italian flair. If desired, substitute fresh or Buffalo mozzarella for the part-skim version, but be aware that the fat content will go up.

Nutritional Analysis (Per Serving)
- Calories: 106
- Protein: 3 g
- Fat: 8 g
- Carbohydrates: 6 g
- Fiber: 1 g
- Sodium: 129 mg
- Cholesterol: 5 mg

Arugula-Bocconcini Salad

2	bunches arugula	2
3 tbsp	extra virgin olive oil	45 mL
2 tbsp	red wine vinegar	25 mL
¼ tsp	salt	1 mL
⅛ tsp	freshly ground black pepper	0.5 mL
8	bocconcini, halved (about 8 oz/250 g)	8

SERVES 4

1. Wash and dry the arugula. Trim 1 inch (2.5 cm) off the stalk and discard, keeping the rest whole. Put in a salad bowl.

2. In a small bottle, shake together oil, vinegar, salt and pepper until slightly emulsified. Drizzle on the arugula; toss well to dress. Add bocconcini halves and fold to distribute, leaving some of them on top. Serve immediately.

Nutritional Analysis (Per Serving)
- Calories: 270
- Protein: 14.3 g
- Fat: 22.7 g
- Carbohydrates: 2.8 g
- Fiber: 0.3 g
- Sodium: 414 mg
- Cholesterol: 32 mg

Insalata Caprese

1 lb	ripe tomatoes, sliced ½ inch (1 cm) thick (about 4 tomatoes)	500 g
¼ cup	thinly sliced red onion	50 mL
¼ cup	thinly sliced green bell peppers	50 mL
¼ cup	extra virgin olive oil	50 mL
2 tbsp	balsamic vinegar	25 mL
	Salt and freshly ground black pepper to taste	
6 oz	bocconcini	175 g
¼ cup	Calamata olives (about 8)	50 mL
12	large leaves fresh basil	12

SERVES 4

1. On a large presentation plate, arrange tomato slices in one layer. Scatter sliced onions and green peppers evenly over the tomatoes.
2. In a small bowl, whisk together oil, vinegar, salt and pepper until emulsified. Pour dressing evenly over the tomatoes.
3. Drain and pat dry the bocconcini. Slice into rounds ¼ inch (0.5 cm) thick. Put at least one slice of cheese on top of each tomato slice.
4. Place olives decoratively among the tomatoes. Garnish with the basil leaves, and serve within 30 minutes.

Nutritional Analysis (Per Serving)
- Calories: 280
- Protein: 12.2 g
- Fat: 21.6 g
- Carbohydrates: 11.1 g
- Fiber: 2.7 g
- Sodium: 284 mg
- Cholesterol: 24 mg

Pear, Lettuce and Feta Cheese Salad

DRESSING

2 tbsp	raspberry vinegar	25 mL
2½ tbsp	olive oil	35 mL
1 tsp	minced garlic	5 mL
1½ tsp	honey	7 mL
1 tsp	sesame oil	5 mL

SALAD

4 cups	red or green leaf lettuce, washed, dried and torn into pieces	1 L
1½ cups	curly endive or escarole, washed, dried and torn into pieces	375 mL
1½ cups	radicchio, washed, dried and torn into pieces	375 mL
1 cup	diced pears (about 1 pear)	250 mL
2 oz	feta cheese, crumbled	50 g
⅓ cup	sliced black olives	75 mL

Sweet fruit and a combination of lettuces make this a perfect salad.

SERVES 4 TO 6

1. *Prepare the dressing:* In a small bowl, whisk together vinegar, olive oil, garlic, honey and sesame oil; set aside.
2. *Make the salad:* In a serving bowl, combine leaf lettuce, curly endive, radicchio, pears, feta and olives. Pour dressing over; toss gently to coat. Serve immediately.

Tips

- Any ripe fruit can replace pears.
- If you don't care for the bitter flavor of curly endive and radicchio, use romaine or Bibb lettuce instead.
- If you don't want the salad to wilt, use a larger amount of romaine lettuce.

Nutritional Analysis (Per Serving)
- Calories: 108
- Protein: 2 g
- Fat: 8 g
- Carbohydrates: 8 g
- Fiber: 2 g
- Sodium: 165 mg
- Cholesterol: 8 mg

Greens with Strawberries

4 cups	assorted lettuce, torn into bite-size pieces	1 L
½ cup	sliced red onion	125 mL
½ cup	alfalfa sprouts	125 mL
DRESSING		
¼ cup	orange juice	50 mL
1 tbsp	lemon juice	15 mL
1 tbsp	chopped fresh mint	15 mL
1 tsp	granulated sugar	5 mL
½ tsp	grated orange zest	2 mL
¼ tsp	grated lemon zest	1 mL
1 cup	sliced fresh strawberries	250 mL

SERVES 6

1. In a salad bowl, combine lettuce, onion and sprouts; cover and refrigerate.
2. *Dressing:* Combine orange and lemon juices, mint, sugar and orange and lemon zest. Pour over sliced strawberries; cover and refrigerate.
3. Just before serving, pour strawberry mixture over salad greens; toss gently.

Nutritional Analysis (Per Serving)
- Calories: 23
- Protein: 1 g
- Fat: 0 g
- Carbohydrates: 5 g
- Fiber: 1 g
- Sodium: 4 mg
- Cholesterol: 0 mg

Lobster Salad

2½ to 3 lbs	lobsters	1.25 to 1.5 kg
½ cup	thinly sliced red onions	125 mL
2	green onions, chopped	2
2 tbsp	lemon juice	25 mL
	Salt and pepper to taste	
3 tbsp	extra virgin olive oil	45 mL
1 tbsp	drained capers	15 mL
1	medium tomato, cut into ½-inch (1 cm) wedges	1
	Several sprigs fresh parsley, chopped	
	Lemon wedges	

SERVES 2 AS A MAIN COURSE OR 4 AS A STARTER

1. Boil lobsters for 10 to 12 minutes in salted water. Rinse and refresh them in cold running water. When cool enough to handle, shell them. Cut the meat in 1-inch (2.5 cm) chunks and put in a working bowl.
2. Add onions, green onions, lemon juice, and salt and pepper to taste. Mix gently but thoroughly to coat. Add olive oil and capers; mix gently but thoroughly once more. Transfer to a serving dish and let marinate, covered and unrefrigerated, for about 15 minutes. (If making in advance, the recipe can be prepared to this point, then kept covered and refrigerated for several hours; let lobster warm to room temperature for 30 minutes and stir before continuing.)
3. Arrange tomato wedges decoratively on the salad. Serve garnished with parsley and lemon wedges.

Tip

- If using shelled lobster meat, use 8 to 12 oz (250 to 375 g).

Nutritional Analysis (Per Serving)
- Calories: 439
- Protein: 16.7 g
- Fat: 14.4 g
- Carbohydrates: 5.3 g
- Fiber: 1.1 g
- Sodium: 68 mg
- Cholesterol: 81 mg

Mussel, Basil and Roasted Pepper Salad

1/3 cup	white wine or water	75 mL
2 lb	mussels	1 kg
3/4 cup	chopped snow peas	175 mL
1/2 cup	chopped roasted red bell peppers	125 mL
3/4 cup	chopped green peppers	175 mL
1/2 cup	chopped carrots	125 mL
1/2 cup	chopped red onions	125 mL
1/2 cup	chopped fresh basil (or 1 1/2 tsp/7 mL dried)	125 mL
2 tbsp	olive oil	25 mL
1 1/2 tbsp	balsamic vinegar	20 mL
1 tsp	minced garlic	5 mL
2 tbsp	fresh lemon juice	25 mL
1/8 tsp	ground black pepper	0.5 mL

Make Ahead

Prepare early in the day. Stir before serving.

SERVES 6

1. Bring the wine to a boil in large heavy saucepan; add mussels and cover. Let cook for approximately 5 minutes, or until shells open. Discard any mussels that do not open. Remove mussels from shells and place in serving bowl.

2. In saucepan of boiling water or in microwave, steam snow peas for 2 minutes or until tender-crisp; drain and rinse with cold water and add to serving bowl along with roasted red peppers, green peppers, carrots, onions, basil, olive oil, vinegar, garlic, lemon juice and pepper. Toss well to mix. Refrigerate until chilled.

Tips

- Clams are an ideal substitute for mussels; or you can use a combination of both, but steam separately. Use water-packed roasted peppers in a jar, or grill your own.
- Other fresh vegetables can be substituted.
- Cilantro, parsley or dill can replace basil.
- To clean mussels, cut off any beards that are visible and discard any that are opened and will not close when you tap them.

Nutritional Analysis (Per Serving)
- Calories: 109
- Protein: 7 g
- Fat: 5 g
- Carbohydrates: 7 g
- Fiber: 1 g
- Sodium: 147 mg
- Cholesterol: 14 mg

Mussel and Sweet Pepper Salad

1/3 cup	white wine or water	75 mL
2 lb	mussels (see tip, page 107)	1 kg
3/4 cup	chopped asparagus	175 mL
1 cup	chopped red peppers	250 mL
3/4 cup	chopped green peppers	175 mL
1/2 cup	chopped red onions	125 mL
1/3 cup	chopped fresh dill (or 2 tsp/10 mL dried)	75 mL
2 tbsp	olive oil	25 mL
1 1/2 tbsp	balsamic vinegar	20 mL
1 tsp	minced garlic	5 mL
2 tbsp	lemon juice	25 mL
1/8 tsp	ground black pepper	0.5 mL

SERVES 6

1. Bring the wine to a boil in large heavy saucepan; add mussels and cover. Let cook for approximately 5 minutes, or until shells open. Discard any mussels that do not open. Remove mussels from shells and place in serving bowl.

2. In saucepan of boiling water or microwave, steam asparagus for 4 minutes or until tender-crisp; add to serving bowl along with red peppers, green peppers, onions, dill, olive oil, vinegar, garlic, lemon juice and pepper. Toss well to mix. Refrigerate until chilled.

Nutritional Analysis (Per Serving)
- Calories: 109
- Protein: 7 g
- Fat: 5 g
- Carbohydrates: 7 g
- Fiber: 1 g
- Sodium: 147 mg
- Cholesterol: 14 mg

Smoked Salmon and Avocado Salad

2 tbsp	lemon juice	25 mL
1	ripe avocado	1
1/4 cup	finely minced red onions	50 mL
1 tbsp	extra virgin olive oil	15 mL
1 tsp	drained capers	5 mL
Pinch	salt	Pinch
4 oz	sliced smoked salmon	125 g
	Freshly ground black pepper, to taste	
1	2-inch (5 cm) piece English cucumber, thinly sliced	1
1	medium tomato, cut into 1/2-inch (1 cm) cubes	1
	Several sprigs fresh coriander and/or parsley, chopped	

SERVES 3 TO 4

1. Put lemon juice into a bowl. Peel and slice (or scoop) avocado into bite-size pieces. Fold into the lemon juice to avoid discoloration. Add red onions, olive oil, capers and salt. Fold all ingredients together carefully until just mixed, taking care not to mash the avocado.

2. Cut the smoked salmon slices into strips 1/2 inch (1 cm) wide. Scatter the pieces onto the avocado. Sprinkle with black pepper. Fold the salmon into the salad carefully.

3. Arrange cucumber slices on the bottom of a serving plate. Heap the salmon-avocado salad onto the middle of the cucumbers, leaving a border of cucumber visible. Garnish with the cubes of tomato and chopped herbs. Serve within 20 minutes.

This salad of pastel colors and summery tastes will please even the most demanding dinner guests. The only caveats are that you use a ripe, unblemished avocado and a really good (which, sad to say, means expensive) smoked salmon.

Nutritional Analysis (Per Serving)
- Calories: 157
- Protein: 6.7 g
- Fat: 12.4 g
- Carbohydrates: 6.8 g
- Fiber: 3.0 g
- Sodium: 324 mg
- Cholesterol: 7 mg

Marinated Salmon with Red Onion and Crème Fraîche

¼ cup	extra virgin olive oil	50 mL
¼ cup	lemon juice	50 mL
12 oz to 1 lb	fillet of fresh salmon, deboned with skin left on	375 to 500 g
	Salt and pepper to taste	
1 cup	thinly sliced red onions	250 mL
1 tbsp	drained capers	15 mL
	Few sprigs fresh parsley, chopped	
1 cup	crème fraîche	250 mL

SERVES 3 OR 4
10-inch (25 cm) ceramic or glass pie plate

1. Put 1 tbsp (15 mL) each oil and lemon juice on the bottom of pie plate and spread to cover the bottom and sides. Take salmon (preferably cold, straight from the refrigerator) and, running your fingers on the surface, make sure all bones are out. Wipe surface of the salmon. Using a very sharp knife, cut the salmon towards the thin end in slices ¼ inch (5 mm) thick — even slightly thinner if you can. The knife will stop on the skin; remove slice from the skin by sliding knife forward. Lay slice on oil-lemon mixture in the pie plate. Continue slicing until you've covered the whole surface of the plate.

2. Sprinkle salmon slices with salt and pepper. Scatter some of the red onions, capers and parsley on top. Drizzle evenly with another 1 tbsp (15 mL) each of lemon and oil.

3. Repeat procedure to make another 2 layers, using all ingredients. (If salmon slices are not thin enough you may only get 1 more layer.) Cover pie plate tightly with plastic wrap and refrigerate for at least 2 hours or up to 24 hours. (For best results, refrigerate 4 to 5 hours.)

4. Take salmon out of the fridge and let it warm to room temperature, about 30 minutes. Carefully pick up salmon slices and distribute among 4 plates. Spoon onions, capers and parsley onto the salmon; moisten each plate with 1 tsp (5 mL) of the marinating juice (discard any leftover juice). Serve with a dollop of crème fraîche in the middle of each portion, and the rest of the crème on the side.

Tip
- Crème fraîche can be faked at home by using 1 cup (250 mL) sour cream, mixing in 1 tbsp (15 mL) lemon juice and enriching it by mixing in 2 tbsp (25 mL) whipping (35%) cream.

Nutritional Analysis (Per Serving)
- Calories: 509
- Protein: 24.2 g
- Fat: 16.9 g
- Carbohydrates: 6.7 g
- Fiber: 0.7 g
- Sodium: 137 mg
- Cholesterol: 148 mg

Fresh Salmon and Leafy Lettuce Salad with Creamy Dill Dressing

8 oz	salmon fillet	250 g
1 tsp	vegetable oil	5 mL
1 tsp	crushed garlic	5 mL
3 cups	mixed torn lettuce (leaf, Boston, radicchio)	750 mL

DRESSING

2 tbsp	buttermilk	25 mL
½ tsp	crushed garlic	2 mL
4 tsp	light mayonnaise	20 mL
2½ tsp	lemon juice	12 mL
1½ tsp	water	7 mL
4 tsp	finely chopped fresh dill	20 mL
2 tsp	finely chopped fresh parsley	10 mL
4 tsp	vegetable oil	20 mL

Make Ahead

Prepare and refrigerate dressing up to a day before. Prepare and refrigerate salmon early in day if serving cold.

SERVES 4

Preheat oven to 400°F (200°C) • Baking sheet sprayed with nonstick vegetable spray

1. Brush salmon with oil and garlic. Place on baking sheet and bake for 10 minutes per inch (2.5 cm) of thickness or until fish flakes easily when tested with fork. Cut into 2-inch (5 cm) pieces.

2. Arrange lettuce on 4 salad plates. Evenly top with salmon.

3. *Dressing:* In small bowl, combine buttermilk, garlic, mayonnaise, lemon juice, water, dill and parsley; gradually whisk in oil until well blended. Drizzle evenly over salmon.

Nutritional Analysis (Per Serving)
- Calories: 145
- Protein: 13 g
- Fat: 9 g
- Carbohydrates: 2 g
- Fiber: 0.5 g
- Sodium: 59 mg
- Cholesterol: 23 mg

Caesar Salad with Baby Shrimp

2 oz	cooked baby shrimp	50 g
1	medium head romaine lettuce, torn into bite-sized pieces	1
1 tbsp	grated Parmesan cheese	15 mL
1 cup	croutons, preferably homemade	250 mL

DRESSING

1	egg	1
1 tsp	crushed garlic	5 mL
1	anchovy, minced	1
4 tsp	lemon juice	20 mL
1 tbsp	red wine vinegar	15 mL
1 tsp	Dijon mustard	5 mL
1 tbsp	grated Parmesan cheese	15 mL
2 tbsp	olive oil	25 mL

SERVES 4 TO 6

1. In large bowl, place shrimp, lettuce, cheese and croutons.

2. *Dressing:* In small bowl, combine egg, garlic, anchovy, lemon juice, vinegar, mustard and cheese; gradually whisk in oil until combined. Pour over salad and toss to coat.

Tip

• To make your own croutons, mix 1 tsp (5 mL) each crushed garlic and melted margarine; brush on both sides of 1 slice whole wheat bread. Broil for 3 minutes until browned, then cut into cubes.

Nutritional Analysis (Per Serving)
- Calories: 99
- Protein: 5 g
- Fat: 7 g
- Carbohydrates: 5 g
- Fiber: 1 g
- Sodium: 117 mg
- Cholesterol: 56 mg

Italian Squid Salad

1 lb	cleaned squid	500 g
3 cups	water	750 mL
Half	lemon, cut in quarters	Half
1	bay leaf	1
1/2 tsp	dried basil	2 mL
2 tbsp	lemon juice	25 mL
1 tbsp	balsamic vinegar	15 mL
	Salt and pepper to taste	
1/4 cup	extra virgin olive oil	50 mL
1/2 cup	thinly sliced red onions	125 mL
Half	green pepper, thinly sliced	Half
1 tbsp	drained capers	15 mL
1	medium tomato, cut into 1/2-inch (1 cm) cubes	1
4	large lettuce leaves	4
	Few sprigs chopped fresh basil and/or parsley	

SERVES 4

1. Slice squid bodies into 1/2-inch (1 cm) rings. Cut tentacles at their base to halve them. Rinse and set aside. In a saucepan bring water to a boil; stir in lemon, bay leaf and basil; boil 2 minutes. Reduce heat to medium and add squid; cook 5 minutes for al dente texture or 8 to 9 minutes if you like squid more tender. Drain, discarding liquid, lemon pieces and bay leaf. Transfer squid to a bowl.

2. Immediately add lemon juice, vinegar, salt and pepper; toss well to coat. Add olive oil, and toss again. Add onions, green pepper and capers; toss to combine. (If time permits, this salad improves if allowed to rest as is, covered and unrefrigerated for 30 minutes to 1 hour.)

3. Add tomato cubes and any tomato juices that have accumulated and toss to combine. Line 4 plates with lettuce leaves and distribute the salad evenly among them, including the dressing. Top with a liberal garnish of herbs and serve.

Variation

- Try a half-and-half combination of squid and shell-on medium shrimp instead of squid alone; cook both seafoods at the same time as described in Step 1, then peel the cooked shrimp; proceed with the recipe, keeping shrimp and squid together.

Nutritional Analysis (Per Serving)
- Calories: 257
- Protein: 19.4 g
- Fat: 15.3 g
- Carbohydrates: 10.6 g
- Fiber: 2.3 g
- Sodium: 119 mg
- Cholesterol: 264 mg

Grilled Tuna with Julienne Vegetables

DRESSING

¼ cup	olive oil	50 mL
2 tbsp	Dijon mustard	25 mL
2 tbsp	lemon juice	25 mL
Pinch	black pepper	Pinch

SALAD

8 oz	yellowfin or other fresh tuna steak	250 g
2	medium carrots, cut into julienne strips	2
1	leek (white part only), cut into julienne strips	1
1	small red onion, cut into julienne strips	1
12	spears asparagus	12

Here's a sophisticated and elegant salad that is easy to make.

SERVES 4

1. *Dressing:* Whisk together oil, mustard, lemon juice and pepper; chill.

2. *Salad:* Grill or broil tuna on greased grill for 3 to 5 minutes per side or until fish flakes easily when tested with fork.

3. Steam or microwave carrots, leek, onion and asparagus just until tender.

4. To serve, divide vegetables among 4 plates. Cut tuna into 4 pieces; place on top of vegetables. Pour 1 tbsp (15 mL) dressing over each salad. Serve warm.

Tips

• If you can't find fresh tuna, try using swordfish or frozen yellowfin tuna, which is available in some supermarkets.

• Many recipes call for extra-virgin olive oil, which comes from the first pressing of the olives. This is the most expensive and flavorful of olive oils. Use extra-virgin olive oil in this recipe, if desired.

• This recipe can be served as a side salad followed by a lighter main meal, or as a meal on its own.

Nutritional Analysis (Per Serving)
• Calories: 193   • Protein: 16 g   • Fat: 10 g
• Carbohydrates: 11 g   • Fiber: 2 g   • Sodium: 122 mg
• Cholesterol: 26 mg

Seafood Salad with Dill Dressing

4 oz	deveined peeled (uncooked) shrimp, chopped	125 g
4 oz	scallops, chopped	125 g
4 oz	squid, chopped	125 g
1/2 cup	chopped sweet red or yellow pepper	125 mL
1/2 cup	chopped sweet green pepper	125 mL
1/2 cup	chopped celery	125 mL
1/2 cup	chopped red onion	125 mL
1	large green onion, sliced	1
	Lettuce leaves	
	Parsley sprigs	

DRESSING

1/2 cup	2% yogurt	125 mL
2 tbsp	light mayonnaise	25 mL
3 tbsp	chopped fresh parsley	45 mL
1/4 cup	chopped fresh dill (or 4 tsp/20 mL dried dillweed)	50 mL
1 tsp	Dijon mustard	5 mL
1 tsp	crushed garlic	5 mL
	Salt and pepper	

Make Ahead

Prepare and refrigerate salad and dressing early in day, but do not combine until 2 hours before eating. Stir just before serving.

SERVES 4

1. In shallow saucepan, bring 2 cups (500 mL) water to boil; reduce heat to simmer. Add shrimp, scallops and squid; cover and poach until shrimp are pink and squid and scallops opaque, approximately 2 minutes. Drain and rinse with cold water; drain well and place in bowl. Add red and green peppers, celery and red and green onions.

2. *Dressing:* In small bowl, combine yogurt, mayonnaise, parsley, dill, mustard, garlic, and salt and pepper to taste, mixing well. Pour over salad and toss well.

3. Line serving bowl with lettuce; top with salad and garnish with parsley.

Tips

- Any combination of seafood is good, but these three work very well.

- Try fresh cilantro or Italian parsley instead of the dill.

Nutritional Analysis (Per Serving)
- Calories: 149
- Protein: 18 g
- Fat: 4 g
- Carbohydrates: 10 g
- Fiber: 2 g
- Sodium: 236 mg
- Cholesterol: 120 mg

Chicken Salad Amandine

¼ cup	mayonnaise	50 mL
2 tbsp	olive oil	25 mL
2 tbsp	lemon juice	25 mL
½ tsp	salt	2 mL
	Freshly ground black pepper	
4 cups	cubed (½ inch/1 cm) cooked chicken	1 L
½ cup	finely chopped celery	125 mL
2 tbsp	finely chopped red or green onion	25 mL
1	bag (10 oz/300 g) washed salad greens, such as hearts of romaine, or 4 cups (1 L) torn lettuce, washed and dried	1
2 tbsp	toasted slivered or sliced almonds (see tip, page 132)	25 mL

SERVES 4

1. In a bowl, combine mayonnaise, olive oil, lemon juice, salt, and black pepper to taste.
2. In a separate bowl, combine chicken, celery and onion. Add mayonnaise mixture. Toss to combine.
3. Spread salad greens over a deep platter. Spoon chicken mixture on top. Garnish with almonds and serve immediately.

Variation

Chicken Salad Sandwich: Omit the salad greens and almonds and use the chicken mixture as a filling for sandwiches. Add sliced tomato, lettuce and/or cucumber slices as desired.

Nutritional Analysis (Per Serving)
- Calories: 368
- Protein: 38.6 g
- Fat: 23.6 g
- Carbohydrates: 3.8 g
- Fiber: 1.7 g
- Sodium: 438 mg
- Cholesterol: 125 mg

Grilled Chicken and Cheese Salad

⅓ cup	olive oil	75 mL
2 tbsp	white wine vinegar	25 mL
¾ tsp	chopped fresh marjoram or (¼ tsp/1 mL) dried	4 mL
¾ tsp	chopped fresh sage or (¼ tsp/1 mL) dried	4 mL
½ tsp	salt	2 mL
¼ tsp	pepper	1 mL
1 tbsp	Dijon mustard	15 mL
3	skinless boneless chicken breasts	3
6 cups	mixed torn greens	1.5 L
1 cup	shredded Swiss cheese	250 mL

Barbecued chicken on simply dressed greens makes a quick, warm main-course salad.

SERVES 4

1. In a small bowl, whisk together oil, vinegar, marjoram, sage, salt and pepper. In a large bowl, combine 2 tbsp (25 mL) of the oil mixture with the mustard. Add chicken, turning to coat thoroughly.
2. On a greased grill, cook chicken over medium-high heat for 12 to 15 minutes, turning once and brushing with any remaining mustard mixture, or until cooked through.
3. Meanwhile, toss the greens and cheese with remaining oil mixture and arrange on 4 dinner plates. Cut the cooked chicken into ½-inch (1 cm) thick strips and arrange on the salad.

Nutritional Analysis (Per Serving)
- Calories: 417
- Protein 38.7 g
- Fat: 27.3 g
- Carbohydrates: 3.8 g
- Fiber: 1.7 g
- Sodium: 490 mg
- Cholesterol: 97 mg

Mustard-Grilled Chicken Salad

DRESSING

1/3 cup	olive oil	75 mL
2 tbsp	white wine vinegar	25 mL
2 tsp	Dijon mustard	10 mL
1	clove garlic, minced	1
	Salt and pepper	
2 tbsp	olive oil	25 mL
2 tbsp	Dijon mustard	25 mL
1 tbsp	white wine vinegar	15 mL
1	clove garlic, minced	1
1 tsp	dried marjoram	5 mL
1 tsp	paprika	5 mL
1/4 tsp	cayenne	1 mL
4	skinless boneless chicken breasts (1 1/2 lbs/750 g total)	4
8 cups	washed and torn mixed salad greens	2 L
2	tomatoes, diced	2

Make Ahead

The greens can be washed and dried and the dressing can be made and refrigerated up to one day ahead. The chicken can be marinated, covered, in the refrigerator up to 4 hours ahead. Warm to room temperature for 30 minutes before grilling.

> *The grilled chicken stays moist and flavorful beneath its mustardy coating for this warm "whole meal" salad.*

SERVES 4

1. *Dressing:* In a bowl, whisk together the oil, vinegar, mustard, garlic and salt and pepper to taste. Set aside.

2. In a non-metallic dish just large enough to hold the chicken in a single layer, combine oil, mustard, vinegar, garlic, marjoram, paprika and cayenne. Add chicken, turning to coat on both sides. Marinate, covered, for 30 minutes at room temperature.

3. Remove chicken from marinade; place on a greased barbecue grill and cook over medium-high heat for 10 to 12 minutes, turning every 4 minutes or until the juices run clear when the chicken is pierced with a skewer and is no longer pink inside. Transfer to a cutting board; cover with foil. Discard any remaining marinade.

4. In a large bowl, toss the greens with just enough dressing to coat the leaves lightly. Divide among 4 plates.

5. Cut chicken crosswise into slices; arrange on top of the greens. Garnish with tomatoes; sprinkle with remaining dressing.

Nutritional Analysis (Per Serving)
- Calories: 451
- Protein: 42.5 g
- Fat: 27.6 g
- Carbohydrates: 8.7 g
- Fiber: 3.7 g
- Sodium: 233 mg
- Cholesterol: 96 mg

Skillet Chicken Salad

4	skinless boneless chicken breasts	4
1	red bell pepper	1
Half	bunch broccoli	Half
¼ cup	vegetable oil	50 mL
¼ cup	chicken stock	50 mL
3 tbsp	white wine vinegar	45 mL
1 tbsp	Dijon mustard	15 mL
1 tsp	dried tarragon	5 mL
¼ tsp	salt	1 mL
¼ tsp	pepper	1 mL
1 cup	tiny whole mushrooms	250 mL
2	green onions, chopped	2
	Boston lettuce leaves	

This hot colorful salad is just the answer for a light supper.

SERVES 4

1. Cut the chicken crosswise into strips ½ inch (1 cm) wide. Seed and core the red pepper; cut into strips. Cut broccoli into small florets; peel and cut stems into ¼-inch (5 mm) thick slices.

2. In a large skillet, heat half the oil over medium-high heat. In 2 batches, add chicken; cook, stirring, for 6 minutes or until golden and no longer pink inside. Using a slotted spoon, transfer to a warmed bowl; cover and keep warm.

3. In the same skillet, heat remaining oil. Add red pepper and broccoli; cook for 2 minutes, stirring occasionally. Stir in stock and reduce heat to low; cover and steam for 2 minutes. Using a slotted spoon, add red pepper and broccoli to chicken.

4. In the same skillet, bring vinegar to a boil, scraping up any brown bits from the bottom of the pan. Stir in mustard, tarragon, salt and pepper. Stir in mushrooms and onions. Return chicken mixture and any juices. Cook for a few seconds or until heated through.

5. Line 4 dinner plates with lettuce, top with the salad and serve.

Nutritional Analysis (Per Serving)
- Calories: 349
- Protein: 42.8 g
- Fat: 16.1 g
- Carbohydrates: 8.6 g
- Fiber: 3.4 g
- Sodium: 352 mg
- Cholesterol: 96 mg

Chicken Salad with Tarragon and Pecans

10 oz	boneless skinless chicken breast, cubed	300 g
¾ cup	chopped sweet red or green pepper	175 mL
¾ cup	chopped carrot	175 mL
¾ cup	chopped broccoli florets	175 mL
¾ cup	chopped snow peas	175 mL
¾ cup	chopped red onion	175 mL
1 tbsp	chopped pecans, toasted	15 mL

DRESSING

½ cup	2% yogurt *	125 mL
2 tbsp	lemon juice	25 mL
2 tbsp	light mayonnaise	25 mL
1 tsp	crushed garlic	5 mL
1 tsp	Dijon mustard	5 mL
¼ cup	chopped fresh parsley	50 mL
2 tsp	dried tarragon (or 3 tbsp/45 mL chopped fresh)	10 mL
	Salt and pepper	

Make Ahead

Prepare and refrigerate salad and dressing separately early in day, but do not mix until ready to serve.

SERVES 4

1. In small saucepan, bring 2 cups (500 mL) water to boil; reduce heat to simmer. Add chicken; cover and cook just until no longer pink inside, 2 to 4 minutes. Drain and place in serving bowl.

2. Add red pepper, carrot, broccoli, snow peas and onion; toss well.

3. *Dressing:* In small bowl, combine yogurt, lemon juice, mayonnaise, garlic, mustard, parsley, tarragon, and salt and pepper to taste; pour over chicken and mix well. Taste and adjust seasoning. Sprinkle with pecans.

Tips

- If tarragon is unavailable, substitute ¼ cup (50 mL) chopped fresh dill.

- Fresh tuna or swordfish are delicious substitutes for chicken.

- Toast pecans in small skillet on medium heat until browned, 2 to 3 minutes.

Nutritional Analysis (Per Serving)
- Calories: 187
- Protein: 20 g
- Fat: 6 g
- Carbohydrates: 13 g
- Fiber: 3 g
- Sodium: 151 mg
- Cholesterol: 42 mg

Smoked Turkey Toss

¼ cup	extra-virgin olive oil	50 mL
2 tbsp	balsamic vinegar	25 mL
1 tbsp	chopped fresh parsley	15 mL
1 tsp	each liquid honey and dried basil	5 mL
Pinch	each salt and black pepper	Pinch
8 cups	thinly sliced romaine lettuce	2 L
4 oz	thinly sliced smoked or cooked turkey breast, cut into strips	125 g
4 oz	part-skim mozzarella cheese, cut into cubes	125 g

For best results, make this tasty salad in the summer when fresh basil is abundant, using 1 tbsp (15 mL) chopped fresh basil instead of the dried.

SERVES 6 AS A SIDE SALAD

1. In a small bowl or measuring cup, mix together oil, vinegar, parsley, honey, basil, salt and pepper. Chill.
2. In a large bowl, toss remaining ingredients. Cover and chill. Add dressing and toss.

Tips

- For variety, replace the romaine lettuce with shredded spinach or red leaf lettuce, or use a combination of lettuces.
- This tasty salad is a good source of protein. To ensure that cheese is lower-fat, look for 20% or less milk fat (M.F.).

Nutritional Analysis (Per Serving)
- Calories: 178
- Protein: 10 g
- Fat: 14 g
- Carbohydrates: 4 g
- Fiber: 1 g
- Sodium: 152 mg
- Cholesterol: 23 mg

Turkey Pesto Salad

2 cups	diced, cooked turkey	500 mL
4 cups	well-packed washed, dried and torn romaine lettuce	1 L
¾ cup	chopped red peppers	175 mL
¾ cup	chopped green peppers	175 mL
½ cup	sliced red onions	125 mL
1	medium green onion, chopped	1
2 oz	feta cheese, crumbled	50 g
PESTO DRESSING		
1 cup	well-packed basil leaves	250 mL
2 tbsp	grated Parmesan cheese	25 mL
2 tbsp	olive oil	25 mL
1 tbsp	toasted pine nuts	15 mL
1 tsp	minced garlic	5 mL
2 tbsp	light sour cream	25 mL
1 tbsp	lemon juice	15 mL

SERVES 4 OR 5

1. In large serving bowl combine turkey, lettuce, red peppers, green peppers, red onions, green onion and feta cheese.
2. Put basil, Parmesan, olive oil, pine nuts and garlic in food processor; process until finely chopped, scraping sides of bowl once. Add sour cream and lemon juice and process until smooth. Pour over salad and toss well to combine. Garnish with a few toasted pine nuts (toast in skillet until browned, approximately 2 minutes).

Tips

- Parsley or spinach leaves can replace basil.

Nutritional Analysis (Per Serving)
- Calories: 215
- Protein: 22 g
- Fat: 11 g
- Carbohydrates: 7 g
- Fiber: 2 g
- Sodium: 219 mg
- Cholesterol: 55 mg

Fish and Seafood

Continued on next page...

Basil and Tomato Fillets

2 tbsp	olive oil, divided	25 mL
1 lb	whitefish, tuna or salmon	500 g
	Salt and freshly ground black pepper	
½ cup	chopped firm tomatoes	125 mL
2 tbsp	chopped fresh basil leaves	25 mL

Tomato and basil are natural partners. Add fish for a fresh delicious meal.

SERVES 4

1. In a nonstick skillet over medium-high heat, heat 1 tbsp (15 mL) oil. Season fish lightly with salt and pepper. Add to skillet.
2. Combine tomatoes, basil and remaining oil. Top fish with spoonfuls of the mixture. Cover skillet tightly and cook on medium-high heat for 10 minutes or until fish is opaque and flakes easily when tested with a fork.

Nutritional Analysis (Per Serving)
- Calories: 225
- Protein: 22.7 g
- Fat: 14.0 g
- Carbohydrates: 1.0 g
- Fiber: 0.3 g
- Sodium: 49 mg
- Cholesterol: 64 mg

Fish with Tomato, Basil and Cheese Topping

1 cup	chopped tomatoes	250 mL
½ cup	grated mozzarella cheese	125 mL
¼ cup	sliced black olives	50 mL
¼ cup	chopped green onions (about 2 medium)	50 mL
2 oz	goat cheese	50 g
1 tsp	minced garlic	5 mL
1½ tsp	dried basil	7 mL
1 lb	fish fillets	500 g

Make Ahead

Tomato mixture can be prepared earlier in the day and refrigerated.

Fatty fish, including salmon, sardines, tuna, mackerel and rainbow trout, are high in omega-3 fatty acids, which are thought to play a role in preventing heart disease. Include fish in your diet 2 to 3 times a week.

SERVES 4

Preheat oven to 425°F (220°C) • Baking dish sprayed with vegetable spray

1. In bowl, combine tomatoes, mozzarella, black olives, green onions, goat cheese, garlic and basil; mix well.
2. Place fish in prepared pan; top with tomato mixture. Bake uncovered approximately 15 minutes for each 1-inch (2.5 cm) thickness of fish fillet, or until fish flakes easily with a fork.

Tips
- This dish suits any type of fish.
- If goat cheese is too intense for you, try ricotta or feta.
- Baking time is increased due to the added sauce, according to fish guidelines.

Nutritional Analysis (Per Serving)
- Calories: 195
- Protein: 27 g
- Fat: 7 g
- Carbohydrates: 5 g
- Fiber: 1 g
- Sodium: 287 mg
- Cholesterol: 63 mg

Fish with Sun-Dried Tomato Pesto, Feta and Black Olives

1½ lbs	fish fillets	750 g
1 oz	feta cheese, crumbled	25 g
2 tbsp	chopped black olives	25 mL
SAUCE		
¼ cup	well-packed, chopped sun-dried tomatoes	50 mL
2 tbsp	chopped fresh basil or parsley	25 mL
1½ tbsp	olive oil	20 mL
1½ tbsp	grated Parmesan cheese	20 mL
1 tbsp	toasted pine nuts	15 mL
1 tsp	minced garlic	5 mL
⅓ cup	chicken stock	75 mL

Make Ahead

Prepare sauce up to 48 hours in advance and keep refrigerated. This sauce can also be frozen for up to 6 weeks.

SERVES 6

Preheat oven to 425°F (220°C) • Baking dish sprayed with vegetable spray

1. *Sauce:* Put sun-dried tomatoes, basil, olive oil, Parmesan, pine nuts and garlic in food processor; process until finely chopped. With machine running, gradually add stock through feed tube; process until smooth.

2. Put fish in single layer in prepared baking dish; spread sun-dried pesto on top. Sprinkle with feta and olives. Bake uncovered for 15 minutes per inch (2.5 cm) thickness of fish or until fish flakes easily when pierced with a fork.

Nutritional Analysis (Per Serving)
- Calories: 172
- Protein: 24 g
- Fat: 7 g
- Carbohydrates: 2 g
- Fiber: 0 g
- Sodium: 295 mg
- Cholesterol: 60 mg

Fish Fillets on Spinach Leaves

8	large fresh spinach leaves	8
3	fish fillets, such as snapper, tilapia or salmon (about 6 oz/175 g each)	3
2	green onions, chopped	2
2 tbsp	chopped oil-packed sun-dried tomatoes	25 mL
1 tbsp	chopped fresh dillweed	15 mL
2 tbsp	dry white wine or water	25 mL
1 tbsp	olive oil	15 mL
1 tbsp	lemon juice	15 mL
¼ tsp	salt	1 mL
¼ tsp	black pepper	1 mL

Make Ahead

Dish can be assembled, covered and refrigerated up to 4 hours before baking.

SERVES 3

1. Remove coarse stems from spinach and shred leaves. Place shredded spinach in bottom of an 8-inch (2 L) square baking dish. Arrange fish fillets over spinach, slightly overlapping if necessary.

2. Sprinkle fish with green onions, sun-dried tomatoes, dill, wine, olive oil, lemon juice, salt and pepper.

3. Cover dish tightly with foil. Bake in preheated 375°F (190°C) toaster oven for 20 to 25 minutes, or until fish flakes when tested with a fork.

Tip

- Swiss chard makes a good substitute for spinach.

Nutritional Analysis (Per Serving)
- Calories: 232
- Protein: 35.6 g
- Fat: 7.5 g
- Carbohydrates: 2.7 g
- Fiber: 0.9 g
- Sodium: 324 mg
- Cholesterol: 60 mg

Fish Fillets with Basil Walnut Sauce

½ cup	fresh parsley, snipped and loosely packed	125 mL
½ cup	fresh basil, snipped and loosely packed	125 mL
3 tbsp	finely chopped walnuts	45 mL
2 tbsp	chicken broth	25 mL
2 tbsp	grated Parmesan cheese	25 mL
1 tbsp	olive oil	15 mL
1 tbsp	balsamic vinegar or malt vinegar	15 mL
1 tsp	granulated sugar	5 mL
1	clove garlic, minced	1
½ tsp	freshly ground black pepper	2 mL
1½ lb	fish fillets (cod, haddock or halibut), 1 inch (2.5 cm) thick	750 g
¼ cup	dry white wine	50 mL
½	lemon	½
1 tbsp	butter or margarine	15 mL
	Salt and black pepper to taste	

SERVES 6
Preheat broiler • Broiler or roasting pan

1. In a food processor or blender, combine parsley, basil, walnuts, chicken broth, cheese, oil, vinegar, sugar, garlic and pepper. Process until smooth; add more broth if thinner sauce is desired.

2. Arrange fish in broiler or roasting pan. Pour wine into pan; squeeze lemon juice over fish. Dot with butter; sprinkle with salt and pepper. Broil for 5 minutes. Spoon sauce over top and broil for another 4 to 5 minutes, allowing total of 10 minutes per inch (2.5 cm) of thickness, or until fish flakes easily with fork.

Tip
• This sauce, like pesto, is quite thick, but it can be thinned with chicken broth if desired.

Nutritional Analysis (Per Serving)
- Calories: 200
- Protein: 25 g
- Fat: 9 g
- Carbohydrates: 3 g
- Fiber: Trace
- Sodium: 126 mg
- Cholesterol: 55 mg

Yogurt-Lime Fish Fillets

1¼ lbs	fish fillets	625 g
1	lime	1
¼ cup	plain yogurt	50 mL
1 tsp	ground cumin	5 mL
	Salt and freshly ground black pepper	

Take any fish fillet, such as salmon, whitefish, sole or turbot, add this easy sauce, and you will quickly have an elegant dinner for guests.

SERVES 4
Preheat oven to 450°F (230°C) • Shallow oblong pan, greased

1. Place fish in prepared baking pan.

2. Grate ½ tsp (2 mL) zest from lime and squeeze out 2 tbsp (25 mL) juice, reserving extra for another use. Place zest and juice in a small bowl. Stir in yogurt, cumin and salt and pepper. Spoon over fish.

3. Bake for 10 minutes per inch (2.5 cm) of thickness or until fish is opaque and flakes easily when tested with a fork.

Nutritional Analysis (Per Serving)
- Calories: 213
- Protein: 29.1 g
- Fat: 9.1 g
- Carbohydrates: 2.1 g
- Fiber: 0.1 g
- Sodium: 73 mg
- Cholesterol: 80 mg

Parmesan Herb Baked Fish Fillets

1	package (1 lb/500 g) frozen fish fillets, thawed and patted dry	1
1/4 cup	light mayonnaise	50 mL
1/4 cup	grated Parmesan cheese	50 mL
2 tbsp	chopped green onions	25 mL
1 tbsp	chopped pimiento or red bell pepper	15 mL
	Cayenne pepper to taste	
1/2 cup	dry bread crumbs	125 mL
1/2 tsp	dried basil	2 mL
	Black pepper to taste	

This elegant entrée is a great dish for entertaining.

SERVES 4
Preheat oven to 400°F (200°C) • 11- by 7-inch (2 L) baking dish, greased

1. Place fish fillets in a single layer in bottom of greased 11- by 7-inch (2 L) baking dish. Set aside.
2. In a small bowl, stir together mayonnaise, Parmesan cheese, onions, pimiento and cayenne. Spread mixture evenly over fish fillets.
3. In a separate bowl, combine bread crumbs, basil, and pepper; sprinkle over top of fish. Bake in preheated oven for 10 to 12 minutes or until fish is opaque and flakes easily with fork.

Nutritional Analysis (Per Serving)
- Calories: 216
- Protein: 23 g
- Fat: 8 g
- Carbohydrates: 12 g
- Fiber: Trace
- Sodium: 397 mg
- Cholesterol: 49 mg

Fish in Mad Water

1/4 cup	olive oil	50 mL
1	large clove garlic, thinly sliced	1
2	ripe tomatoes, peeled and thickly sliced	2
	Salt and freshly ground black pepper	
4	fish fillets (each 6 to 8 oz/175 to 250 g), such as sea bass, grouper or salmon	4
8	whole basil leaves	8

"Mad water" refers to the quick and furious boil to which the fish is treated.

SERVES 4 TO 6

1. In a large skillet, heat olive oil over medium-low heat. Add garlic and cook for 3 minutes or until just beginning to brown. Sprinkle tomato slices with salt and add to skillet; cook, shaking the pan occasionally, for 4 minutes or until tomatoes are warmed through and their juices start to run.
2. Add fish fillets along with 1 cup (250 mL) water; bring to a boil. Reduce heat to medium-high, cover and cook, turning once, for 4 minutes or until fish is cooked through. Lift fish onto serving plates. Season sauce with salt and pepper; pour over fish. Garnish with basil and serve immediately.

Nutritional Analysis (Per Serving)
- Calories: 351
- Protein: 34.4 g
- Fat: 21.8 g
- Carbohydrates: 3.3 g
- Fiber: 0.9 g
- Sodium: 192 mg
- Cholesterol: 96 mg

Fish in White Wine

1/2 cup	olive oil	125 mL
1/4 cup	chopped flat-leaf parsley	50 mL
2	cloves garlic, finely chopped	2
1 lb	plum tomatoes, peeled and chopped, or 4 cups (1 L) canned plum tomatoes, drained and chopped	500 g
1 tbsp	coarsely grated lemon zest	15 mL
1	whole red mullet or red snapper (about 2 lbs/1 kg) scaled, gutted and rinsed	1
	Salt and freshly ground black pepper	
1 cup	dry white wine	250 mL
	Lemon wedges	

SERVES 4 TO 6

1. In a large skillet, heat olive oil over low heat. Add parsley and garlic; cook for 2 minutes. Stir in tomatoes and lemon zest, increase heat to medium and cook, stirring occasionally, for 10 minutes or until slightly thickened.

2. Lay the fish in the sauce; sprinkle with salt and pepper. Reduce heat to medium-low. Cook 10 minutes; turn fish and cook 6 to 10 minutes longer or until cooked through.

3. Transfer fish to a warm serving platter. Add wine to the sauce in the skillet; increase heat and boil for 1 minute. Season to taste with salt and pepper; pour over fish. Serve immediately with lemon wedges.

Nutritional Analysis (Per Serving)
- Calories: 420
- Protein: 36.4 g
- Fat: 24.2 g
- Carbohydrates: 7.1 g
- Fiber: 1.9 g
- Sodium: 236 mg
- Cholesterol: 60 mg

Fish with Smoked Salmon and Green Peas

1 lb	fish fillets or steaks	500 g
1/4 cup	chopped green onions (about 2 medium)	50 mL
2 oz	smoked salmon, diced	50 g
SAUCE		
2 tsp	margarine or butter	10 mL
4 tsp	all-purpose flour	20 mL
1/2 cup	fish or chicken stock	125 mL
1/2 cup	2% milk	125 mL
1/3 cup	frozen peas	75 mL
3 tbsp	chopped fresh dill (or 2 tsp/10 mL dried)	50 mL

Make Ahead

Prepare sauce up to 24 hours ahead. Add more stock or milk if too thick.

SERVES 4
Preheat oven to 425°F (220°C) • Baking dish sprayed with vegetable spray

1. *Sauce:* Melt the margarine in small saucepan over medium-low heat; add the flour and cook, stirring, for 1 minute. Add stock and milk, stirring or whisking constantly, until mixture starts to simmer and thicken slightly, 5 to 7 minutes. Stir peas and dill into sauce, and pour over fish.

2. Bake until fish is just done at center, and flakes easily with a fork, 10 minutes for every inch (2.5 cm) thickness. Remove fish from oven.

3. Sprinkle with green onions and smoked salmon pieces and serve.

Nutritional Analysis (Per Serving)
- Calories: 175
- Protein: 26 g
- Fat: 5 g
- Carbohydrates: 6 g
- Fiber: 1 g
- Sodium: 376 mg
- Cholesterol: 60 mg

Stuffed Fish with Garlic Herb Topping

3 to 3½ lbs	whole fish, such as red snapper, red fish or other similar fish	1.5 to 1.75 kg
1	lime or lemon	1
2½ tsp	salt or to taste	12 mL

STUFFING

1½ tbsp	vegetable oil	22 mL
4 cups	finely sliced onions (about 4)	1 L
1 tbsp	minced peeled gingerroot	15 mL
2 tsp	minced garlic	10 mL
1 tsp	cayenne pepper	5 mL
¾ tsp	salt or to taste	4 mL
1 cup	mint leaves, chopped	250 mL
1 cup	cilantro leaves, chopped	250 mL

TOPPING

1 tbsp	vegetable oil	15 mL
⅓ cup	coarsely chopped garlic (about 1 large head)	75 mL
¾ cup	sliced green onions (3 to 4)	175 mL
2 cups	mint leaves, loosely packed	500 mL
2 cups	cilantro, loosely packed	500 mL

Get the freshest fish possible for this heavenly dish. Sweet caramelized onions balanced with a healthy dose of cayenne make a stuffing that is the essence of simplicity yet complex in its flavors.

SERVES 6 TO 8

Preheat oven to 375°F (190°C) • Baking sheet, lined with foil

1. Scale and clean fish, removing center bone. Do not remove head and tail. Score skin on both sides of fish. Rub all over with lime and salt. Cover and refrigerate for at least 1 hour or up to 2 hours.

2. *Stuffing:* In a skillet, heat oil over medium-high heat. Sauté onions, stirring occasionally, until deep brown, 15 to 20 minutes. Stir in ginger, garlic, cayenne and salt. Cook for 2 minutes. Remove from heat. Stir in mint and cilantro.

3. Place fish on prepared baking sheet. Stuff with mixture. Bake in preheated oven for 30 minutes or until fish flakes easily with a fork. Peel off skin from top of fish. Transfer to serving platter and keep warm.

4. *Topping:* In a small saucepan, heat oil over medium heat. Sauté garlic until golden and fragrant, about 2 minutes. Stir in green onions and cook for 2 minutes. Add mint and cilantro and cook for 2 minutes longer. Spoon over fish and serve immediately.

Nutritional Analysis (Per Serving)
- Calories: 298
- Protein: 44.5 g
- Fat: 7.8 g
- Carbohydrates: 11.2 g
- Fiber: 1.8 g
- Sodium: 1221 mg
- Cholesterol: 74 mg

Poached Fish Jardinière

1	small onion, chopped	1
6 to 8	bay leaves	6 to 8
6 to 8	portions (4 oz/125 g each) fresh or frozen halibut or haddock	6 to 8
6 to 8	thin slices lemon	6 to 8
1 cup	dry white wine	250 mL
½ cup	water	125 mL

SAUCE

4	large tomatoes, chopped	4
2	cloves garlic, minced	2
¼ cup	plain yogurt	50 mL
2 tbsp	olive oil	25 mL
2 tbsp	chopped fresh parsley	25 mL
1 tbsp	Dijon mustard	15 mL
2 tsp	each dried chervil and tarragon	10 mL
1 tsp	Worcestershire sauce	5 mL
¼ tsp	salt	1 mL
	Black pepper	

SERVES 8
Preheat oven to 425°F (220°C)

1. Spread onion on bottom of a large shallow baking dish. Place bay leaves in dish; top each with piece of fish and lemon slice. Pour wine and water over top. Cover and chill for at least 1 hour.

2. *Sauce:* In a saucepan, combine tomatoes, garlic, yogurt, oil, parsley, mustard, chervil, tarragon, Worcestershire sauce, salt, and pepper to taste; cook over low heat for 10 to 15 minutes to blend flavors. (Do not boil.)

3. Bake fish in preheated oven for 10 to 15 minutes or until fish flakes easily when tested with fork. Remove fish from liquid and arrange on plates, adding some liquid to sauce for desired consistency if necessary. Pour sauce over fish.

Nutritional Analysis (Per Serving)
- Calories: 204
- Protein: 26 g
- Fat: 8 g
- Carbohydrates: 7 g
- Fiber: 2 g
- Sodium: 170 mg
- Cholesterol: 36 mg

Lemon and Dill Fish Kabobs

⅓ cup	lemon juice	75 mL
¼ cup	chopped fresh dillweed	50 mL
2 tbsp	olive oil	25 mL
1 tbsp	Russian-style mustard	15 mL
½ tsp	salt	2 mL
¼ tsp	black pepper	1 mL
2 lbs	salmon, halibut or cod, cut in 1-inch (2.5 cm) pieces	1 kg
1	large red bell pepper, seeded and cut in 1-inch (2.5 cm) pieces	1

SERVES 6

1. In a large non-metallic bowl, combine lemon juice, dill, olive oil, mustard, salt and pepper.

2. Add fish to marinade and toss gently to coat. Marinate for 10 minutes.

3. Thread fish and pepper pieces onto six 6- to 8-inch (15 to 20 cm) skewers. Arrange on a lightly greased broiler pan. Spoon over any remaining marinade.

4. Place fish about 4 inches (10 cm) from the heat and convection broil under a preheated broiler for 4 minutes. Turn and cook for 4 to 5 minutes longer, or until fish flakes easily with a fork.

Nutritional Analysis (Per Serving)
- Calories: 199
- Protein 22.8 g
- Fat: 10.7 g
- Carbohydrates: 2.0 g
- Fiber: 0.5 g
- Sodium: 215 mg
- Cholesterol: 64 mg

Preeti's Grilled Fish

3 lbs	catfish fillets or any other fish fillets	1.5 kg
8 to 10	cloves garlic	8 to 10
1 tbsp	cumin seeds	15 mL
8	dried red chilies, seeds removed	8
	Juice of 1 large lime or lemon	
2½ tsp	salt or to taste	12 mL

TOPPING

1 tbsp	vegetable oil	15 mL
2 tbsp	chopped green chilies, preferably serranos	25 mL
1¼ cups	chopped tomatoes	300 mL
1 cup	sliced green onions, including some green part	250 mL
½ cup	cilantro, chopped	125 mL
	Lemon wedges or slices, for garnish	

SERVES 8
Preheat broiler

1. Rinse fish and pat dry.

2. In a blender, grind together garlic, cumin seeds, red chilies and lime juice until a paste forms. Coat fish with paste and place on a baking sheet. Set aside for 15 minutes.

3. Grill fish in preheated broiler until it flakes easily with a fork, 6 to 8 minutes, depending on thickness of fillet. Sprinkle with salt.

4. *Topping:* Meanwhile, in a skillet, heat oil over medium heat. Sauté chilies for 1 minute. Add tomatoes and green onions. Sauté for 2 minutes. Stir in cilantro and remove from heat. Arrange fish on serving platter. Top with vegetables. Garnish with lemon wedges.

Nutritional Analysis (Per Serving)
- Calories: 210
- Protein: 36.2 g
- Fat: 4.4 g
- Carbohydrates: 5.7 g
- Fiber: 1.9 g
- Sodium: 843 mg
- Cholesterol: 60 mg

Oriental Fish Fillets

4	green onions, diagonally sliced	4
2	cloves garlic, minced	2
1 tbsp	canola oil	15 mL
4	fish fillets (turbot, cod, haddock or halibut)	4
1 tbsp	finely chopped gingerroot	15 mL
½ cup	dry sherry	125 mL
2 tbsp	soy sauce	25 mL
¼ cup	coarsely chopped fresh cilantro	50 mL

SERVES 4

1. In a heavy skillet over high heat, cook green onions and garlic in hot oil for about 2 minutes. Remove onion mixture and add fish to skillet.

2. Combine onion mixture, ginger root, sherry and soy sauce; pour over fish. Sprinkle with cilantro. Cook, covered, over medium heat for about 5 minutes or until fish flakes easily when tested with fork. Transfer fillets to preheated platter. Cook sauce over high heat until reduced and slightly thickened. Pour sauce over fish and serve.

In this recipe, the oriental flavors of ginger root, soy sauce and cilantro give ordinary fish fillets a new lease on life.

Nutritional Analysis (Per Serving)
- Calories: 214
- Protein: 25 g
- Fat: 10 g
- Carbohydrates: 5 g
- Fiber: Trace
- Sodium: 361 mg
- Cholesterol: 54 mg

Baked Fish and Vegetables en Papillote

4	fish fillets (each about ¼ lb/125 g)	4
4	large white mushrooms, sliced	4
2	green onions, sliced	2
20	snow peas, trimmed	20
	Salt and freshly ground black pepper	

SERVES 4

Nonstick cooking spray • Preheat oven to 450°F (230°C)

1. Cut four pieces of parchment paper or foil 4 inches (10 cm) larger than fish fillets. Lightly spray with cooking spray. Place each fillet in center of paper. Top each with 1 sliced mushroom, half the onions and 5 snow peas. Season lightly with salt and pepper.
2. Fold long ends of paper or foil twice so mixture is tightly enclosed. Lift short ends, bring together on top and fold twice. Place seam-side up on baking pan.
3. Bake for 20 minutes or until fish is opaque and flakes easily when tested with a fork and vegetables are tender. Open each package and serve contents on dinner plates.

Nutritional Analysis (Per Serving)
- Calories: 135
- Protein: 25.3 g
- Fat: 1.7 g
- Carbohydrates: 4.1 g
- Fiber: 1.3 g
- Sodium: 77 mg
- Cholesterol: 40 mg

Arshi's Fish Curry

3 cups	plain nonfat yogurt, at room temperature	750 mL
2 tbsp	cornstarch	25 mL
1 tbsp	vegetable oil	15 mL
1 tsp	nigella seeds (kalaunji)	5 mL
¾ tsp	fenugreek seeds (methi)	4 mL
3 lbs	fish fillets, such as catfish, sea bass, red snapper or tilapia	1.5 kg
2½ tsp	salt or to taste	12 mL
15 to 20	fresh curry leaves, chopped (optional)	15 to 20

SERVES 8

1. Stir yogurt until it has a creamy consistency. Stir in cornstarch and set aside.
2. In a large skillet, heat oil over medium heat. Add nigella and fenugreek seeds and stir-fry for 20 to 30 seconds. Pour yogurt mixture into skillet and bring to a gentle boil over medium heat.
3. Place fish in a single layer in skillet. Sprinkle salt and curry leaves, if using, on top. Cover and return to a gentle boil. Simmer until fish flakes when tested with a fork, 6 to 8 minutes, depending on the fish used.

Nutritional Analysis (Per Serving)
- Calories: 245
- Protein: 40.3 g
- Fat: 4.2 g
- Carbohydrates: 9.3 g
- Fiber: 0.2 g
- Sodium: 907 mg
- Cholesterol: 62 mg

Thai Fish Parcels

6	fish fillets (each 6 oz/175 g), thawed if frozen	6
1¹/₂ cups	sliced shiitake mushrooms, stems removed (about 6 oz/175 g with stems)	375 mL
1 tbsp	minced ginger root	15 mL
2	cloves garlic, minced	2
¹/₂ tsp	salt	2 mL
¹/₂ tsp	black pepper	2 mL
2 tbsp	sesame oil	25 mL
	Hot pepper sauce to taste	
¹/₃ cup	chopped fresh coriander	75 mL
12	large fresh basil leaves	12
1	small lemon, cut into 6 slices	1
2 tbsp	finely chopped green onion	25 mL

Make Ahead

If using parchment, fish and flavorings can be wrapped and refrigerated for up to 8 hours before cooking. If using foil, cook fish as soon as it's wrapped to prevent the acid in the lemon juice from reacting with the aluminum foil.

SERVES 6

Preheat oven to 450°F (230°C) • Six 15- by 10-inch (37.5 by 25 cm) rectangles of parchment paper or aluminum foil, lightly oiled • Baking sheet

1. Place 1 fish fillet on one half of each piece of parchment. Top fish with shiitake mushrooms, dividing evenly. Sprinkle with ginger, garlic, salt and pepper. Drizzle with sesame oil; add a dash of hot pepper sauce. Sprinkle with coriander; top each with 2 basil leaves and 1 lemon slice.

2. Fold parchment in half to enclose ingredients. Starting at a corner near fold, turn in edges all around, pleating and pinching to seal well. Place packages on baking sheet. Bake in preheated oven for 10 to 12 minutes or until fish is opaque and flakes easily with a fork.

3. Open packages carefully, avoiding steam. Discard basil and lemon slices. Spoon fish and cooking juices onto dinner plates. Garnish with green onion; serve at once.

Tip

• Any type of fish fillets can be used in this recipe — salmon, orange roughy, cod or red snapper, for instance.

Nutritional Analysis (Per Serving)
• Calories: 293   • Protein: 34.6 g   • Fat: 15.4 g
• Carbohydrates: 2.6 g   • Fiber: 0.5 g   • Sodium: 268 mg
• Cholesterol: 96 mg

Fish Roll-Ups

½	package (10 oz/300 g) fresh spinach	½
1	small onion, chopped	1
1 tbsp	butter or margarine	15 mL
1 cup	chopped mushrooms	250 mL
¼ cup	whole-wheat bread crumbs	50 mL
1 lb	sole fillets	500 g
	Salt, black pepper and dried thyme to taste	
½	lemon	½
	Paprika	

In combination with onions and mushrooms, spinach makes a tasty filling for fish.

SERVES 4

Preheat oven to 425°F (220°C) • Baking pan, lightly greased

1. Steam spinach until tender; drain well. In a small skillet over medium-high heat, cook onion in butter for about 5 minutes or until browned. Add mushrooms; cook for 3 minutes. In a food processor, combine spinach, mushroom mixture and bread crumbs. Process using on/off motion until coarsely chopped.

2. Season fish fillets with salt, pepper and thyme. (If fish fillets are too wide, cut in half down center.) Spoon spinach filling over each fillet; roll up and secure with toothpicks. Place fish seam side down in nonstick or lightly greased baking pan. Squeeze lemon over fish; sprinkle with paprika. Bake, uncovered, in preheated oven for 10 minutes per inch (2.5 cm) of thickness or until fish flakes easily with fork. Remove toothpicks and serve.

Nutritional Analysis (Per Serving)
- Calories: 144
- Protein: 19 g
- Fat: 4 g
- Carbohydrates: 8 g
- Fiber: 1 g
- Sodium: 177 mg
- Cholesterol: 64 mg

Baked Cajun Catfish

½ tsp	chili powder	2 mL
½ tsp	garlic powder	2 mL
¼ tsp	dried oregano leaves	1 mL
¼ tsp	dried thyme leaves	1 mL
¼ tsp	paprika	1 mL
¼ tsp	salt	1 mL
¼ tsp	black pepper	1 mL
Pinch	cayenne pepper	Pinch
2	catfish fillets (about 12 oz/375 g total)	2
1 tbsp	olive oil	15 mL
1 tbsp	lime juice or lemon juice	15 mL

SERVES 2

1. In a small bowl, combine chili powder, garlic powder, oregano, thyme, paprika, salt, pepper and cayenne.

2. Place fillets in a shallow dish. Sprinkle fish with oil and lime juice.

3. Rub seasoning mix over fish to coat all sides.

4. Place fillets in a single layer on lightly greased broiler rack placed over oven pan. Bake in preheated 400°F (200°C) toaster oven for 12 to 14 minutes, or until fish is opaque and flakes easily when tested with a fork.

Nutritional Analysis (Per Serving)
- Calories: 296
- Protein: 26.8 g
- Fat: 19.7 g
- Carbohydrates: 2.1 g
- Fiber: 0.5 g
- Sodium: 381 mg
- Cholesterol: 78 mg

Cod with Almonds and Lemon Sauce

1 lb	cod, cut into 4 serving-sized pieces	500 g
2 tbsp	chopped fresh dill (or 1 tsp/5 mL dried dillweed)	25 mL
4 tsp	margarine, melted	20 mL
4 tsp	lemon juice	20 mL
1 tsp	crushed garlic	5 mL
2 tbsp	sliced almonds, toasted	25 mL

SERVES 4

Preheat oven to 425°F (220°C) • Baking dish sprayed with nonstick vegetable spray

1. Place fish in baking dish large enough to arrange in single layer. Combine dill, margarine, lemon juice and garlic; pour over fish.

2. Bake until fish flakes easily when tested with fork, approximately 10 minutes. Sprinkle with almonds.

Tips

• Pecans also suit this dish.

• Toast nuts in skillet on top of stove on high, or in 450°F (230°C) oven for 2 minutes or until golden.

Nutritional Analysis (Per Serving)
- Calories: 152
- Protein: 22 g
- Fat: 6 g
- Carbohydrates: 1 g
- Fiber: 0 g
- Sodium: 146 mg
- Cholesterol: 60 mg

Baked Cod with Pistou

½ cup	packed fresh basil leaves	125 mL
1	clove garlic, chopped	1
3 tbsp	olive oil	45 mL
2 tbsp	grated Parmesan cheese	25 mL
½ tsp	salt	2 mL
¼ tsp	black pepper	1 mL
1 lb	cod, cut in 4 pieces	500 g
1	large tomato, halved lengthwise, cored and cut in 6 slices per side	1

Make Ahead

Assemble dish completely. Cover with plastic and refrigerate for up to four hours before baking.

SERVES 4

1. To prepare pistou, place basil, garlic, olive oil, cheese, salt and pepper in food processor. Blend until smooth.

2. Arrange cod pieces in one layer on a parchment-lined baking sheet. Spoon pistou evenly over fish. Turn fish to coat in pistou. Place 3 tomato slices over each piece of fish.

3. Convection bake in a preheated 400°F (200°C) oven for 10 to 12 minutes, or until fish is opaque and just flakes with a fork.

Tip

• Pistou is basically the Provençal version of pesto, without the pine nuts. If you have pesto on hand, it can be used instead.

Nutritional Analysis (Per Serving)
- Calories: 206
- Protein: 21.7 g
- Fat: 11.7 g
- Carbohydrates: 2.7 g
- Fiber: 0.6 g
- Sodium: 399 mg
- Cholesterol: 50 mg

Cod with Mushrooms and Tomato

1	package (14 oz/400 g) frozen cod, sole, turbot or haddock fillets, defrosted	1
	Salt and freshly ground black pepper	
1 1/2 cups	sliced mushrooms	375 mL
1	large tomato, seeded and diced	1
2	green onions, sliced	2
2 tbsp	chopped fresh dill or parsley	25 mL
1/3 cup	dry white wine or fish stock	75 mL
1 tbsp	cornstarch	15 mL
1/3 cup	half-and-half (10%) cream	75 mL

No trip to the fish market is required to make this quick main-course dish. Packaged frozen fish fillets work just fine. And here's an extra bonus — even with a small amount of light cream added, this dish is low in fat.

SERVES 4

Preheat oven to 375°F (190°C) • 8-inch (2 L) square baking dish

1. Arrange fish fillets in a single layer in baking dish; season with salt and pepper. Layer with mushrooms, tomato, green onions and dill. Pour wine over top. Bake for 20 to 25 minutes or until fish is opaque and flakes when tested with a fork.

2. Remove from oven; carefully pour juices from dish into small saucepan. (Place a large plate or lid over dish.) Return fish to turned-off oven to keep warm.

3. In a bowl, blend cornstarch with 2 tbsp (25 mL) cold water; stir in cream. Add to saucepan. Place over medium heat; cook, whisking, until sauce comes to a boil and thickens. Season with salt and pepper to taste. (Sauce will be thick.) Pour over fish and serve.

Tip

• To defrost a package of frozen fish fillets, remove package wrapping; place fish on plate. Microwave on Medium for 3 minutes. Shield ends with thin strips of foil to prevent them from cooking before the rest of the fish has defrosted. Microwave on Defrost for 3 minutes more or until fish separates into fillets. Let stand for 10 minutes to complete defrosting. Pat dry with paper towels to absorb excess moisture.

Nutritional Analysis (Per Serving)
• Calories: 190   • Protein: 19.7 g   • Fat: 8.2 g
• Carbohydrates: 6.4 g   • Fiber: 1.2 g   • Sodium: 66 mg
• Cholesterol: 69 mg

Cod Provençal

1¼ lbs	cod or halibut, cut into 4 pieces	625 g
	Salt and freshly ground black pepper	
2	ripe tomatoes, diced	2
2	green onions, sliced	2
1	clove garlic, minced	1
¼ cup	Kalamata olives, rinsed, cut into slivers	50 mL
2 tbsp	chopped fresh parsley or basil leaves	25 mL
1 tbsp	capers, drained and rinsed	15 mL
Pinch	hot pepper flakes (optional)	Pinch
2 tbsp	olive oil	25 mL

SERVES 4
Preheat oven to 425°F (220°C) • Shallow baking dish

1. Arrange cod in a single layer in baking dish. Season with salt and pepper.

2. In a bowl, combine tomatoes, green onions, garlic, olives, parsley, capers and hot pepper flakes, if using; season with salt and pepper. Spoon tomato-olive mixture over fish fillets; drizzle with oil.

3. Bake in preheated oven for 15 to 20 minutes or until fish flakes when tested with a fork. Serve in warmed wide shallow bowls and spoon pan juices over top.

Nutritional Analysis (Per Serving)
- Calories: 224
- Protein: 31.5 g
- Fat: 8.6 g
- Carbohydrates: 5.0 g
- Fiber: 1.6 g
- Sodium: 199 mg
- Cholesterol: 72 mg

Halibut with Chunky Tomato Sauce and Black Olives

1 tbsp	margarine	15 mL
1 tsp	crushed garlic	5 mL
1 cup	sliced mushrooms	250 mL
⅔ cup	chopped onions	150 mL
2	large tomatoes, diced	2
1 tsp	each dried basil and oregano (or 2 tbsp/25 mL each chopped fresh)	5 mL
⅓ cup	sliced black olives	75 mL
1 lb	halibut, cut into 4 serving-sized pieces	500 g
1 tbsp	grated Parmesan cheese	15 mL

SERVES 4
Preheat oven to 425°F (220°C) • Baking dish sprayed with nonstick vegetable spray

1. In large nonstick skillet, melt margarine; sauté garlic, mushrooms and onions until softened, approximately 3 minutes.

2. Add tomatoes, basil, oregano and olives; simmer for 3 minutes.

3. Place fish in baking dish large enough to arrange in single layer; pour sauce over top. Bake for 10 to 15 minutes or until fish flakes easily when tested with fork. Serve sprinkled with Parmesan cheese.

Nutritional Analysis (Per Serving)
- Calories: 184
- Protein: 23 g
- Fat: 6 g
- Carbohydrates: 8 g
- Fiber: 2 g
- Sodium: 262 mg
- Cholesterol: 61 mg

Halibut with Lemon and Pecans

½ cup	bread crumbs	125 mL
1 tsp	dried parsley	5 mL
½ tsp	dried basil	2 mL
½ tsp	crushed garlic	2 mL
1½ tsp	grated Parmesan cheese	7 mL
1 lb	halibut, cut into serving-sized pieces	4 500 g
1	egg white	1
2 tbsp	margarine	25 mL
2 tbsp	white wine	25 mL
4 tsp	lemon juice	20 mL
1 tbsp	chopped fresh parsley	15 mL
1	green onion, chopped	1
1 tbsp	chopped pecans, toasted	15 mL

SERVES 4

Preheat oven to 400°F (200°C) • Baking dish sprayed with nonstick vegetable spray

1. In shallow dish, combine bread crumbs, dried parsley, basil, garlic and cheese. Dip fish pieces into egg white, then into bread crumb mixture.

2. In large nonstick skillet, melt 1 tbsp (15 mL) of the margarine; add fish and cook just until browned on both sides. Transfer fish to baking dish and bake for 5 to 10 minutes or until fish flakes easily when tested with fork. Remove to serving platter and keep warm.

3. To skillet, add remaining margarine, wine, lemon juice, parsley, onions and pecans; cook for 1 minute. Pour over fish.

Tips

- Other white fish, such as sole, flounder or turbot, can be substituted.

- If using a thin piece of fish, you can probably skip the baking time. The fish will cook through in the skillet.

- Toast pecans either in 400°F (200°C) oven or in skillet on top of stove for 2 minutes or until brown.

Nutritional Analysis (Per Serving)
- Calories: 231
- Protein: 24 g
- Fat: 9 g
- Carbohydrates: 10 g
- Fiber: 1 g
- Sodium: 302 mg
- Cholesterol: 61 mg

Rosemary Smoked Halibut with Balsamic Vinaigrette

2 or 3	sprigs fresh rosemary	2 or 3
1½ lb	halibut fillets	750 g
BALSAMIC VINAIGRETTE		
¼ cup	olive oil	50 mL
2 tbsp	balsamic vinegar	25 mL
¼ tsp	coarsely crushed black pepper	1 mL
⅛ tsp	salt	0.5 mL
½ cup	diced seeded tomato	125 mL
1 tsp	finely chopped shallot	5 mL

It's hard to believe this impressive-sounding recipe is so easy to make. Just lighting the sprigs of rosemary gives the fish a tantalizing herb flavor and aroma.

SERVES 6

Preheat oven to 425°F (220°C) • Baking dish

1. In a baking dish, place rosemary beside halibut; light rosemary with match (rosemary may not remain lit). Cover tightly with foil. Bake in preheated oven for 8 to 12 minutes or until fish flakes easily when tested with fork.
2. *Balsamic Vinaigrette:* Meanwhile, in a small bowl, whisk together oil, balsamic vinegar, pepper and salt; stir in tomato and shallot. Serve with halibut.

Nutritional Analysis (Per Serving)
- Calories: 208
- Carbohydrates: 1 g
- Cholesterol: 36 mg
- Protein: 24 g
- Fiber: Trace
- Fat: 12 g
- Sodium: 111 mg

Cumin-Crusted Halibut Steaks

1 tbsp	cumin seeds	15 mL
½ tsp	salt	2 mL
¼ tsp	freshly ground black pepper	1 mL
1 lb	halibut or other fish steaks	500 g
2 tsp	olive oil	10 mL
	Chopped fresh parsley, optional	

SERVES 4

Preheat oven to 450°F (230°C)

1. In a nonstick skillet over medium heat, toast cumin seeds, stirring, for 2 minutes or until golden. Place seeds, salt and pepper in a coffee or spice grinder. Pulse until finely ground. Rub mixture into both sides of fish.
2. Heat olive oil in a large nonstick skillet over medium-high heat. Add fish, in batches, if necessary, and cook for 2 minutes per side or until browned.
3. Return all fish to skillet and wrap handle with foil. Bake in preheated oven for 5 minutes or until fish is opaque and flakes easily when tested with a fork. Sprinkle with parsley, if using, and serve.

Nutritional Analysis (Per Serving)
- Calories: 150
- Carbohydrates: 0.8 g
- Cholesterol: 36 mg
- Protein: 23.9 g
- Fiber: 0.2 g
- Fat: 5.2 g
- Sodium: 354 mg

Broiled Halibut with Black Butter

2	halibut steaks (about 1 lb/500 g), ¾-inch (2 cm) thick	2
1 tsp	butter	5 mL
¼ cup	salted butter	50 mL
⅛ tsp	salt	0.5 mL
⅛ tsp	freshly ground black pepper	0.5 mL
1 tsp	black or white sesame seeds	5 mL
1 tbsp	balsamic vinegar	15 mL
	Few sprigs fresh parsley, chopped	

SERVES 2
Baking sheet • Preheat broiler

1. Rub 1 tsp (5 mL) butter on both sides of the halibut steaks. Put them on a baking sheet. Broil for 4 to 5 minutes each side or until cooked through.

2. Meanwhile, in a small pot, combine ¼ cup (50 mL) butter, salt and pepper. Cook over medium-high heat, stirring, for about 8 minutes or until browned. (It'll foam during the last 2 minutes, so you have to watch and stir actively to make sure it isn't burning; despite its name, beurre noir is ruined if it turns black.) Remove from heat. Add sesame seeds and vinegar in quick succession (careful, it'll splutter). Set aside.

3. Put halibut steaks in the centers of 2 warm plates. Pour portions of black butter (including its solids) over, allowing it to pool around the fish. Garnish with chopped parsley and serve immediately.

Nutritional Analysis (Per Serving)
- Calories: 479
- Protein: 47.9 g
- Fat: 30.9 g
- Carbohydrates: 0.8 g
- Fiber: 0.1 g
- Sodium: 520 mg
- Cholesterol: 139 mg

South Side Halibut

1	clove garlic, minced	1
⅓ cup	finely chopped onion	75 mL
1 tsp	vegetable oil	5 mL
2 tbsp	chopped fresh parsley	25 mL
½ tsp	grated orange zest	2 mL
⅛ tsp	black pepper	0.5 mL
¼ cup	orange juice	50 mL
1 tbsp	lemon juice	15 mL
4	halibut steaks (4 oz/125 g each) or 1 lb (500 g) halibut or Pacific snapper fillets	4

SERVES 4
Preheat oven to 400°F (200°C) • Baking dish

1. In a small skillet, sauté garlic and onion in oil over medium heat until tender. Remove from heat; stir in parsley, orange zest and pepper. Combine orange juice and lemon juice.

2. Arrange fish in baking dish. Spread onion mixture over fish; pour juice over top. Cover tightly with foil. Bake in preheated oven for 8 to 10 minutes or until fish flakes easily when tested with fork.

Nutritional Analysis (Per Serving)
- Calories: 149
- Protein: 24 g
- Fat: 4 g
- Carbohydrates: 4 g
- Fiber: Trace
- Sodium: 62 mg
- Cholesterol: 36 mg

Halibut Provençal

SAUCE

2 tbsp	olive oil	25 mL
1	small onion, chopped	1
2	cloves garlic, finely chopped	2
½ cup	dry white wine	125 mL
1 cup	chopped tomato	250 mL
1 tsp	grated orange zest	5 mL
½ tsp	dried thyme leaves	2 mL
½ tsp	salt	2 mL
½ tsp	black pepper	2 mL

FISH

1 tbsp	olive oil	15 mL
1 tbsp	lemon juice	15 mL
¼ tsp	salt	1 mL
¼ tsp	black pepper	1 mL
1½ lbs	halibut fillets, cut in 4 pieces	750 g
⅓ cup	pitted black olives	75 mL
2 tsp	capers	10 mL
2 tbsp	chopped fresh basil or parsley	25 mL

SERVES 4

1. To make sauce, in a medium skillet, heat oil over medium-high heat. Add onion and garlic. Cook, stirring occasionally, for 3 minutes. Add wine, tomato, orange zest, thyme, salt and pepper. Bring to a boil, reduce heat and simmer for 8 minutes.

2. Meanwhile, lightly grease broiler rack and place over oven pan (add ¼ cup/50 mL water to pan). To prepare fish, in a shallow dish, combine olive oil, lemon juice, salt and pepper. Dip fish into marinade, then place on broiler rack.

3. Place rack under preheated broiler in top position of convection toaster oven. Leave door ajar. Broil for 6 to 8 minutes per side, or until fish flakes lightly with a fork (timing depends on thickness of fish). Place fish on a serving platter. Spoon sauce over fish and top with olives, capers and basil.

Nutritional Analysis (Per Serving)
- Calories: 333
- Protein: 36.5 g
- Fat: 14.8 g
- Carbohydrates: 7.7 g
- Fiber: 1.5 g
- Sodium: 621 mg
- Cholesterol: 54 mg

Halibut Burgers with Dijon Mustard Glaze

1 lb	halibut or seabass, cut into chunks	500 g
3 tbsp	seasoned bread crumbs	45 mL
1	egg	1
2 tsp	minced garlic	10 mL
⅓ cup	finely chopped red peppers	75 mL
¼ cup	finely chopped fresh basil (or 1 tsp/5 mL dried)	50 mL
1 tsp	vegetable oil	5 mL
3 tbsp	2% yogurt	45 mL
1 tbsp	Dijon mustard	15 mL

Make Ahead

Prepare mustard sauce up to a day before serving. Stir before serving.

SERVES 4 OR 5

1. Put fish, bread crumbs, egg, garlic, red peppers and basil in food processor; pulse on and off until fish is chunky. Do not purée. Form into 4 or 5 burgers.

2. In nonstick skillet sprayed with vegetable spray, heat oil (or heat barbecue); cook patties over medium-high heat for about 3 or 4 minutes; turn and cook another 3 minutes until browned.

3. In small bowl whisk together yogurt and mustard. Serve burgers with mustard sauce drizzled on top.

Nutritional Analysis (Per Serving)
- Calories: 144
- Protein: 21 g
- Fat: 5 g
- Carbohydrates: 3 g
- Fiber: 0 g
- Sodium: 145 mg
- Cholesterol: 82 mg

Pan-Seared Mahi Mahi with Papaya Mint Relish

PAPAYA MINT RELISH

1½ cups	diced peeled papaya (1 large)	375 mL
⅓ cup	finely diced shallots or green onions	75 mL
3 tbsp	finely chopped fresh mint	45 mL
2 tbsp	lime juice	25 mL
Pinch	each salt, black pepper and granulated sugar	Pinch

FISH

2 tbsp	all-purpose flour	25 mL
Pinch	each salt and black pepper	Pinch
4	mahi mahi fillets (30 oz/90 g each)	4
1 tbsp	extra-virgin olive oil	15 mL

SERVES 4

1. *Papaya Mint Relish:* In a small bowl, mix papaya, shallots, mint, lime juice, salt, pepper and sugar; set aside.

2. *Fish:* Mix together flour, salt and pepper; dip fish fillets into flour to coat both sides. In a nonstick pan, heat oil over medium-high heat; cook fish for 1½ to 3 minutes per side or until fish flakes easily when tested with fork. Serve topped with Papaya Mint Relish.

Tip

- Substitute sea bass or halibut if mahi mahi is not available. If papaya is not in season, use fresh or canned pineapple or mango instead.

Nutritional Analysis (Per Serving)
- Calories: 149
- Protein: 17 g
- Fat: 4 g
- Carbohydrates: 11 g
- Fiber: 1 g
- Sodium: 260 mg
- Cholesterol: 158 mg

Red Snapper with Dill Tomato Sauce

1 tbsp	vegetable oil	15 mL
1 tsp	crushed garlic	5 mL
½ cup	sliced sweet red pepper	125 mL
½ cup	sliced sweet green pepper	125 mL
½ cup	sliced onions	125 mL
½ cup	sliced mushrooms	125 mL
1 cup	puréed drained canned tomatoes	250 mL
½ tsp	dried oregano	2 mL
3 tbsp	chopped fresh dill (or 1 tsp/5 mL dried dillweed)	45 mL
1 lb	red snapper, divided into 4 portions	500
1 tbsp	grated Parmesan cheese	15 mL

SERVES 4

Preheat oven to 425°F (220°C) • Baking dish sprayed with nonstick vegetable spray

1. In large nonstick skillet, heat oil; sauté garlic, red and green peppers, onions and mushrooms until softened, approximately 5 minutes.

2. Add tomatoes and oregano; simmer for 5 minutes. Add dill; cook for 1 more minute.

3. Place red snapper in single layer in baking dish; pour sauce over top. Bake for 18 to 25 minutes or until fish flakes easily when tested with fork. Sprinkle Parmesan over top.

Nutritional Analysis (Per Serving)
- Calories: 170
- Protein: 23 g
- Fat: 5 g
- Carbohydrates: 7 g
- Fiber: 2 g
- Sodium: 216 mg
- Cholesterol: 61 mg

Red Snapper with Broccoli and Dill Cheese Sauce

2 cups	chopped broccoli florets	500 mL
1 lb	red snapper (or any firm fish fillets)	500 g
1 tbsp	margarine	15 mL
1 tbsp	all-purpose flour	15 mL
1 cup	2% milk	250 mL
1/3 cup	shredded Cheddar cheese	75 mL
2 tbsp	chopped fresh dill (or 1/2 tsp/2 mL dried dillweed)	25 mL
	Salt and pepper	

SERVES 4
Preheat oven to 425°F (220°C)

1. In boiling water, blanch broccoli until still crisp and color brightens; drain and place in baking dish. Place fish in single layer over top.

2. In small saucepan, melt margarine; add flour and cook, stirring, for 1 minute. Add milk and cook, stirring constantly, until thickened, approximately 3 minutes. Stir in cheese, dill, and salt and pepper to taste until cheese has melted; pour over fish.

3. Bake, uncovered, for 15 to 20 minutes or until fish flakes easily when tested with fork.

Nutritional Analysis (Per Serving)
- Calories: 217
- Protein: 27 g
- Fat: 8 g
- Carbohydrates: 7 g
- Fiber: 1 g
- Sodium: 232 mg
- Cholesterol: 74 mg

Herb-Roasted Salmon

1	large salmon fillet (about 2 lbs/1 kg)	1
1 tbsp	olive oil	15 mL
2 tbsp	chopped fresh chives	25 mL
1 tbsp	chopped fresh tarragon or 1 tsp (5 mL) dried	15 mL
	Salt and freshly ground black pepper	

Salmon has such a marvelous flavor that little else is needed in the way of seasoning. This simple herb-oil mixture makes it easy.

SERVES 6
Preheat oven to 450°F (230°C) • Shallow oblong pan, greased

1. Place fish skin-side down in prepared pan.

2. In a small bowl, combine oil, chives and tarragon. Rub half into flesh of salmon.

3. Bake for 10 minutes per inch (2.5 cm) of thickness or until fish is opaque and flakes easily when tested with a fork.

4. To serve, cut salmon in half crosswise. Lift flesh from skin with a spatula. Transfer to a platter. Discard skin, and then drizzle fish with remaining herbs and oil. Season lightly with salt and pepper.

Nutritional Analysis (Per Serving)
- Calories: 181
- Protein: 22.6 g
- Fat: 9.5 g
- Carbohydrates: 0.2 g
- Fiber: 0 g
- Sodium: 48 mg
- Cholesterol: 64 mg

Perfectly Poached Salmon

POACHING LIQUID

6 cups	water	1.5 L
1 cup	dry white wine	250 mL
2	stalks celery, sliced	2
2	sprigs parsley	2
1	onion, peeled and cut in wedges	1
1	carrot, peeled and sliced	1
1 tsp	dried thyme leaves	5 mL
1/2 tsp	salt	2 mL
1/2 tsp	whole black peppercorns	2 mL
1	bay leaf	1

SALMON

1	salmon fillet (about 3 to 4 lbs/1.5 to 2 kg)	1

CUCUMBER DILL SAUCE

1 cup	mayonnaise	250 mL
1 cup	sour cream	250 mL
1/2 cup	finely chopped cucumber	125 mL
1 tsp	chopped fresh dillweed	5 mL
1/2 tsp	salt	2 mL
1/4 tsp	black pepper	1 mL

Make Ahead

Poaching liquid can be made up to 24 hours in advance. Refrigerate until ready to use and reheat on the stove before placing in slow cooker.

SERVES 4 TO 6

3 1/2 to 6 qt slow cooker

1. To prepare poaching liquid, in a saucepan, combine water, wine, celery, parsley, onion, carrot, thyme, salt, peppercorns and bay leaf. Bring to a boil on the stove, reduce heat and simmer for 30 minutes. Strain through a sieve and discard solids. Reserve liquid.

2. To prepare salmon, preheat slow cooker on High for 15 minutes. Line slow cooker stoneware with a double thickness of cheesecloth or fold a 2-foot (60 cm) piece of foil in half lengthwise and lay on bottom of slow cooker. Place salmon on top of cheesecloth or foil and pour hot poaching liquid over salmon.

3. Cover and cook on High for 1 hour.

4. With oven mitts, remove stoneware from slow cooker and let salmon cool in poaching liquid for 20 minutes. If serving cold, stoneware can be stored in refrigerator to allow salmon to chill in liquid.

5. Lift salmon out of stoneware using cheesecloth or foil handles and gently place on a platter.

6. To prepare sauce, in a bowl, combine mayonnaise, sour cream, cucumber, dill, salt and pepper. Serve salmon with sauce.

Tip

- Serve the salmon hot or cold as part of a buffet, and garnish with slices of lemon and sprigs of parsley and dill.

Nutritional Analysis (Per Serving)
- Calories: 730
- Protein: 46.8 g
- Fat: 57.6 g
- Carbohydrates: 3.3 g
- Fiber: 0.1 g
- Sodium: 361 mg
- Cholesterol: 170 mg

Salmon with Spinach

1	package (10 oz/300 g) frozen chopped spinach, thawed	1
1 tbsp	grated gingerroot	15 mL
2	large white mushrooms, thickly sliced	2
	Salt and freshly ground black pepper	
4	salmon steaks or fillets (see variation, at right)	4

Salmon will remain moist using this cooking procedure. Layer spinach and mushrooms, then top with salmon. Bake on high heat for the recommended 10 minutes per inch (2.5 cm) thickness of the fish. Due to the extra thickness of fish and vegetables, you may need a few extra minutes of baking time.

SERVES 4

Preheat oven to 450°F (230°C) • Shallow oblong pan, greased

1. In a sieve, drain spinach, pressing with a spoon to remove excess liquid. Discard liquid. Spread spinach in bottom of prepared pan in a shape resembling the size of the fish. Arrange gingerroot and mushrooms evenly over spinach. Season lightly with salt and pepper. Add fish. Sprinkle lightly with salt and pepper.
2. Cover pan loosely with a tent of foil. Bake for 15 minutes or until fish is opaque and flakes easily when tested with a fork.

Variations

- As well as salmon, any white or firm-fleshed fish will do. These are turbot, swordfish, halibut or tuna. For ease of serving fish fillets, cut them into serving-size pieces before baking.
- *Crusty Layered Salmon:* Sprinkle toasted sesame seeds over the fish before baking to give it a crusty crunch.

Nutritional Analysis (Per Serving)
- Calories: 194
- Protein: 26.2 g
- Fat: 7.5 g
- Carbohydrates: 6.2 g
- Fiber: 2.3 g
- Sodium: 131 mg
- Cholesterol: 64 mg

Salmon with Pesto

1 lb	salmon steaks or fillet, cut into 4 serving-sized portions	500 g
1 tsp	vegetable oil	5 mL
1 tsp	lemon juice	5 mL
1 tsp	crushed garlic	5 mL
¼ cup	Pesto Sauce (see recipe, page 59)	50 mL

SERVES 4

Preheat oven to 425°F (220°C) • Baking sheet sprayed with nonstick vegetable spray

1. Place salmon on baking sheet; brush with oil, lemon juice and garlic. Bake approximately 10 minutes or just until fish flakes easily when tested with fork.
2. Top each serving with 1 tbsp (15 mL) Pesto Sauce.

Nutritional Analysis (Per Serving)
- Calories: 209
- Protein: 25 g
- Fat: 11 g
- Carbohydrates: 1 g
- Fiber: 0.5 g
- Sodium: 70 mg
- Cholesterol: 44 mg

Smothered Salmon with Spinach

12	large spinach leaves	12
2 lb	whole salmon	1 kg
1 tbsp	chopped fresh dill (or 1 tsp/5 mL dried dillweed)	15 mL
1/2 tsp	each salt and black pepper	2 mL
1 cup	cold water	250 mL
1 1/2 tsp	margarine, melted	7 mL
1	bunch green onions, sliced (about 2/3 cup/ 150 mL)	1
1	clove garlic, minced	1

In this elegant recipe, salmon is smothered with seasoning, green onion and minced garlic, then poached in the oven on spinach leaves. Serve with a medley of fresh vegetables, if desired.

SERVES 8
Preheat oven to 325°F (160°C) • 13- by 9-inch (3 L) baking dish

1. Arrange spinach leaves on bottom of 13- by 9-inch (3.5 L) baking dish. Top with salmon; sprinkle with dill, salt and pepper. Pour water and margarine over salmon. Top with green onions and garlic. Cover tightly with foil.

2. Bake in preheated oven for 25 to 30 minutes or until salmon flakes easily when tested with fork, basting twice. Arrange salmon with spinach on serving platter with pan juices.

Nutritional Analysis (Per Serving)
- Calories: 157
- Protein: 21 g
- Fat: 7 g
- Carbohydrates: 1 g
- Fiber: Trace
- Sodium: 226 mg
- Cholesterol: 96 mg

Salmon Fillets with Black Bean Sauce

1 lb	salmon fillets	500 g
1/4 cup	chopped green onions (about 2 medium)	50 mL

SAUCE

1/2 cup	chicken stock	125 mL
5 tsp	brown sugar	25 mL
1 tbsp	black bean sauce	15 mL
2 tsp	rice wine vinegar	10 mL
2 tsp	soya sauce	10 mL
2 tsp	sesame oil	10 mL
1 1/4 tsp	cornstarch	6 mL
3/4 tsp	minced ginger root	4 mL
1/2 tsp	minced garlic	2 mL

Make Ahead

Prepare sauce up to 48 hours ahead and keep refrigerated. Stir again before using.

SERVES 4
Preheat oven to 425°F (220°C) • Baking dish sprayed with vegetable spray

1. Put salmon fillets in single layer in prepared baking dish.

2. *Sauce:* In saucepan whisk together stock, brown sugar, black bean sauce, vinegar, soya sauce, sesame oil, cornstarch, ginger and garlic; cook over medium heat, stirring, for 4 minutes or until sauce thickens slightly. Pour over fish and bake uncovered 10 minutes per inch (2.5 cm) thickness of fish, or until fish flakes easily when pierced with a fork. Serve sprinkled with green onions.

Nutritional Analysis (Per Serving)
- Calories: 196
- Protein: 23 g
- Fat: 8 g
- Carbohydrates: 7 g
- Fiber: 0 g
- Sodium: 417 mg
- Cholesterol: 56 mg

Salmon with Lemon-Ginger Sauce

4	salmon fillets, each 5 oz (150 g)	4
MARINADE		
2	green onions	2
1½ tsp	minced fresh gingerroot	7 mL
1	clove garlic, minced	1
2 tbsp	soy sauce	25 mL
1 tbsp	fresh lemon juice	15 mL
1 tsp	grated lemon zest	5 mL
1 tsp	granulated sugar	5 mL
1 tsp	sesame oil	5 mL

Fresh gingerroot gives a sparkling flavor to salmon — or any fish, for that matter. Dried ground ginger doesn't come close to imparting the same crisp taste as fresh gingerroot, which is available in most supermarkets and produce stores.

SERVES 4

Preheat oven to 425°F (220°C) • Shallow baking dish

1. Place salmon fillets in a single layer in baking dish.
2. *Marinade:* Chop green onions; set aside chopped green tops for garnish. In a bowl, combine white part of green onions, ginger, garlic, soy sauce, lemon juice and zest, sugar and sesame oil. Pour marinade over salmon; let stand at room temperature for 15 minutes or in the refrigerator for up to 1 hour.
3. Bake, uncovered, in preheated oven for 13 to 15 minutes or until salmon turns opaque. Arrange on serving plates, spoon sauce over and sprinkle with reserved green onion tops.

Nutritional Analysis (Per Serving)
- Calories: 237
- Protein: 31 g
- Fat: 11 g
- Carbohydrates: 3 g
- Fiber: 0 g
- Sodium: 293 mg
- Cholesterol: 83 mg

Salmon with Cranberry and Caper Vinaigrette

½ cup	red wine vinegar	125 mL
¼ cup	vegetable oil	50 mL
¼ cup	water	50 mL
¼ cup	sliced cranberries	50 mL
2 tbsp	capers	25 mL
1 tbsp	finely chopped shallots	15 mL
1 tsp	minced fresh or dried chives	5 mL
1 tsp	minced garlic	5 mL
½ tsp	pink peppercorns	2 mL
½	each small lemon and lime, peeled and cut into 4 wedges	1/2
¼ to ½ tsp	cayenne pepper	1 to 2 mL
Pinch	dried thyme	Pinch
6	salmon fillets (4 oz/125 g each), skin on	6

SERVES 6

Preheat barbecue or broiler

1. In a jar, combine vinegar, oil, water, cranberries, capers, shallots, chives, garlic, pink peppercorns, lemon and lime wedges, cayenne and thyme; shake well and let stand for 6 to 8 hours.
2. Broil or grill salmon fillets over medium-high heat for 3 to 4 minutes per side or until fish flakes easily when tested with fork.
3. Warm vinaigrette on stove or in microwave; remove lemon and lime wedges. Remove skin from salmon. Serve with vinaigrette spooned over fillets.

Nutritional Analysis (Per Serving)
- Calories: 237
- Protein: 21 g
- Fat: 16 g
- Carbohydrates: 3 g
- Fiber: Trace
- Sodium: 134 mg
- Cholesterol: 34 mg

Broiled Salmon with Green Tapenade and Endive

8 to 16	green olives, pitted and chopped (about 1/3 cup/75 mL)	8 to 16
1/4 cup	chopped packed fresh dill	50 mL
1/4 cup	grated onions, with juices	50 mL
1 tbsp	pine nuts	15 mL
2 tbsp	lemon juice	25 mL
2 tbsp	extra virgin olive oil	25 mL
1/4 tsp	freshly ground black pepper	1 mL
1 tbsp	extra virgin olive oil	15 mL
1	Belgian endive, sliced lengthwise into 1/4 -inch (5 mm) strips	1
1 1/2 lbs	skinless boneless salmon fillet, cut into 4 equal pieces	750 g
	Few sprigs fresh dill	
	Few thin strips red bell pepper	

A tapenade made with green olives is sweeter than its black-olive counterpart — and it works as wonderfully with fish as the black variety works with meat and chicken.

SERVES 4

Baking sheet • Preheat broiler

1. In a food processor combine olives, dill, onions, pine nuts, lemon juice, 2 tbsp (25 mL) olive oil and black pepper. Process, scraping down sides of bowl once, for 1 minute or until coarse but well blended. You should have 1/2 cup (125 mL) green tapenade.

2. Smear 1 tbsp (15 mL) olive oil on baking sheet. Add endive strips and turn them in the oil until thoroughly coated. Push the endive to the sides. Place salmon pieces in the vacated middle. Spread 1 tbsp (15 mL) tapenade thinly on each piece of salmon to cover top surface.

3. On the middle rack of the oven, broil (without turning) 8 to 10 minutes if fillets are from the tail end (which is thinner) and 10 to 12 minutes if they are from the head end. (The minimum times will leave a moist center; the maximum times will give you fish that is well-cooked right through.)

4. Distribute the endive strips (which should be wilted and somewhat charred) in the center of 4 warmed plates. Place the salmon pieces on the beds of endive. Add 1 tbsp (15 mL) fresh tapenade on the center of each nugget and garnish with sprigs of dill and criss-crossed strips of red pepper. Serve immediately.

Tip

• Use large, meaty green olives. The much milder supermarket variety are generally smaller, and you'll need twice as many.

Nutritional Analysis (Per Serving)
• Calories: 371 • Protein: 34.8 g • Fat: 24.0 g
• Carbohydrates: 2.9 g • Fiber: 1.0 g • Sodium: 447 mg
• Cholesterol: 96 mg

Salmon Medallions with Two Purées

CHERRY TOMATO PURÉE

10	cherry tomatoes	10
1 tbsp	sliced green onion	15 mL
1 1/2 tsp	soy sauce	7 mL
1/4 tsp	Worcestershire sauce	1 mL
1/4 tsp	salt	1 mL

BEET PURÉE

3/4 cup	chopped cooked beets	175 mL
2 tbsp	water	25 mL
1 tbsp	chopped onion	15 mL
1 tbsp	red wine vinegar	15 mL
1/4 tsp	salt	1 mL
1 1/4 lb	salmon fillets	625 g
	Black pepper	
1 tbsp	vegetable oil	15 mL
	Chopped fresh chives	

At first glance, this recipe may sound complicated, but it is actually very easy. The two purées — cherry tomato and beet — are easily made in a food processor or blender, then chilled. The slices of salmon are quickly fried in a small amount of oil.

SERVES 6

1. *Cherry Tomato Purée:* In a food processor or blender, process tomatoes, green onion, soy sauce, Worcestershire sauce and salt until smooth. Pour into a small bowl and chill.

2. *Beet Purée:* In a food processor or blender, process beets, water, onion, vinegar and salt until smooth. Pour into a small bowl and chill.

3. Place salmon in freezer for 30 minutes to aid slicing. Slice diagonally into 6 thin medallions. Sprinkle with pepper to taste. In a skillet, heat oil over medium-high heat; quickly cook salmon, about 1 minute per side.

4. To serve, place salmon on plate; spoon purées around salmon. Garnish with chives.

Tips

- When puréeing a small quantity of food, such as these two sauces, use a hand-held blender for convenience.

- These vegetable purées add elegance, color, flavor and nutrients to this dish, but no fat. Enjoy this salmon with a side salad for a special lunch.

Nutritional Analysis (Per Serving)
- Calories: 174
- Protein: 19 g
- Fat: 8 g
- Carbohydrates: 4 g
- Fiber: 1 g
- Sodium: 292 mg
- Cholesterol: 53 mg

Barbecued Stuffed Salmon

1	small onion, finely chopped	1
2	cloves garlic, minced	2
1	stalk celery, finely chopped	1
1 tbsp	butter or margarine	15 mL
1	can (4 1/2 oz/128 g) crabmeat, drained	1
1 cup	cooked rice	250 mL
2 tbsp	lemon juice	25 mL
1 tbsp	finely chopped parsley	15 mL
1 tsp	grated lemon zest	5 mL
1/2 tsp	salt	2 mL
1/4 tsp	black pepper	1 mL
2	salmon fillets (1 1/2 lb/750 g)	2
1/2	lemon, sliced	1/2

This quick and easy-to-make dish is perfect for entertaining. Your guests will be impressed, and you'll be relaxed at serving time.

SERVES 6
Preheat barbecue or oven to 450°F (230°C)

1. In a medium skillet over high heat, cook onion, garlic and celery in butter until softened. Stir in crabmeat, rice, lemon juice, parsley, lemon peel and seasonings.

2. Place stuffing over 1 fish fillet; top with second fillet. Secure with string or toothpicks. Arrange lemon slices on top. Wrap loosely in several thicknesses of aluminum foil.

3. Place on barbecue grill. Cook for about 45 minutes or until fish flakes easily with fork, or bake in preheated oven for 10 minutes per inch (2.5 cm) of thickness.

Tips

- To cook fish on the barbecue, put it in a fish cooker or wrap it loosely in foil left open at the top. This way, the fish will remain moist yet will have that great barbecue flavor.

- Make this recipe the centerpiece of a summer dinner on the deck. Roast an assortment of vegetables on the grill with the salmon. Serve a cold, refreshing bowl of Babsi's Broccoli Soup (see recipe, page 73) while the main course is cooking.

Nutritional Analysis (Per Serving)
- Calories: 238
- Protein: 28 g
- Fat: 9 g
- Carbohydrates: 9 g
- Fiber: Trace
- Sodium: 328 mg
- Cholesterol: 83 mg

Cedar-Baked Salmon

1½ lb	salmon fillets	750 g
	Grated zest and juice of 1 lime	
1½ cups	diagonally sliced asparagus	375 mL
¼ cup	julienned leek	50 mL
4	thin slices red onion	4
¼ cup	diagonally sliced celery	50 mL
½ cup	thickly sliced shiitake mushrooms	125 mL
2	medium tomatoes, seeded and cut into strips	2
8	fresh basil leaves, slivered	8
1	bag (10 oz/300 g) fresh spinach, trimmed	1
	Salt and black pepper	

> *Cedar shingles and shims, available at lumberyards, impart a unique flavor to salmon when baking. For this recipe, you'll need to soak 2 untreated cedar shingles or 1 package of cedar shims in water for at least 2 hours or preferably overnight.*

SERVES 6

Soaked cedar shingles or shims • Preheat oven to 425°F (220°C) • Steamer basket

1. Place soaked shingles or shims on baking sheet; lightly brush with oil. Remove skin and any bones from salmon; cut into 6 serving-size pieces and place on cedar. Sprinkle with lime zest and juice. Bake in preheated oven for 10 to 15 minutes or until fish flakes easily when tested with fork.

2. Meanwhile, in steamer basket, combine asparagus, leek, onion and celery; steam until partially cooked. Add mushrooms, tomatoes, basil and spinach; steam just until tender-crisp and spinach has wilted. Place on 6 individual plates; season with salt and pepper to taste. Top each with salmon.

Tips

- Wood or wood chips, such as mesquite or grape vine, are often used in barbecuing to add flavor to foods. Soaking the wood ensures that it is damp enough to produce lots of aromatic smoke.

- When soaking shingles or shims, weight them down. Otherwise they will float to the surface.

- Salmon is a source of omega-3 fatty acids. Accompanied by an array of vegetables, this recipe is a winner.

Nutritional Analysis (Per Serving)
- Calories: 181
- Protein: 23 g
- Fat: 7 g
- Carbohydrates: 7 g
- Fiber: 3 g
- Sodium: 89 mg
- Cholesterol: 64 mg

Salmon Burgers with Mango Salsa

1/3 cup	finely chopped green peppers	75 mL
1/4 cup	finely chopped fresh dill (or 1 tsp/5 mL dried)	50 mL
3 tbsp	chopped chives	45 mL
3 tbsp	bread crumbs	45 mL
1	egg	1
2 tsp	minced garlic	10 mL
1 lb	salmon, cut into chunks	500 g
SALSA		
3/4 cup	finely diced mangoes or peaches	175 mL
1/2 cup	finely diced red peppers	125 mL
1/4 cup	finely diced green peppers	50 mL
1/4 cup	finely diced red onions	50 mL
2 tbsp	chopped fresh coriander	25 mL
1 tbsp	lemon juice	15 mL
1 tsp	olive oil	5 mL
1/2 tsp	minced garlic	2 mL

SERVES 4 OR 5

1. Put peppers, dill, chives, bread crumbs, egg, garlic and salmon in food processor; process on and off until chunky. Do not purée. Form into 4 or 5 burgers.
2. *Salsa:* In bowl combine mango, red peppers, green peppers, red onions, coriander, lemon juice, olive oil and garlic; mix thoroughly.
3. In nonstick skillet sprayed with nonstick vegetable spray, or on the barbecue, cook patties over medium-high heat for 2 to 3 minutes; turn and cook another 1 minute or until just done at the center. Serve with salsa.

Nutritional Analysis (Per Serving)
- Calories: 186
- Protein: 21 g
- Fat: 6 g
- Carbohydrates: 4 g
- Fiber: 0 g
- Sodium: 145 mg
- Cholesterol: 88 mg

Creamy Salmon Quiche

1/4 cup	dry whole-wheat bread crumbs	50 mL
1 tbsp	100% bran cereal, crushed	15 mL
1	can (7.5 oz/213 g) salmon	1
1/4 cup	chopped green onion	50 mL
1/4 cup	cubed light cream cheese	50 mL
1 tbsp	chopped fresh parsley	15 mL
1 1/4 cups	2% milk	300 mL
3	eggs	3
1/2 tsp	white pepper	2 mL
	Paprika	

SERVES 6
Preheat oven to 350°F (180°C) • 9-inch (23 cm) pie plate, lightly greased

1. Combine bread crumbs and crushed cereal; sprinkle over bottom of prepared pie plate. Break salmon into chunks; arrange chunks over bread crumbs. Top with onion, cream cheese cubes and parsley.
2. Whisk together milk, eggs and pepper. Pour over salmon. Sprinkle lightly with paprika. Bake in preheated oven for 40 minutes or until knife inserted in center comes out clean. Let stand for 5 minutes before cutting into wedges.

Nutritional Analysis (Per Serving)
- Calories: 153
- Protein: 14 g
- Fat: 8 g
- Carbohydrates: 7 g
- Fiber: Trace
- Sodium: 386 mg
- Cholesterol: 148 mg

> *This crustless quiche is prepared in a pie plate and cut into wedges. For a more elegant presentation, bake it in small tart tins and serve as an appetizer.*

Cheesy Salmon Loaf

2	eggs	2
1 cup	rolled oats	250 mL
2	cans (each 7.5 oz/213 g) salmon	2
1 cup	shredded part-skim mozzarella cheese	250 mL
1/4 cup	chopped onion	50 mL
1	stalk celery, chopped	1
1	large carrot, grated	1
2 tbsp	lemon juice	25 mL

Salmon loaf is a perennial favorite for no-fuss family dinners. Grated carrot and part-skim mozzarella add new interest in this tasty version, which is a great standby to make from pantry ingredients.

SERVES 6
Preheat oven to 350°F (180°C) • 9- by 5-inch (2 L) loaf pan, lightly greased

1. In a large bowl, beat eggs. Stir in rolled oats, salmon, cheese, onion, celery, carrot and lemon juice until well combined. Turn salmon mixture into nonstick or lightly greased 9- by 5-inch (2 L) loaf pan. Bake in preheated oven for about 35 minutes. Let stand for 5 minutes before slicing.

Tip

- There is something from all the food groups in this recipe, which provides generous amounts of high-quality protein, niacin, vitamin A and calcium.

Nutritional Analysis (Per Serving)
- Calories: 235
- Protein: 23 g
- Fat: 10 g
- Carbohydrates: 12 g
- Fiber: 2 g
- Sodium: 449 mg
- Cholesterol: 115 mg

Sole with Spinach and Cream Sauce

2 tsp	vegetable oil	10 mL
3/4 cup	chopped onions	175 mL
1 tsp	crushed garlic	5 mL
Half	package (10 oz/300 g) fresh spinach, cooked and drained	Half
	Salt and pepper	
1/3 cup	white wine	75 mL
1 tbsp	lemon juice	15 mL
1 lb	sole fillets	500 g
1 1/2	tsp margarine	7 mL
1 tbsp	all-purpose flour	15 mL
1/3 cup	2% milk	75 mL
2 tbsp	grated Parmesan cheese	25 mL

SERVES 4

1. In small skillet, heat oil; sauté onions and garlic for 3 minutes. Add spinach and cook for 2 minutes. Season with salt and pepper to taste. Spread over flat serving dish. Set aside.

2. In large skillet, bring wine, lemon juice and fish fillets to boil. Reduce heat, cover and simmer just until fish is barely opaque, approximately 3 minutes. With slotted spoon, carefully place fish over spinach mixture, reserving poaching liquid.

3. In small pan, melt margarine; stir in flour and cook for1 minute. Add milk and reserved poaching liquid; simmer, stirring, until thickened. Stir in 1 tbsp (15 mL) cheese; pour over fish. Sprinkle with remaining cheese.

Nutritional Analysis (Per Serving)
- Calories: 188
- Protein: 22 g
- Fat: 6 g
- Carbohydrates: 7 g
- Fiber: 1 g
- Sodium: 182 mg
- Cholesterol: 56 mg

Filet of Sole with Coriander Pesto

PESTO

1 cup	packed roughly chopped coriander	250 mL
1/2 cup	grated strong Italian cheese, such as Asiago, Crotonese or aged Provolone (about 2 oz/50 g)	125 mL
1/4 cup	pine nuts	50 mL
2 tbsp	lime juice	25 mL
1 to 2 tbsp	minced fresh hot chilies or 1/4 to 1/2 tsp (1 to 2 mL) cayenne pepper	15 to 25 mL
1/4 tsp	salt	1 mL
1/8 tsp	freshly ground black pepper	0.5 mL
1/4 cup	extra virgin olive oil	50 mL
1 tsp	olive oil	5 mL
1 lb	filet of sole (about 4 fillets)	500 g
8	thin strips red bell pepper	8

In this dish, the sunbelt tastes of the pesto come from fresh coriander, lime juice and hot chilies.

SERVES 4

Preheat oven to 425°F (220°C) • Baking sheet

1. *Make the pesto:* In a food processor combine coriander, cheese, pine nuts, lime juice, chilies, salt and pepper; process until finely chopped. With machine running, add 1/4 cup (50 mL) olive oil through the feed tube; continue to process until smooth, scraping down sides of bowl once. You should have about 1 cup (250 mL) of a bright green, dense paste. Divide in half. Store one half for another use, tightly covered, in refrigerator for up to 3 days. Set other half aside.

2. Brush the underneath (darker side) of the fillets with a little oil. Lay on baking sheet, oiled side down. Spread about 1 tbsp (15 mL) of the pesto on each filet covering the entire surface. Bake for 6 minutes, without turning. Remove from oven and divide fillets between 4 warmed plates. Heap 1 tbsp (15 mL) pesto on the middle of each fillet. Decorate with 2 red pepper strips making an "x" on each fillet. Serve immediately, accompanied by a vegetable of your choice.

Nutritional Analysis (Per Serving)
- Calories: 349
- Protein: 29.3 g
- Fat: 24.3 g
- Carbohydrates: 3.4 g
- Fiber: 1.0 g
- Sodium: 344 mg
- Cholesterol: 50 mg

Sole with Oriental Peanut Sauce

1 lb	sole fillets	500 g
	Salt and pepper	
⅓ cup	Oriental Peanut Sauce (see recipe, below right)	75 mL
1 tbsp	chopped peanuts	15 mL

SERVES 4
Preheat oven to 425°F (220°C) • Baking dish sprayed with nonstick vegetable spray

1. Season fillets with salt and pepper to taste; place in single layer in baking dish.
2. Pour Oriental Peanut Sauce over fish. Cover and bake for 10 to 15 minutes or just until fish flakes easily when tested with fork. Sprinkle nuts over top.

Tips

- This intense sauce goes well with lighter-flavored fish. Try it over boneless chicken breasts as well.

- Substitute cashews or almonds for the peanuts for a change.

Nutritional Analysis (Per Serving)
- Calories: 149
- Protein: 20 g
- Fat: 7 g
- Carbohydrates: 1 g
- Fiber: 0 g
- Sodium: 251 mg
- Cholesterol: 53 mg

ORIENTAL PEANUT SAUCE

2 tbsp	vegetable oil	25 mL
2 tbsp	rice wine vinegar	25 mL
2 tbsp	water	25 mL
1 tbsp	soya sauce	15 mL
1 tbsp	lemon juice	15 mL
1 tbsp	red wine vinegar	15 mL
4 tsp	peanut butter	20 mL
1 tbsp	hoisin sauce	15 mL
2 tsp	sesame oil	10 mL

MAKES ⅔ CUP (150 ML)

1. In small saucepan, combine vegetable oil, rice wine vinegar, water, soya sauce, lemon juice, red wine vinegar, peanut butter, hoisin sauce and sesame oil; bring to boil and remove immediately.

Nutritional Analysis (Per 1 tbsp/15 mL Serving)
- Calories: 63
- Protein: 1 g
- Fat: 6 g
- Carbohydrates: 1 g
- Fiber: 0 g
- Sodium: 213 mg
- Cholesterol: 0 mg

Stuffed Sole

1 tbsp	butter	15 mL
1/4 cup	chopped green onions	50 mL
1 cup	chopped mushrooms	250 mL
1	red bell pepper, cut into very thin 1-inch (2.5 cm) strips	1
1 tsp	dried tarragon	5 mL
	Salt and white pepper	
8	small sole fillets (about 1 1/2 pounds/750 g)	8
1/3 cup	white wine or fish stock	75 mL
2 tsp	cornstarch	10 mL
1/3 cup	whipping (35%) cream	75 mL

Want to wow your guests? Put this on your menu. Tender sole fillets with vibrant red pepper stuffing marry well in a light wine and cream sauce. It makes an attractive fish dish that never fails to impress.

SERVES 4

Preheat oven to 425°F (220°C) • 8-inch (2 L) square baking dish

1. In a nonstick skillet, heat butter over medium heat. Add green onions, mushrooms, pepper and tarragon; cook, stirring, for 3 minutes or until softened. Let cool.

2. Lay sole fillets, skinned side down, on work surface with smaller tapered ends closest to you; season with salt and pepper. Spoon a generous tablespoonful (15 mL) on bottom ends of fillets. Roll up and place fillets seam-side down in baking dish. Pour wine over top. (Recipe can be prepared up to this point earlier in day, then covered and refrigerated.)

3. To bake, cover with lid or foil; place in preheated oven for 16 to 20 minutes or until fish turns opaque.

4. Using a slotted spoon, remove fillets and arrange on serving plate; cover and keep warm.

5. Strain fish juices through a fine sieve into a medium saucepan; bring to a boil over high heat and reduce to about 1/2 cup (125 mL). In a bowl, blend cornstarch with 1 tbsp (15 mL) cold water; stir in cream. Pour into saucepan, whisking constantly, until sauce comes to a boil and thickens. Adjust seasoning with salt and pepper to taste. Spoon sauce over fish and serve.

Tip

- In the past, fish dishes were adorned with silky rich sauces loaded with cream and butter. Adding only a small amount of whipping cream still gives this sauce its luxurious and creamy appeal, but keeps the calorie count way down.

Nutritional Analysis (Per Serving)
- Calories: 297
- Protein: 33.7 g
- Fat: 12.4 g
- Carbohydrates: 8.2 g
- Fiber: 1.2 g
- Sodium: 178 mg
- Cholesterol: 119 mg

Sole Fillets with Mushroom Stuffing

1 lb	fish fillets, cut into serving-sized pieces	4 500 g
1/3 cup	shredded mozzarella cheese	75 mL
1 tbsp	margarine, melted	15 mL
1 tbsp	lemon juice	15 mL
2 tbsp	chicken stock or white wine	25 mL
2 tbsp	chopped fresh parsley	25 mL

STUFFING

1 tsp	margarine	5 mL
1/2 cup	chopped mushrooms	125 mL
1/3 cup	chopped onions	75 mL
1 tsp	crushed garlic	5 mL
2 tbsp	dry bread crumbs	25 mL
2 tbsp	chopped fresh dill (or 1/2 tsp/2 mL dried dillweed)	25 mL
1 tbsp	water	15 mL

Make Ahead

Prepare stuffing early in the day, but roll up in fillets just before baking.

SERVES 4
Preheat oven to 425°F (220°C) • Baking dish sprayed with nonstick vegetable spray

1. *Stuffing:* In small nonstick skillet, melt margarine; sauté mushrooms, onions and garlic for 5 minutes. Add crumbs, dill and water; mix well.

2. Divide stuffing among fillets; sprinkle with cheese. Roll up fillets and fasten with toothpicks. Place in single layer in baking dish.

3. Combine margarine, lemon juice and stock; pour over fish. Bake for approximately 10 minutes or until fish flakes easily when tested with fork. Garnish with parsley.

Tips

- When working with sole, be gentle. It breaks quite easily.
- A firmer yet still light white fish, such as white fish or orange roughy, can be substituted.

Nutritional Analysis (Per Serving)
- Calories: 175
- Protein: 22 g
- Fat: 7 g
- Carbohydrates: 5 g
- Fiber: 1 g
- Sodium: 233 mg
- Cholesterol: 58 mg

Grilled Swordfish

1 1/2 lb	swordfish steaks	750 g
1/3 cup	minced onion	75 mL
2 tbsp	white wine vinegar	25 mL
1 tbsp	liquid honey	15 mL
Pinch	white pepper	Pinch
	Lime wedges	

In this recipe, a tangy, fat-free marinade adds zest to swordfish, which is particularly well suited to grilling as its flesh is very dense. Since you don't need to worry about tenderizing fish, the marinating time is short.

SERVES 6

1. Cut swordfish into 6 pieces; place in plastic bag. Combine onion, vinegar, honey and pepper; pour over fish. Seal bag and marinate, refrigerated, for 30 minutes, rotating bag occasionally.

2. Remove steaks from marinade. Grill on greased grill or broil for 3 to 5 minutes per side or until fish flakes easily when tested with fork. Garnish with lime wedges.

Nutritional Analysis (Per Serving)
- Calories: 132
- Protein: 24 g
- Fat: 3 g
- Carbohydrates: 2 g
- Fiber: Trace
- Sodium: 104 mg
- Cholesterol: 44 mg

Greek Swordfish with Tomatoes and Feta

2 tbsp	olive oil	25 mL
1	large onion, halved and thinly sliced	1
2	cloves garlic, minced	2
1	can (28 oz/796 mL) diced tomatoes	1
1/3 cup	chopped fresh basil or oregano (or 2 tsp/ 10 mL dried)	75 mL
1/4 cup	dry white wine	50 mL
2 tbsp	tomato paste	25 mL
1 tsp	liquid honey	5 mL
1/4 tsp	salt	1 mL
1/4 tsp	black pepper	1 mL
1	bay leaf	1
6	swordfish steaks, each about 6 oz (175 g)	6
1 cup	crumbled feta cheese (about 5 oz/150 g)	250 mL
	Fresh basil, oregano or parsley	

Make Ahead

Tomato sauce can be refrigerated, covered, for up to 3 days. Reheat until piping hot before pouring over swordfish steaks.

SERVES 6

Preheat oven to 400°F (200°C) • 13- by 9-inch (3 L) baking dish, lightly oiled

1. In a large skillet, heat oil over medium-high heat. Add onion and garlic; cook, stirring, for 3 to 5 minutes or until onion is soft but not brown.

2. Stir in tomatoes, basil, wine, tomato paste, honey, salt, pepper and bay leaf. Increase heat to high; bring to a boil. Reduce heat to medium; simmer, uncovered and stirring occasionally, for 8 to 10 minutes or until sauce has thickened slightly. Discard bay leaf.

3. In the baking dish, arrange swordfish steaks in a single layer; cover evenly with tomato mixture. Bake, uncovered, in preheated oven for 10 to 15 minutes or until sauce is bubbly; sprinkle with feta cheese. Bake for another 5 to 10 minutes or until steaks are opaque, flake easily with a fork, and feta has melted and is starting to brown. Serve garnished with basil.

Variation

• If swordfish is unavailable, substitute halibut, tuna or marlin steaks.

Nutritional Analysis (Per Serving)
• Calories: 368   • Protein: 39.0 g   • Fat: 16.7 g
• Carbohydrates: 13.3 g • Fiber: 2.1 g   • Sodium: 551 mg
• Cholesterol: 88 mg

Swordfish with Gazpacho

2 tbsp	olive oil	25 mL
2	cloves garlic, minced	2
4	swordfish or shark steaks (4 oz/125 g each)	4
1	small onion, chopped	1
3	tomatoes, peeled and chopped (about 2 cups/500 mL)	3
1 cup	chopped seeded peeled cucumber	250 mL
2	green onions, sliced	2
2 tbsp	lemon juice	25 mL
2 tsp	dried basil (or 2 tbsp/ 25 mL chopped fresh)	10 mL
½ tsp	ground cumin	2 mL
Pinch	each dried thyme and black pepper	Pinch

This recipe works well with both swordfish and shark, which are available at many seafood counters or fish shops. Gazpacho, a cold soup made with tomatoes, is given a twist as a warm topping for the fish.

SERVES 4

1. In a large skillet, heat oil over medium-high heat; cook garlic, stirring, for a few seconds. Add fish; lightly brown on both sides. Add onion; cook for 1 to 2 minutes.

2. Add tomatoes, cucumber, green onions, lemon juice, basil, cumin, thyme and pepper. Reduce heat and simmer until fish flakes easily when tested with fork, about 5 minutes.

Tips

• Substitute drained canned tomatoes if ripe fresh tomatoes are not available.

• There are many different varieties of basil, a leafy herb known for its heady aroma. Basil goes so well with tomatoes that it is often referred to as "the tomato herb."

Nutritional Analysis (Per Serving)
- Calories: 219
- Protein: 22 g
- Fat: 11 g
- Carbohydrates: 8 g
- Fiber: 2 g
- Sodium: 123 mg
- Cholesterol: 44 mg

Swordfish Parmigiana

1½ tsp	margarine	7 mL
1 cup	sliced mushrooms	250 mL
½ cup	sliced sweet green pepper	125 mL
½ cup	sliced onions	125 mL
1 tsp	crushed garlic	5 mL
½ tsp	dried basil	2 mL
½ tsp	dried oregano	2 mL
1 cup	tomato sauce	250 mL
1 lb	swordfish, cut into serving-sized pieces	4 500 g
½ cup	shredded mozzarella cheese	125 mL

SERVES 4
Preheat oven to 425°F (220°C)

1. In nonstick skillet, melt margarine; sauté mushrooms, green pepper, onions and garlic for 5 minutes or until softened. Add basil, oregano and tomato sauce; simmer for 5 minutes. Pour half of mixture into baking dish. Place fish over top. Pour remaining sauce over top. Sprinkle with cheese.

2. Bake for 10 to 15 minutes or until fish flakes easily when tested with fork.

Nutritional Analysis (Per Serving)
- Calories: 217
- Protein: 24 g
- Fat: 9 g
- Carbohydrates: 8 g
- Fiber: 2 g
- Sodium: 520 mg
- Cholesterol: 67 mg

Swordfish with Balsamic Vinegar

1 lb	swordfish steak, ³⁄₄-inch (2 cm) thick, cut into 2 pieces	500 g
1 tbsp	olive oil	15 mL
1	bay leaf, crumbled	1
1 tbsp	balsamic vinegar	15 mL
2 tbsp	extra virgin olive oil	25 mL
¹⁄₈ tsp	salt	0.5 mL
¹⁄₈ tsp	freshly ground black pepper	0.5 mL
2	softened sun-dried tomatoes, cut into quarters	2
4	black olives, pitted and chopped into small bits	4
2 tbsp	finely minced red onions	25 mL
	Few sprigs fresh parsley, chopped	

SERVES 2
Preheat grill or broiler

1. Wash and wipe swordfish steaks. Brush both sides with 1 tbsp (15 mL) olive oil. Sprinkle bay leaf crumbles over top sides of the fish. Grill or broil the fish with the bay leaf side facing up for 3 to 5 minutes. Turn over and cook second side for 2 to 4 minutes. (Cook the maximum times if you prefer medium-well done; the shorter times will leave a pink middle.)

2. *Meanwhile prepare the sauce:* In a bowl whisk together vinegar, olive oil, salt and pepper until emulsified, about 1 minute. Stir in sun-dried tomatoes, olives and red onions.

3. When the fish is ready, transfer each steak to a warm plate. Pick off leftover bay leaf pieces. Heap half the sauce on the middle of each steak. Sprinkle chopped parsley over the whole plate and serve immediately.

Swordfish, when fresh (as is desirable), is often very expensive. The frozen variety is substantially cheaper, but expect a 25% loss of quality in texture, tenderness and flavor.

Nutritional Analysis (Per Serving)
- Calories: 501
- Protein: 45.9 g
- Fat: 32.0 g
- Carbohydrates: 6.2 g
- Fiber: 1.3 g
- Sodium: 469 mg
- Cholesterol: 88 mg

Swordfish with Mango Coriander Salsa

1¹⁄₂ lbs	swordfish steaks	750 g
1 tsp	vegetable oil	5 mL
SALSA		
1¹⁄₂ cups	finely diced mango or peach	375 mL
³⁄₄ cup	finely diced red peppers	175 mL
¹⁄₂ cup	finely diced green peppers	125 mL
¹⁄₂ cup	finely diced red onions	125 mL
¹⁄₄ cup	chopped fresh coriander	50 mL
2 tbsp	lemon juice	25 mL
2 tsp	olive oil	10 mL
1 tsp	minced garlic	5 mL

SERVES 6
Start barbecue or preheat oven to 425°F (220°C)

1. Brush fish with 1 tsp (5 mL) of oil on both sides. Barbecue or bake fish for 10 minutes per inch (2.5 cm) thickness, or until it flakes easily when pierced with a fork.

2. Meanwhile, in bowl combine mango, red peppers, green peppers, red onions, coriander, lemon juice, olive oil and garlic; mix thoroughly. Serve over fish.

Nutritional Analysis (Per Serving)
- Calories: 197
- Protein: 22 g
- Fat: 7 g
- Carbohydrates: 11 g
- Fiber: 2 g
- Sodium: 101 mg
- Cholesterol: 43 mg

Swordfish Kabobs with Lime and Garlic Marinade

1 lb	swordfish, cut into 16 cubes	500 g
16	pieces (2-inch/5 cm) sweet red pepper	16
16	pieces (2-inch/5 cm) sweet green pepper	16
16	medium mushroom caps	16
16	pieces (2-inch/5 cm) onion	16
MARINADE		
3 tbsp	lime or lemon juice	45 mL
2 tbsp	vegetable oil	25 mL
3 tbsp	chopped fresh coriander or parsley	45 mL
2 tbsp	water	25 mL
1 tsp	crushed garlic	5 mL
1 tsp	Dijon mustard	5 mL

SERVES 4

1. Alternately thread 2 pieces each of swordfish, red pepper, green pepper, mushrooms and onion onto 8 barbecue skewers.

2. *Marinade:* Combine lime juice, oil, coriander, water, garlic and mustard; pour into shallow dish large enough to hold kabobs. Add kabobs; marinate for 30 minutes, turning occasionally.

3. Barbecue kabobs, brushing with marinade and turning carefully, for 10 to 15 minutes or until fish flakes easily when tested with fork.

Nutritional Analysis (Per Serving)
- Calories: 250
- Protein: 22 g
- Fat: 12 g
- Carbohydrates: 12 g
- Fiber: 3 g
- Sodium: 80 mg
- Cholesterol: 60 mg

Swordfish Kebabs with Parsley Sauce

3 tbsp	extra virgin olive oil	45 mL
2 tbsp	finely chopped fresh parsley	25 mL
1 tbsp	lemon juice	15 mL
1 tsp	balsamic vinegar	5 mL
1/4 tsp	salt	1 mL
1/8 tsp	freshly ground black pepper	0.5 mL
1 1/2 lbs	boneless skinless swordfish, cut into 1-inch (2.5 cm) cubes	750 g
Half	red bell pepper, cut into 1-inch (2.5 cm) squares	Half
Half	green or yellow pepper, cut into 1-inch (2.5 cm) squares	Half
1	onion, cut into 1-inch (2.5 cm) chunks	1
1 tsp	olive oil	5 mL
2	bay leaves, crumbled	2
	Tomato wedges	

SERVES 4

Eight 8-inch (20 cm) metal skewers or wooden skewers soaked in water • Preheat grill or broiler

1. *Make the parsley sauce:* In a small bowl, whisk together 3 tbsp (45 mL) olive oil, parsley, lemon juice, vinegar, salt and pepper. Set aside.

2. Skewer swordfish, alternating it with pieces of red pepper, green pepper and onion. Brush the skewers with a little oil and scatter crumbled bay leaves over everything.

3. Grill or broil the skewers for 3 to 5 minutes; turn over and cook 2 to 4 minutes. (Cook the maximum times if you prefer medium-well done; the shorter times will leave a pink middle.)

4. Garnish with wedges of tomato and serve immediately with parsley sauce on the side for spooning at table.

Nutritional Analysis (Per Serving)
- Calories 352
- Protein 35.1 g
- Fat 18.2 g
- Carbohydrates 11.4 g
- Fiber 2.2 g
- Sodium 308 mg
- Cholesterol 66 mg

Lemon Dill Tilapia

2	tilapia fillets (about 12 oz/375 g total)	2
2 tbsp	lemon juice	25 mL
1 tbsp	olive oil	15 mL
2 tbsp	chopped fresh dillweed	25 mL
1/4 tsp	salt	1 mL

Tilapia is a mild and delicate fish similar to snapper. Haddock, sole or snapper can also be used in this recipe.

SERVES 2

1. Place fillets in a shallow baking dish. Sprinkle fish with lemon juice, oil, dill and salt. Turn fish to coat all sides. Marinate for 10 minutes.
2. Place fillets on lightly greased broiler rack placed over oven pan.
3. Broil under preheated toaster oven broiler for 10 minutes, or until fish flakes easily when tested with a fork.

Tip

- The fillets should be about 1/2 inch (1 cm) thick; otherwise adjust the cooking time. (Check the oven manufacturer's manual to see whether the door should be left ajar during broiling.)

Nutritional Analysis (Per Serving)
- Calories: 232
- Protein: 34.9 g
- Fat: 9.0 g
- Carbohydrates: 0.9 g
- Fiber: 0.1 g
- Sodium: 399 mg
- Cholesterol: 60 mg

Lake Trout with Red Pepper Sauce

1 lb	lake or salmon trout fillets	500 g
1 tsp	vegetable oil	5 mL
	Salt and pepper	
SAUCE		
1 1/2 tsp	margarine	7 mL
1 tsp	crushed garlic	5 mL
1/4 cup	chopped onion	50 mL
1	medium sweet red pepper, diced	1
1/2 cup	chicken stock	125 mL
1 1/2 tsp	vegetable oil	7 mL

Make Ahead

Prepare and refrigerate sauce up to a day before.

SERVES 4
Preheat oven to 425°F (220°C) • Baking dish sprayed with nonstick vegetable spray

1. Brush fish with oil; season with salt and pepper to taste and place in single layer in baking dish.
2. *Sauce:* In nonstick skillet, heat margarine; sauté garlic and onion for 2 minutes. Add red pepper and stock; simmer for 5 minutes.
3. Pour sauce into food processor; add oil and purée until smooth. Pour over fish. Bake for 12 to 15 minutes or just until fish flakes easily when tested with fork.

Tip

- This fish can also be broiled and the sauce served alongside.

Nutritional Analysis (Per Serving)
- Calories: 204
- Protein: 25 g
- Fat: 10 g
- Carbohydrates: 2 g
- Fiber: 0.5 g
- Sodium: 168 mg
- Cholesterol: 42 mg

Trout with Fresh Tomato Herb Sauce

2	ripe tomatoes, seeded and diced	2
2 tbsp	chopped fresh basil or chives	25 mL
2 tbsp	chopped fresh parsley	25 mL
1 tbsp	balsamic vinegar	15 mL
2 tbsp	olive oil, divided	25 mL
	Salt and freshly ground black pepper	
4	trout fillets (each 5 oz/150 g)	4
¼ cup	white wine or chicken stock	50 mL

Here's a summery no-fuss cooking technique for trout or salmon or any of your favorite fish, including red snapper or tilapia. Serve with green beans.

SERVES 4

10-cup (2.5 L) shallow rectangular baking dish or 11- by 7-inch (2 L) baking dish

1. In a bowl, combine tomatoes, basil, parsley, vinegar and 1 tbsp (15 mL) of the oil. Season with salt and pepper to taste. Set aside.

2. Place trout in baking dish. Season fillets with salt and pepper. Drizzle with remaining olive oil and wine.

3. Cover with plastic wrap and turn back one corner to vent. Microwave on Medium (50%) for 3½ to 5 minutes or until fish is opaque. Let stand, covered, for 2 minutes. To serve, arrange fish on serving plates and top with a spoonful of the tomato sauce.

Nutritional Analysis (Per Serving)
- Calories: 298
- Protein: 30.3 g
- Fat: 16.3 g
- Carbohydrates: 4.2 g
- Fiber: 1.2 g
- Sodium: 154 mg
- Cholesterol: 80 mg

Crab, Bok Choy and Cheddar Egg Foo Yung

6	large eggs	6
1 cup	milk	250 mL
2	green onions, finely sliced	2
4 oz	crab meat	125 g
1 cup	finely chopped bok choy	250 mL
	Salt and pepper to taste	
1 tbsp	vegetable oil	15 mL
1 cup	shredded Cheddar cheese	250 mL
1 tsp	sesame oil	5 mL

This is a great dish for a special brunch or when you're entertaining house guests.

SERVES 4

Preheat oven to 350°F (180°C) • Ovenproof skillet

1. In a medium bowl, whisk eggs and milk together until well blended. Add onions, crab and bok choy. Season with salt and pepper; stir to combine.

2. In an ovenproof skillet, heat oil over medium heat for 30 seconds. Add egg mixture and stir with a spatula until the egg begins to scramble but is still fairly moist. Spread Cheddar over top and bake for 7 to 8 minutes or until the egg is firmly set and the cheese is melted. Remove from oven; drizzle with sesame oil and serve straight from pan.

Nutritional Analysis (Per Serving)
- Calories: 337
- Protein: 24.0 g
- Fat: 24.0 g
- Carbohydrates: 5.4 g
- Fiber: 0.5 g
- Sodium: 397 mg
- Cholesterol: 380 mg

Zucchini Stuffed with Crabmeat, Tomatoes and Dill

4	zucchini	4
2 tsp	margarine or butter	10 mL
1 tsp	minced garlic	5 mL
1/3 cup	chopped onions	75 mL
6 oz	chopped crabmeat	150 g
1/3 cup	chopped tomatoes	75 mL
3 tbsp	seasoned bread crumbs	45 mL
3 tbsp	chopped fresh dill (or 2 tsp/10 mL dried)	45 mL
2 tbsp	light sour cream	25 mL
2 tbsp	chopped green onions (about 1 medium)	25 mL
1 tbsp	grated Parmesan cheese	15 mL

Make Ahead

Shells can be filled up to a day ahead, covered and kept in refrigerator. Bake for 20 minutes to heat thoroughly.

SERVES 4

Preheat oven to 400°F (200°C) • Baking sheet

1. Trim ends of zucchini. Cook in boiling water, covered, for 5 minutes or until tender. Rinse with cold water and drain. Cut in half lengthwise; scoop out pulp, leaving shell intact. Chop pulp and squeeze out moisture. Set aside. Place shells on baking sheet.

2. In nonstick saucepan, heat margarine over medium heat; cook garlic and onions for 4 minutes or until softened. Add zucchini pulp and cook for 4 minutes more.

3. Place vegetable mixture in food processor along with crabmeat, tomatoes, bread crumbs, dill, sour cream and green onions. Pulse on and off just until finely chopped. Divide among shells. Sprinkle with Parmesan.

4. Bake for 10 minutes or until heated through.

Tips

- Try yellow zucchini if available.
- Diced, cooked shrimp can substitute for crabmeat. Imitation crab (surimi) can also be used.
- When using margarine, choose a soft (non-hydrogenated) version to limit consumption of trans fats.

Nutritional Analysis (Per Serving)
- Calories: 113
- Protein: 10 g
- Fat: 3 g
- Carbohydrates: 12 g
- Fiber: 3 g
- Sodium: 756 mg
- Cholesterol: 4 mg

Mussels with Tomatoes, Basil and Garlic

2 lb	mussels	1 kg
1½ tsp	vegetable oil	7 mL
½ cup	finely diced onions	125 mL
2 tsp	crushed garlic	10 mL
1	can (14 oz/398 mL) tomatoes, drained and chopped	1
⅓ cup	dry white wine	75 mL
1 tbsp	chopped fresh basil (or ½ tsp/2 mL dried)	15 mL
1½ tsp	chopped fresh oregano (or ¼ tsp/1 mL dried)	7 mL

SERVES 4

1. Scrub mussels under cold water; pull off hairy beards. Discard any that do not close when tapped. Set aside.

2. In large nonstick saucepan, heat oil; sauté onions and garlic for 2 minutes. Add tomatoes, wine, basil and oregano; cook for 3 minutes, stirring constantly.

3. Add mussels; cover and cook until mussels fully open, 4 to 5 minutes. Discard any that do not open. Arrange mussels in bowls; pour sauce over top.

Tips

- When you're buying mussels, the shells should be tightly closed.
- Fresh juicy tomatoes are excellent when in season.
- Substitute clams for the mussels.

Nutritional Analysis (Per Serving)
- Calories: 108
- Protein: 10 g
- Fat: 2 g
- Carbohydrates: 8 g
- Fiber: 2 g
- Sodium: 351 mg
- Cholesterol: 22 mg

Mussels with Sweet Bell Peppers and Garlic

1 cup	white wine	250 mL
⅓ cup	thinly sliced carrots	75 mL
½ cup	thinly sliced celery	125 mL
½ cup	thinly sliced yellow peppers	125 mL
½ cup	thinly sliced red peppers	125 mL
2 tsp	crushed garlic	10 mL
2 lb	mussels (see tip, page 163)	1 kg
⅓ cup	freshly chopped parsley or dill	75 mL

SERVES 4

1. Put wine in a large saucepan; add carrots, celery, yellow peppers and red peppers. Add garlic and mussels. Cover and cook just until mussels are open, approximately 3 minutes. Discard any mussels that do not open.

2. Pour into serving dish and sprinkle with parsley.

Tips

- Use clams for a change.
- Steam with fish or vegetable stock.

Nutritional Analysis (Per Serving)
- Calories: 190
- Protein: 11 g
- Fat: 4 g
- Carbohydrates: 9 g
- Fiber: 0 g
- Sodium: 320 mg
- Cholesterol: 30 g

Mussels with Basil and Parsley Pesto

PESTO

1 cup	packed fresh basil	250 mL
1/4 cup	packed fresh parsley	50 mL
3 tbsp	olive oil	45 mL
2 tbsp	pine nuts, toasted	25 mL
2 tbsp	grated Parmesan cheese	25 mL
1 tsp	minced garlic	5 mL
1/4 cup	water	50 mL
1/4 cup	white wine	50 mL
2 lbs	cleaned mussels	1 kg

Make Ahead

Prepare pesto earlier in the day, cover and refrigerate. Pesto can also be frozen for up to 2 weeks.

SERVES 4

1. *Pesto:* Put basil, parsley, olive oil, pine nuts, Parmesan and garlic in food processor; process until finely chopped, scraping down sides of bowl once. With machine running, gradually add water through feed tube; process until smooth.

2. Put pesto and wine in large heavy-bottomed saucepan. Bring to a boil; add mussels and cover. Cook, shaking the saucepan for 2 minutes, or just until mussels open. Discard any that do not open.

Tip

- To clean mussels, cut off any beards that are visible and check the condition of the shells — discard any with cracked or broken shells, as well as any that are opened and will not close when you tap them.

Nutritional Analysis (Per Serving)
- Calories: 201
- Protein: 11 g
- Fat: 15 g
- Carbohydrates: 4 g
- Fiber: 1 g
- Sodium: 240 mg
- Cholesterol: 23 mg

Mussels with Pesto

1/4 cup	white wine or chicken stock	50 mL
2 lbs	cleaned mussels (see tip, in recipe above)	1 kg

PESTO

1 1/4 cups	packed fresh basil	300 mL
3 tbsp	olive oil	45 mL
2 tbsp	toasted pine nuts	25 mL
2 tbsp	grated Parmesan cheese	25 mL
1 tsp	minced garlic	5 mL
1/4 cup	chicken stock	50 mL

Make Ahead

Prepare pesto earlier in the day, cover and refrigerate. Pesto can also be frozen for up to 2 weeks.

SERVES 4

1. *Pesto:* Put basil, olive oil, pine nuts, Parmesan and garlic in food processor; process until finely chopped, scraping down sides of bowl once. With machine running, gradually add stock through feed tube; process until smooth.

2. Put pesto and wine in large heavy-bottomed saucepan. Bring to a boil; add mussels and cover. Cook, shaking the saucepan for 2 minutes, or just until mussels open. Discard any that do not open.

Nutritional Analysis (Per Serving)
- Calories: 201
- Protein: 11 g
- Fat: 15 g
- Carbohydrates: 4 g
- Fiber: 1 g
- Sodium: 312 mg
- Cholesterol: 23 mg

Broiled Scallops on Eggplant Purée

1	large eggplant (about 1½ lbs/750 g)	1
1 tsp	vegetable oil	5 mL
1	medium onion, coarsely grated, with juices	1
½ tsp	salt	2 mL
¼ tsp	freshly ground black pepper	1 mL
½ tsp	ground nutmeg	2 mL
2 tbsp	extra virgin olive oil	25 mL
2 tbsp	lemon juice	25 mL
1 tbsp	melted butter (optional)	15 mL
1 tbsp	finely chopped fresh basil (or ½ tsp/2 mL dried)	15 mL
1 lb	large sea scallops (about 12 to 16)	500 g
1 tbsp	olive oil	15 mL
	Few sprigs fresh basil and parsley, chopped	

SERVES 4

Baking sheet • Preheat oven to 450°F (230°C)

1. Brush eggplant lightly with vegetable oil. Using a fork, pierce the skin lightly at 1-inch (2.5 cm) intervals. Place on baking sheet. Bake for 1 hour or until eggplant is very soft and the skin is dark brown and caved in. Remove from oven and let cool for 15 minutes.

2. Meanwhile, in a nonstick frying pan, combine grated onion with its juices, salt, pepper and ground nutmeg; cook, stirring, over high heat for 2 minutes or until liquid has evaporated. Add 2 tbsp (25 mL) olive oil and cook, stirring, for 1 minute or until just beginning to brown, Remove from heat and set aside in the frying pan.

3. When cool enough to handle, cut off and discard stem and bottom 1 inch (2.5 cm) of eggplant. Peel the eggplant (the peel should come off easily), scraping pulp from the inside of the peel (discard peels). Cut open the peeled eggplant to reveal its many dark seed pods. Using a small spoon, remove and discard as many seed pods as you can. Transfer the remaining pulp to a colander and let excess liquid drain. (Do not push down on solids.)

4. Transfer the drained eggplant to a small bowl. Add lemon juice. Using a wooden spoon, mash and stir the pulp until puréed. Add purée to onion in the frying pan. Add melted butter, if using, and chopped basil; mix and fold until everything is well integrated. Set aside in the frying pan. (The recipe can be prepared in advance to this point, then kept up to 2 hours, covered and unrefrigerated.)

5. Roll scallops in 1 tbsp (15 mL) olive oil and arrange in a single layer on baking sheet. Broil on one side only for 7 to 9 minutes or to your liking (at 7 minutes, scallops will be firm to the touch and moist inside). During the last minutes of broiling, place frying pan with eggplant purée over high heat; cook, stirring, for 1 to 2 minutes or until bubbling.

6. Put pillows of purée in the center of 4 warmed plates. Portion the broiled scallops directly on each purée. Garnish with chopped basil and serve immediately.

Nutritional Analysis (Per Serving)
- Calories: 298
- Protein: 21.2 g
- Fat: 16.4 g
- Carbohydrates: 17.5 g
- Fiber: 4.8 g
- Sodium: 520 mg
- Cholesterol: 46 mg

Shrimp and Scallops with Cheesy Cream Sauce

1 tbsp	margarine	15 mL
1 tsp	crushed garlic	5 mL
1/3 cup	chopped green onions	75 mL
1 lb	seafood (shrimp, scallops or combination)	500 g
1/4 cup	chopped fresh parsley	50 mL
2 oz	goat or feta cheese, crumbled	50 g

SAUCE

1 tbsp	margarine	15 mL
2 1/2 tsp	all-purpose flour	12 mL
1/3 cup	dry white wine	75 mL
1/2 cup	2% milk	125 mL

SERVES 4

1. *Sauce:* In small saucepan, melt margarine; stir in flour and cook, stirring, for 1 minute. Add wine and milk; cook, stirring, until thickened and smooth, approximately 2 minutes. Set aside and keep warm.

2. In nonstick skillet, melt margarine; sauté garlic, green onions and seafood just until seafood is opaque. Remove from stove; add sauce and mix well.

3. Pour into serving dish; sprinkle parsley and cheese over top.

Nutritional Analysis (Per Serving)
- Calories: 234
- Protein: 25 g
- Fat: 10 g
- Carbohydrates: 6 g
- Fiber: 0.5 g
- Sodium: 498 mg
- Cholesterol: 113 mg

Garlic Shrimp with Mushrooms

3 tbsp	olive oil	45 mL
1/4 tsp	salt	1 mL
1/4 tsp	freshly ground black pepper	1 mL
8 oz	raw large shrimp, peeled and deveined	250 g
6 oz	wild or button mushrooms, trimmed and halved	175 g
1 tbsp	minced garlic	15 mL
1 tbsp	lemon zest, cut into thin ribbons	15 mL
3 tbsp	white wine	45 mL
1 tbsp	lemon juice	15 mL
	Few sprigs fresh parsley, chopped	

SERVES 2 AS A MAIN COURSE OR 4 AS A STARTER

1. In a large frying pan, heat olive oil, salt and pepper over high heat for 1 minute. Add shrimp and mushrooms; stir-fry actively for 3 minutes or until the shrimp are pink on both sides and the mushrooms are soft.

2. Immediately add garlic and zest; stir-fry for under 1 minute or until the garlic is beginning to color. Add wine and lemon juice; cook, stirring, for 1 minute or until the liquid bubbles. Reduce heat to medium; cook, stirring, for 1 to 2 minutes or until a thick sauce has formed, but before it reduces too much. Remove from heat.

3. Transfer to a serving dish, garnish liberally with parsley and serve immediately.

Nutritional Analysis (Per Serving)
- Calories: 348
- Protein: 26.4 g
- Fat: 22.6 g
- Carbohydrates: 7.0 g
- Fiber: 1.6 g
- Sodium: 467 mg
- Cholesterol: 172 mg

Spanish Shrimp with Paprika

1 lb	raw medium shrimp	500 g
⅓ cup	olive oil	75 mL
Half	green pepper, thinly sliced	Half
1 tbsp	sweet paprika	15 mL
¼ tsp	salt	1 mL
Pinch	cayenne pepper	Pinch
2 tbsp	finely chopped garlic	25 mL
½ tsp	dried oregano	2 mL
	Few sprigs fresh parsley, chopped	
	Lemon wedges	

These shrimp make for a messy but entertaining nosh. The shells (minus the legs) are left on for a reason: the shrimp end up more succulent, so you're free to enjoy them just as they are once shelled at table or, more richly, by dipping them in their cooking sauce — a lusty concoction of oil, garlic and spices.

SERVES 2 AS A MAIN COURSE OR 4 AS A STARTER

1. Wash shrimp. As carefully as possible, peel off the little legs and belly shell on the underside of the shrimps without removing either the main part of the shell on the topside or the tail. Set aside.

2. In a large frying pan, heat olive oil over high heat for 1 minute. Add green peppers, paprika, salt and cayenne; stir-fry for 1 to 2 minutes or until the green pepper has wilted. Immediately add reserved shrimp; stir-fry for 2 minutes. Add garlic and oregano; stir-fry for 2 more minutes or until the garlic has started to brown and the shrimps are bright pink and springy. Remove from heat.

3. Transfer to a serving dish, garnish with chopped parsley and fit lemon wedges around the dish for squeezing at table. Serve immediately.

Nutritional Analysis (Per Serving)
- Calories: 588
- Protein: 47.1 g
- Fat: 40.2 g
- Carbohydrates: 9.0 g
- Fiber: 2.1 g
- Sodium: 631 mg
- Cholesterol: 344 mg

Shrimp in Tomato Sauce with Feta

2 tbsp	vegetable oil	25 mL
1 lb	peeled and deveined shrimp, thawed if frozen	500 g
2 tbsp	minced garlic	25 mL
	Freshly ground black pepper	
¼ cup	lemon juice	50 mL
1 cup	tomato sauce	250 mL
4 oz	crumbled feta cheese (about 1 cup/250 mL)	125 g

SERVES 4
Preheat broiler • 6-cup (1.5 L) shallow baking or gratin dish

1. In a skillet, heat oil over medium-high heat. Add shrimp and cook, stirring, until they firm up and turn pink, 3 to 5 minutes. Using a slotted spoon, transfer to baking dish. Reduce heat to medium-low and return pan to element.

2. Add garlic, and black pepper to taste. Cook, stirring, for 1 minute. Add lemon juice and stir. Add tomato sauce and bring to a simmer.

3. Pour mixture over shrimp. Sprinkle with cheese. Place under preheated broiler until cheese begins to melt and turn brown, about 3 minutes.

Nutritional Analysis (Per Serving)
- Calories: 304
- Protein: 29.3 g
- Fat: 16.8 g
- Carbohydrates: 8.5 g
- Fiber: 1 g
- Sodium: 957 mg
- Cholesterol: 206 mg

Shrimp with Tomato and Feta

3 tbsp	olive oil	45 mL
¼ tsp	freshly ground black pepper	1 mL
Pinch	salt	Pinch
1 cup	thinly sliced onions	250 mL
1 tbsp	lemon zest, cut into ribbons	15 mL
12 oz	plum tomatoes, peeled and quartered, with juices	375 g
1 tsp	dried oregano	5 mL
2 tbsp	lemon juice	25 mL
1 tsp	drained capers	5 mL
1 lb	raw medium shrimp, peeled and deveined	500 g
5 oz	feta cheese, finely crumbled	150 g
	Few sprigs fresh parsley, chopped	

SERVES 3 OR 4

8- or 9-inch (20 or 22.5 cm) round ovenproof dish • Preheat broiler

1. In a large frying pan, heat olive oil with pepper and salt over high heat for 1 minute. Add onions and stir-fry for 2 minutes or until softened and starting to brown. Add lemon zest and stir-fry for 30 seconds. Immediately add tomatoes and oregano; stir-fry 2 minutes or until the tomatoes begin to break up and a sauce starts to form.

2. Add lemon juice, capers and the shrimp; stir-fry for exactly 1 minute, turning the shrimp so that they are light pink on both sides and all the ingredients are well mixed together.

3. Transfer contents of the pan to an ovenproof dish, spreading everything into a flat layer. Sprinkle feta crumbles evenly to cover the entire surface. Broil 6 to 7 minutes until the feta is quite brown and the juices are bubbling up around the perimeter of the dish.

4. Bring the dish immediately to table and scoop out portions, garnishing them with chopped parsley.

Nutritional Analysis (Per Serving)
- Calories: 345
- Protein: 29.6 g
- Fat: 20.3 g
- Carbohydrates: 11.0 g
- Fiber: 1.6 g
- Sodium: 690 mg
- Cholesterol: 206 mg

Shrimp and Zucchini in Buttermilk Herb Sauce

	Fish stock or water	
24	shrimp, peeled and deveined	24
2	medium zucchini	2
½ cup	buttermilk	125 mL
¼ cup	light sour cream	50 mL
¼ cup	lower-fat plain yogurt	50 mL
1 tbsp	each chopped fresh basil, chives and dill	15 mL
Pinch	coarsely ground black pepper	Pinch

Here's an unusual recipe that uses thin strips of zucchini to replace pasta. Serve cold for a summer lunch, garnished with a basil leaf or sprig of dill.

SERVES 4

1. In a skillet of gently simmering fish stock, poach shrimp until pink; drain and chill.
2. Cut zucchini in half lengthwise; place flat side down and slice into thin ribbons resembling fettuccine. Steam until just tender-crisp. Chill.
3. In a bowl, combine buttermilk, sour cream, yogurt, basil, chives, dill and pepper; stir in zucchini. Divide among plates; top with shrimp.

Tip

- Many people have the misconception that buttermilk is fattening, but, in fact, it has less fat than 2% milk! Traditionally, it came from milk that was used to make butter and that soured naturally. Today's buttermilk is artificially soured. It has a longer shelf life than regular milk because its higher acid content helps to inhibit the growth of most spoilage-causing bacteria.

Nutritional Analysis (Per Serving)
- Calories: 142
- Protein: 21 g
- Fat: 3 g
- Carbohydrates: 8 g
- Fiber: 1 g
- Sodium: 215 mg
- Cholesterol: 174 mg

Poached Jumbo Shrimp

½ cup	dry white wine	125 mL
2	sprigs fresh parsley	2
2	shallots, sliced	2
36	jumbo shrimp	36

Grilled or baked fish truly benefits when served with mango salsa. For extra heat, add some finely chopped jalapeño pepper.

SERVES 6

1. In a large saucepan, bring wine, ½ cup (125 mL) water, parsley and shallots to a boil. Add shrimp. Reduce heat to medium and cook slowly for 4 minutes or until shrimp turn pink.
2. Remove with a slotted spoon to a bowl. Serve 6 shrimp per person with Fresh Mango Salsa (see recipe, below).

Tip

- To check a mango's ripeness, hold it in your hand — it should feel like a good handshake, firm with a little give. To ripen further, store unripe mangoes at room temperature for 2 to 4 days in a paper bag, then store them in the refrigerator.

Nutritional Analysis (Per Serving)
- Calories: 245
- Protein: 35.0 g
- Fat: 5.2 g
- Carbohydrates: 9.9 g
- Fiber: 1.0 g
- Sodium: 257 mg
- Cholesterol: 258 mg

FRESH MANGO SALSA

1	large ripe mango, peeled and finely diced (see tip, above)	1
2	green onions, sliced	2
1 tbsp	extra virgin olive oil	15 mL
2 tsp	freshly squeezed lemon juice	10 mL
	Salt and freshly ground black pepper	

MAKES 2 CUPS (500 ML)

1. In a small bowl, stir together mango, onions, oil, lemon juice and salt and pepper to taste.
2. Cover and refrigerate for up to 2 days.

Golden Shrimp with Cilantro and Lime

8	cloves garlic	8
2 tsp	salt	10 mL
3 lbs	shrimp, peeled and deveined	1.5 kg
1	bay leaf	1
½ cup	lime juice, divided	125 mL
2¼ tsp	turmeric, divided	11 mL
1 tsp	cayenne pepper	5 mL
½ cup	cilantro leaves, divided	125 mL

SERVES 8

1. Mash garlic and salt to a paste with a mortar and pestle and rub into shrimp. Set aside for 15 minutes.

2. In a large saucepan over medium-high heat, combine 8 cups (2 L) water, bay leaf, 1 tbsp (15 mL) of the lime juice and 2 tsp (10 mL) of the turmeric. Bring to a boil. When water is boiling, stir in shrimp and cook just until opaque, 2 to 3 minutes. Do not overcook. Drain and transfer shrimp to a bowl.

3. Stir together remaining turmeric, cayenne pepper and remaining lime juice. Pour over warm shrimp. Toss until well combined.

4. Chop half of the cilantro leaves and add to cooled shrimp. Add remaining whole leaves and toss. Adjust seasonings and refrigerate for at least 3 hours before serving.

Tip

- Serve over a bed of greens as a first course or as an entrée. I also like to serve it as a cocktail appetizer or as part of a buffet.

Nutritional Analysis (Per Serving)
- Calories: 192
- Protein: 34.9 g
- Fat: 3.0 g
- Carbohydrates: 4.7 g
- Fiber: 0.3 g
- Sodium: 834 mg
- Cholesterol: 258 mg

Charcoal-Grilled Spiced Squid with Ginger and Mint-Tomato Dip

MINT-TOMATO DIP

2 tsp	canola oil	10 mL
1	small onion, thinly sliced	1
1 tbsp	minced ginger root	15 mL
2	cloves garlic, minced	2
2	large tomatoes, chopped	2
1 tbsp	sugar	15 mL
1 tbsp	rice vinegar	15 mL
1 tbsp	lime juice	15 mL
1 tbsp	lemon juice	15 mL
2 tsp	finely chopped green onions	10 mL
2 tsp	finely chopped basil	10 mL
2 tsp	finely chopped mint	10 mL

SPICED SQUID

4	whole star anise (or 1 tsp/5 mL ground anise)	4
1 tsp	white pepper	5 mL
1 tsp	cinnamon	5 mL
1 tsp	cayenne pepper	5 mL
1 tsp	coarse Hungarian paprika	5 mL
1 tsp	ground cloves	5 mL
Pinch	salt	Pinch
1½ lbs	squid bodies and tentacles (fresh or frozen)	750 g

SERVES 6

Preheat barbecue or grill • 12 long bamboo skewers soaked in water

1. *Mint-tomato dip:* In a large nonstick skillet, heat oil over medium heat. Add onion and sauté 4 to 6 minutes or until brown. Stir in ginger and garlic; sauté for another minute. Add tomatoes; reduce heat to low and cook, stirring constantly, until slightly thickened. Add sugar and rice vinegar; cook, stirring constantly for an another 2 minutes. Transfer mixture to a bowl to cool. Stir in lime juice, lemon juice, green onions, basil and mint.

2. *Spiced squid:* In a blender or spice mill, grind star anise to a powder. Add anise powder to a bowl and mix with white pepper, cinnamon, cayenne, paprika, ground cloves and salt. Rub squid all over with spices.

3. Thread skewers through squid and grill over charcoal fire for 2 minutes on one side, turn over and cook 1 to 2 minutes more. Do not overcook or the squid will be tough.

4. Before serving, remove tentacles from skewers; if desired, slice squid bodies into rings. Serve with mint-tomato dip.

Tip

- Many fish markets will clean the squid upon request, but here's how to prepare it yourself: Separate the tentacles from the body by pulling firmly. Then take out the transparent quill from inside the body and discard. Cut the tentacles off just above the eyes and squeeze out the hard beak from the center of the tentacles. Finally, peel off the skin from the body.

Nutritional Analysis (Per Serving)
- Calories: 155
- Protein: 18.7 g
- Fat: 3.3 g
- Carbohydrates: 12.8 g
- Fiber: 1.8 g
- Sodium: 54 mg
- Cholesterol: 264 mg

Calamari Fricassee

1 lb	cleaned squid, including tentacles (about 6)	500 g
3 tbsp	olive oil	45 mL
4	cloves	4
1/2 tsp	salt	2 mL
1/4 tsp	freshly ground black pepper	1 mL
1 cup	thinly sliced onions	250 mL
1	stalk celery with leaves, finely chopped	1
1 tbsp	finely chopped garlic	15 mL
2 tbsp	balsamic vinegar	25 mL
1 cup	fish stock or white wine	250 mL
1 tsp	dried basil	5 mL
1 tbsp	softened butter	15 mL
Pinch	sweet paprika	Pinch
1/4 cup	finely diced red bell peppers	50 mL
	Few sprigs fresh basil or parsley, chopped	

This dish provides a subtle taste with feathery textures, but it satisfies and comforts along with the best of them.

SERVES 3 OR 4

1. Slice squid bodies into 1/4-inch (5 mm) rings. Cut tentacles at their base to halve them. Rinse and set aside.

2. In a large nonstick frying pan, heat oil with cloves, salt and pepper over high heat for 1 minute. Add onions, celery and celery leaves; stir-fry for 2 minutes or until wilted and beginning to color. Add garlic and stir-fry for 1 minute. Add vinegar and stir-fry for 30 seconds or until sizzling. Add fish stock and basil; cook, stirring, for 1 minute or until bubbling actively.

3. Immediately add the reserved squid and reduce heat to low. Cook, stirring, for 4 to 5 minutes for an al dente texture or 7 to 9 minutes for a tender texture. Remove from heat and immediately stir in the butter until it is melted.

4. Portion squid, with plenty of sauce. Sprinkle with a little paprika, garnish with red peppers and chopped basil. Serve immediately.

Nutritional Analysis (Per Serving)
- Calories: 385
- Protein: 24.8 g
- Fat: 19.7 g
- Carbohydrates: 14.6 g
- Fiber: 2.0 g
- Sodium: 534 mg
- Cholesterol: 362 mg

Calamari, Two Ways

3 tbsp	extra virgin olive oil	45 mL
2 tbsp	minced red onions	25 mL
1 tbsp	drained capers	15 mL
1 tbsp	finely chopped lemon zest	15 mL
2 tbsp	lemon juice	25 mL
	Salt and pepper to taste	
1 lb	cleaned squid, including tentacles (about 6)	500 g
1 tbsp	extra virgin olive oil	15 mL
2 tbsp	all-purpose flour	25 mL
¼ cup	vegetable oil	50 mL
	Few sprigs fresh basil or parsley, chopped	
	Tomato wedges	

> *This recipe combines grilled calamari with a small amount of fried (for a little sinfulness) to create a double whammy of textures. It is dressed with a simple sauce that doesn't drown the subtle flavor of the main ingredient.*

SERVES 2 OR 3
Preheat grill or broiler

1. In a small bowl, combine 3 tbsp (45 mL) olive oil, red onions, capers, lemon zest, lemon juice, salt and pepper. Mix to distribute, cover and set aside. (The sauce can sit for up to 3 hours, unrefrigerated.)

2. Separate the tentacles from the bodies of the squid. Wash, drain and set aside the tentacles. Slit the bodies as if they were envelopes. Flatten out, wash both sides and dry them. Roll the bodies in 1 tbsp (15 mL) olive oil on both sides until thoroughly coated.

3. Now you must perform two operations in quick succession:

   (a) Dredge the tentacles in flour, shaking off excess through a strainer. In a medium frying pan, heat vegetable oil over high heat for 1 to 2 minutes or until just about to smoke. Fry the tentacles for about 1 minute, turning them to cook all sides (watch out for spluttering). With a slotted spoon, remove tentacles from oil and transfer them to drain on a plate lined with paper towels.

   (b) Grill or broil the squid bodies, on one side only for 2 to 3 minutes or until a skewer pierces them easily and they have lost their shine. (When picked off the grill, they will curl; don't worry, this is normal.)

4. Arrange the grilled bodies and fried tentacles on warm plates. Decorate with basil and tomato wedges. Stir the sauce and drizzle some on the squid, offering the rest for additional spooning at table. Serve immediately, providing serrated knives for easy slicing.

Nutritional Analysis (Per Serving)
- Calories: 490
- Protein: 24.6 g
- Fat: 38.2 g
- Carbohydrates: 11.3 g
- Fiber: 0.8 g
- Sodium: 152 mg
- Cholesterol: 352 mg

Poultry

Continued on next page...

Basic Whole Roast Chicken

1	roasting chicken (about 5 lbs/2.5 kg)	1
Half	lemon	Half
	Salt and pepper	
1	onion, quartered	1
1 tbsp	butter, softened	15 mL
1 tbsp	Dijon mustard	15 mL
1/2 tsp	dried thyme	2 mL
1/2 tsp	crushed dried sage	2 mL

Leftovers from a Sunday roast chicken provide the basis for many quick and wonderful dishes throughout the week — so much so that you might even want to roast two chickens, one for Sunday and one for other days.

SERVES 6

Preheat oven to 325°F (160°C)

1. Remove giblets and neck from chicken. Rinse and pat dry inside and out; rub inside and out with lemon. Sprinkle inside and out with salt and pepper. Place onion in cavity. Tie legs together with string; tuck wings under back. Place, breast-side up, on rack in roasting pan.

2. Combine butter, mustard, thyme and sage; spread over chicken. Roast in preheated oven for about 2 hours or until juices run clear when chicken is pierced and a meat thermometer inserted in the thigh registers 185°F (85°C).

3. Transfer chicken to a platter; tent with foil and let stand for 10 to 15 minutes before carving for juices to settle into meat.

Tip

- You can roast chickens smaller than called for here (anything from about 3 1/2 lbs/1.75 kg and up is fine); just adjust the time, allowing 20 to 30 minutes per pound (500 g).

Nutritional Analysis (Per Serving)
- Calories: 384
- Protein: 32.5 g
- Fat: 25.5 g
- Carbohydrates: 4.5 g
- Fiber: 0.8 g
- Sodium: 166 mg
- Cholesterol: 128 mg

One-Hour Roast Chicken with Sage and Garlic

1	chicken (about 3½ lbs/1.75 kg)	1
1 tbsp	butter, softened	15 mL
2	cloves garlic, minced	2
1 tbsp	minced fresh sage or 1 tsp (5 mL) dried sage leaves	15 mL
1½ tsp	grated lemon zest	7 mL
½ tsp	salt	2 mL
½ tsp	freshly ground black pepper	2 mL
2 tsp	olive oil	10 mL
¼ tsp	paprika	1 mL

SERVES 4

Preheat oven to 400°F (200°C) • Broiler pan, greased

1. Remove giblets and neck from chicken. Rinse and pat chicken dry inside and out with paper towels. Using heavy-duty kitchen scissors, cut chicken open along backbone; press down on breast bone to flatten slightly and arrange skin-side up on rack of a broiler pan.

2. In a bowl, blend butter with garlic, sage, lemon zest, salt and pepper. Gently lift breast skin; using a knife or spatula, spread butter mixture under skin to coat breasts and part of legs. Press down on outside skin to smooth and spread butter mixture.

3. In a small bowl, combine olive oil and paprika; brush over chicken.

4. Roast chicken for 1 hour or until juices run clear and a meat thermometer inserted in the thickest part of the thigh registers 185°F (85°C). Transfer chicken to a platter. Tent with foil; let rest 5 minutes before carving.

Tip

- Take an hour off the roasting time by cutting the bird open along the backbone, placing it flat on the broiler pan and then boosting the oven temperature.

Nutritional Analysis (Per Serving)
- Calories: 514
- Protein: 42.9 g
- Fat: 36.5 g
- Carbohydrates: 1.1 g
- Fiber: 0.4 g
- Sodium: 476 mg
- Cholesterol: 172 mg

Thyme-Roasted Chicken with Garlic Gravy

1	chicken (about 3½ lbs/1.75 kg)	1
10	cloves garlic, peeled	10
1 tsp	dried thyme leaves	5 mL
¼ tsp	salt	1 mL
¼ tsp	freshly ground black pepper	1 mL
1⅓ cups	chicken stock, divided (approx.)	325 mL
½ cup	white wine or additional chicken stock	125 mL
1 tbsp	all-purpose flour	15 mL

Roast chicken conjures up a homey smell and feel. Here, herbs and seasonings are placed under the bird's skin to produce a succulent, flavorful chicken. Slow roasting with lots of garlic creates a wonderful aroma — yet, surprisingly, imparts only a subtle flavor to the gravy.

SERVES 4

Preheat oven to 325°F (160°C) • Roasting pan with rack

1. Remove giblets and neck from chicken. Rinse and pat chicken dry inside and out. Place 2 cloves garlic inside cavity. Starting at cavity opening, gently lift skin and rub thyme, salt and pepper over breasts and legs. Tie legs together with string; tuck wings under back.

2. Add remaining garlic, ⅔ cup (150 mL) chicken stock and wine to roasting pan; place chicken, breast side up, on rack in pan.

3. Roast in preheated oven, basting every 30 minutes, adding additional stock if pan juices evaporate, for 1¾ to 2 hours or until pan juices run clear when chicken is pierced and meat thermometer inserted in thigh registers 185°F (85°C).

4. Transfer to a platter; tent with foil and let stand for 10 minutes before carving. Meanwhile, strain pan juices into measure, pressing down firmly to mash garlic into juices; skim off fat. Add enough of remaining stock to make ¾ cup (175 mL).

5. In a small saucepan, stir together 2 tbsp (25 mL) of pan juices and flour; cook, stirring, over medium heat for 1 minute. Gradually whisk in remaining pan juices; cook, stirring, until boiling and thickened. Serve with chicken.

Nutritional Analysis (Per Serving)
- Calories: 507
- Protein: 44.1 g
- Fat: 31.4 g
- Carbohydrates: 4.8 g
- Fiber: 0.5 g
- Sodium: 493 mg
- Cholesterol: 164 mg

Roasted Flat Chicken

2 tbsp	Dijon mustard	25 mL
1 tbsp	soy sauce	15 mL
2	cloves garlic, finely chopped	2
2 tsp	chopped fresh rosemary, or 1/2 tsp (2 mL) dried	10 mL
1/4 tsp	black pepper	1 mL
1	3-lb (1.5 kg) chicken, rinsed and patted dry	1

SERVES 4 TO 6

1. In a small bowl, combine mustard, soy sauce, garlic, rosemary and pepper.

2. With kitchen shears or a sharp knife, cut carefully along both sides of backbone. Remove backbone. Cut off wing tips (freeze backbone and wing tips for stock). Spread chicken open and press firmly to flatten.

3. Spoon mustard mixture over both sides of chicken. Arrange chicken, skin side up, on a foil- and parchment-lined baking sheet (this will make cleanup easier).

4. Convection roast in a preheated 325°F (160°C) oven for 55 to 60 minutes, or until juices run clear when thigh is pierced or meat thermometer registers 180°F (82°C) when inserted into thigh. If chicken is browning too quickly, cover loosely with foil, tucking edges under chicken, during last half of roasting time. Transfer to a carving board or serving platter and cut into serving pieces.

Nutritional Analysis (Per Serving)
- Calories: 473
- Protein: 43.1 g
- Fat: 31.5 g
- Carbohydrates: 1.5 g
- Fiber: 0.5 g
- Sodium: 330 mg
- Cholesterol: 164 mg

Grilled Whole Chicken with Lime or Lemon Butter

1	chicken (about 4 lbs/2 kg), patted dry	1
1	lime or lemon, halved	1
1 tsp	dried thyme	5 mL
¼ cup	butter, softened	50 mL
1 tsp	grated lime or lemon zest	5 mL
¼ cup	fresh lime or lemon juice	50 mL

This may not be an under-30-minute recipe, but it's a good way to have chicken on hand for speedy recipes such as salads, soups and the like throughout the week. Grill 2 chickens — one to enjoy on Sunday and the other one for leftovers. Or grill one while you have the barbecue on for something else.

SERVES 6
Grease barbecue grill and preheat to medium-high

1. Rub chicken all over, inside and out, with cut side of lime. Sprinkle with thyme.
2. Place chicken, breast-side up, on grill; cook, turning often, for 10 to 15 minutes or until browned. Turn off one burner and place the chicken over the turned-off burner. Increase heat to high on remaining burner; cook, covered, for 1 hour, turning halfway through.
3. Meanwhile, whisk together the butter, lime zest and juice. Brush chicken with mixture. Cook, turning and basting occasionally, for 30 minutes to 1 hour longer or until meat thermometer registers 185°F (85°C).

Nutritional Analysis (Per Serving)
- Calories: 421
- Protein: 32.2 g
- Fat: 31.2 g
- Carbohydrates: 1.5 g
- Fiber: 0.1 g
- Sodium: 195 mg
- Cholesterol: 144 mg

Mustard-Thyme Grilled Breasts

⅓ cup	Dijon mustard	75 mL
1 tbsp	vegetable oil	15 mL
1 tbsp	white wine vinegar	15 mL
1 tsp	cayenne pepper	5 mL
1 tsp	dried thyme	5 mL
4	skin-on bone-in chicken breasts	4

Make Ahead

The chicken can be marinated, covered and refrigerated for up to 4 hours ahead. Bring to room temperature for 30 minutes before cooking.

With only a handful of ingredients, this marinade keeps the bone-in breasts moist and delicious.

SERVES 4
Grease barbecue grill and preheat to medium-high

1. In a bowl combine half the mustard, the oil, vinegar, half the cayenne and half the thyme. Place chicken in a glass dish and spread mixture over the breasts. Cover and let sit for 15 to 30 minutes at room temperature. In a small bowl, stir together the remaining mustard, cayenne and thyme and set aside.
2. Place chicken, skin-side down on the grill and cook for 15 minutes, turning often.
3. Turn chicken skin-side up and brush with reserved mustard mixture. Cook for 10 to 15 minutes longer or until chicken is no longer pink inside.

Nutritional Analysis (Per Serving)
- Calories: 340
- Protein: 36.4 g
- Fat: 19.8 g
- Carbohydrates: 2.3 g
- Fiber: 0.9 g
- Sodium: 332 mg
- Cholesterol: 108 mg

Broiled Cilantro Garlic Chicken Breasts

4	boneless, skinless chicken breasts (about 6 oz/175 g each)	4
4	cloves garlic, peeled	4
2	shallots or 1 small onion, peeled	2
1 cup	loosely packed fresh cilantro leaves	250 mL
1/4 cup	lemon juice or lime juice	50 mL
1 tbsp	granulated sugar	15 mL
1 tbsp	fish sauce or soy sauce	15 mL
1 tsp	black pepper	5 mL

This may sound like a lot of garlic and cilantro, but the result is a tangy, moist chicken.

SERVES 4

1. Place one chicken breast between sheets of parchment paper or plastic wrap (I cut open a plastic bag). With a meat pounder or rolling pin, flatten chicken until about 1/2 inch (1 cm) thick. Place in a shallow glass or ceramic dish. Repeat with remaining chicken breasts.

2. In a food processor or blender, finely chop garlic, shallots and cilantro. Blend in lemon juice, sugar, fish sauce and pepper. Pour over chicken, turning to coat on all sides. Cover and refrigerate for 1 to 12 hours.

3. To cook, arrange chicken breasts with marinade on a lightly greased broiler pan. Place under a preheated broiler about 4 inches (10 cm) from heat. Convection broil for 4 minutes. Turn and broil for 4 to 6 minutes longer, or until chicken is no longer pink inside. Do not overcook or chicken will be dry.

Tips

- You can also use the marinade on thick slices of extra-firm tofu, but reduce the cooking time by at least half.

- Serve with sliced tomato and cucumber.

- This chicken is also good chilled and thinly sliced. Add to a salad with diced mango.

Nutritional Analysis (Per Serving)
- Calories: 213
- Protein: 40.0 g
- Fat: 2.1 g
- Carbohydrates: 6.6 g
- Fiber: 0.4 g
- Sodium: 243 mg
- Cholesterol: 96 mg

Chicken with Red Pepper and Onions

| 4 | chicken breasts or legs | 4 |
| | All-purpose flour for dusting | |

SAUCE

1 tbsp	margarine	15 mL
1½ tsp	crushed garlic	7 mL
¾ cup	diced onion	175 mL
1½ cups	diced sweet red pepper	375 mL
1 tbsp	all-purpose flour	15 mL
1⅓ cups	chicken stock	325 mL
	Parsley sprigs	

SERVES 4

Preheat oven to 400°F (200°C) • Baking dish sprayed with nonstick vegetable spray

1. Dust chicken with flour. In large nonstick skillet sprayed with nonstick vegetable spray, brown chicken on both sides, approximately 10 minutes. Place in baking dish; cover and bake for 20 to 30 minutes or until no longer pink inside and juices run clear when chicken is pierced.

2. *Sauce:* Meanwhile, in small saucepan, melt margarine; sauté garlic, onion and red pepper for 5 minutes or until softened. Add flour and cook, stirring, for 1 minute. Add stock and cook, stirring, just until thickened, approximately 3 minutes.

3. Place chicken on serving dish; pour sauce over top. Garnish with parsley. Remove skin before eating.

Tips

- This red pepper sauce can also be puréed.
- Cut down on foods that have been fried or deep-fried and those that contain hydrogenated vegetable oils.
- When using margarine, choose a soft (non-hydrogenated) version to limit consumption of trans fats.

Nutritional Analysis (Per Serving)
- Calories: 250
- Protein: 35 g
- Fat: 8 g
- Carbohydrates: 13 g
- Fiber: 0 g
- Sodium: 383 mg
- Cholesterol: 84 mg

Chicken Breasts Rolled with Roasted Red Peppers and Cheese

1 lb	skinless, boneless chicken breasts (about 4)	500 g
3 tbsp	finely chopped chives	45 mL
3 tbsp	finely chopped roasted red peppers	45 mL
2 oz	brick or Havarti cheese, at room temperature	50 g
3 tbsp	all-purpose flour	45 mL
1	egg	1
2 tbsp	2% milk	25 mL
½ cup	seasoned bread crumbs	125 mL
1 tbsp	vegetable oil	15 mL

Make Ahead

Prepare chicken breasts early in the day, sauté, then refrigerate. Bake for an extra 5 minutes just prior to serving.

SERVES 4

Preheat oven to 425°F (220°C) • Baking sheet sprayed with vegetable spray

1. Between sheets of waxed paper, pound breasts to ¼-inch (5 mm) thickness. Spread with chives and peppers. Place cheese at short end of each breast. Roll up tightly; secure edge with a toothpick. Dust with flour. Mix egg and milk.

2. Dip each chicken roll in egg wash, then in bread crumbs. Heat oil in large nonstick skillet sprayed with vegetable spray, cook over high heat for 3 minutes, turning often, or until browned on all sides. Put on prepared baking sheet and bake for 10 minutes or until just done at center. Remove toothpicks before serving.

Tips

- Instead of serving each breast whole, slice each crosswise into medallions and fan out on plates.
- Replace chicken with turkey, veal or pork scaloppine.
- Use roasted red peppers packed in water in a jar.
- A stronger-tasting cheese can replace the brick cheese.

Nutritional Analysis (Per Serving)
- Calories: 300
- Protein: 33 g
- Fat: 12 g
- Carbohydrates: 12 g
- Fiber: 0 g
- Sodium: 617 mg
- Cholesterol: 134 g

Brie-Stuffed Breast of Chicken

4	boneless skinless chicken breasts (4 oz/125 g each)	4
4 tsp	pesto sauce	20 mL
2 oz	Brie cheese, rind removed and diced (1/2 cup/125 mL)	60 g
3/4 cup	chicken broth	175 mL
1/4 cup	white wine	50 mL
2 tbsp	lemon juice	25 mL
1/2 cup	2% evaporated milk	125 mL

> *Stuffed chicken breasts are easier to make than you may think. They add a touch of elegance and surprise at serving time.*

SERVES 4

Preheat oven to 350°F (180°C) • 4-cup (1 L) covered casserole

1. With meat mallet, pound chicken between plastic wrap to 1/4-inch (5 mm) thickness. Spread 1 tsp (5 mL) pesto over each breast; place Brie cheese in middle. Fold up sides and ends, overlapping to cover cheese completely; secure with toothpick if necessary. Place seam side down in 4-cup (1 L) covered casserole.

2. In a saucepan, bring chicken broth, wine and lemon juice just to a boil; pour over chicken. Cover and bake in preheated oven for 15 to 20 minutes or until no longer pink.

3. Reduce temperature to 200°F (100°C). Drain liquid from breasts into rinsed saucepan; return covered breasts to oven to keep warm. Boil liquid until reduced by half. Stir in evaporated milk; simmer until hot.

4. Slice chicken breasts and fan on warmed plates; drizzle with sauce.

Tips

- Prepared pesto sauce can be found in supermarkets near fresh pasta or in the deli.

- Lean and tender boneless chicken breasts are a great convenience food and a valuable asset in a program of healthy eating. Evaporated milk is an excellent substitute for cream in this rich-tasting, velvety sauce. Add a serving of Spinach Fancy (see recipe, page 335), and you have a special-occasion meal.

Nutritional Analysis (Per Serving)
- Calories: 234
- Protein: 33 g
- Fat: 8 g
- Carbohydrates: 5 g
- Fiber: Trace
- Sodium: 329 mg
- Cholesterol: 84 mg

Chicken Breasts with Chili Butter

¼ cup	unsalted butter, softened	50 mL
1 tbsp	chili powder	15 mL
½ tsp	salt	2 mL
¼ tsp	hot pepper flakes	1 mL
2	cloves garlic, minced	2
4	bone-in skin-on chicken breasts	4

This simple, but delicious recipe produces moist chicken with nice crisp skin and is easily halved or doubled.

SERVES 4
Preheat oven to 400°F (200°C)

1. In a small bowl, cream together butter, chili powder, salt, hot pepper flakes and garlic until well blended. Divide into 4 portions.
2. Gently poke your fingers under the skin of each breast and lift the skin slightly. Being careful not to tear the membrane that connects the skin to the chicken, gently stuff one portion of the chili butter between, massaging to even out.
3. Arrange breasts skin-side up on a rack in a large shallow roasting pan. Roast in preheated oven for 30 minutes or until chicken is no longer pink inside, brushing once or twice with melted butter from the bottom of the pan.

Nutritional Analysis (Per Serving)
- Calories: 402
- Protein: 35.9 g
- Fat: 27.3 g
- Carbohydrates: 1.6 g
- Fiber: 0.5 g
- Sodium: 516 mg
- Cholesterol: 139 mg

Grilled Chicken with Lemon-Herb Sauce

¼ cup	freshly squeezed lemon juice	50 mL
¼ cup	chopped fresh oregano leaves	50 mL
¼ cup	chopped fresh chives	50 mL
	Salt and freshly ground black pepper	
8	chicken pieces, such as breasts or drumsticks	8

SERVES 6 TO 8

1. Stir together lemon juice, oregano, chives and salt and pepper. Pour into a serving dish large enough to hold all chicken pieces.
2. Rinse and wipe chicken with paper towel. Grill at medium-high heat or roast until meat is no longer pink inside, about 20 minutes.
3. When chicken is cooked, transfer to bowl with lemon mixture. Turn to coat and serve.

Tip
- The chicken may be grilled on the barbecue or baked in the oven. Immersing the cooked chicken in the lemon-herb sauce provides an after-cooking marinated approach that is absolutely delicious.

Nutritional Analysis (Per Serving)
- Calories: 304
- Protein: 35.8 g
- Fat: 15.9 g
- Carbohydrates: 2.0 g
- Fiber: 0.9 g
- Sodium: 108 mg
- Cholesterol: 108 mg

Chicken Breasts Stuffed with Red Pepper Purée in Creamy Sauce

4	boneless skinless chicken breasts	4
1 tbsp	vegetable oil	15 mL
1/2 tsp	crushed garlic	2 mL
3/4 cup	diced sweet red pepper	175 mL
1 tbsp	water	15 mL
2 tbsp	chopped fresh dill (or 1/2 tsp/2 mL dried dillweed)	25 mL
2 tbsp	dry bread crumbs	25 mL
1 1/2 tsp	grated Parmesan cheese	7 mL
1 tbsp	toasted pine nuts	15 mL
	Salt and pepper	
1/4 cup	chicken stock or water	50 mL

SAUCE

1 1/2 tsp	margarine	7 mL
1 1/2 tsp	all-purpose flour	7 mL
3/4 cup	2% milk	175 mL
1 tbsp	grated Parmesan cheese	15 mL
1 tbsp	chopped fresh dill (or 1/4 tsp/1 mL dried dillweed)	15 mL
Pinch	paprika	Pinch

Make Ahead

Assemble stuffed breasts early in day and refrigerate. Bake just before serving. Prepare sauce early in day and reheat gently, adding a little more milk if too thick.

SERVES 4

Preheat oven to 375°F (190°C) • Baking dish sprayed with nonstick vegetable spray

1. Place chicken between 2 sheets of waxed paper; pound until flattened. Set aside.

2. In nonstick skillet, heat oil; sauté garlic and red pepper for 3 minutes; stir in water. Transfer to food processor and purée; pour into bowl. Stir in dill, bread crumbs, cheese, pine nuts, and salt and pepper to taste, mixing well and adding a little water if too dry.

3. Divide purée among chicken breasts; roll up and fasten with toothpicks. Place in baking dish; pour in stock. Cover and bake for about 15 minutes or until chicken is no longer pink inside. Transfer to serving dish.

4. *Sauce:* Meanwhile, in saucepan, melt margarine; add flour and cook, stirring, for 1 minute. Gradually add milk and cook, stirring, until thickened, approximately 3 minutes. Stir in cheese, dill and paprika. Pour over chicken.

Tips

- Try yellow pepper instead of the red.
- Fresh herbs will last longer if placed in a glass with some water covering the stems and plastic wrap to cover the glass. Store in the refrigerator.

Nutritional Analysis (Per Serving)
- Calories: 251
- Protein: 30 g
- Fat: 11 g
- Carbohydrates: 7 g
- Fiber: 1 g
- Sodium: 211 mg
- Cholesterol: 71 mg

Chicken Breasts Stuffed with Spinach and Cheese with Tomato Garlic Sauce

4	boneless skinless chicken breasts	4
1 1/2 tsp	vegetable oil	7 mL
1/2 tsp	crushed garlic	2 mL
1	medium green onion, finely chopped	1
1/4 cup	drained cooked chopped spinach	50 mL
1/4 cup	diced mushrooms	50 mL
1/4 cup	shredded mozzarella	50 mL
1/4 cup	chicken stock	50 mL

SAUCE

1 1/2 tsp	margarine	7 mL
1 tsp	crushed garlic	5 mL
1 1/2 cups	diced tomatoes	375 mL
1/3 cup	chicken stock	75 mL
1 tbsp	chopped fresh parsley	15 mL

Make Ahead

Assemble and refrigerate stuffed breasts early in day, but bake just before eating.

SERVES 4

Preheat oven to 400°F (200°C) • Baking dish sprayed with nonstick vegetable spray

1. Place chicken between 2 sheets of waxed paper; pound until flattened. Set aside.

2. In nonstick skillet, heat oil; sauté garlic, onion, spinach and mushrooms until softened. Spoon evenly over breasts; sprinkle with cheese. Roll up and fasten with toothpicks.

3. Place chicken in baking dish; pour in stock. Cover and bake for 10 minutes or until chicken is no longer pink. Remove chicken to serving dish and keep warm.

4. *Sauce:* Meanwhile, in small saucepan, melt margarine; sauté garlic for 1 minute. Stir in tomatoes and chicken stock; cook for 3 minutes or until heated through. Add parsley and serve over chicken.

Tips

- Be sure not to overcook the chicken or it will become dry.
- If using fresh spinach, use 1 1/2 cups (375 mL). Cook, drain well and chop.

Nutritional Analysis (Per Serving)
- Calories: 216
- Protein: 30 g
- Fat: 8 g
- Carbohydrates: 4 g
- Fiber: 1 g
- Sodium: 247 mg
- Cholesterol: 70 mg

Pepper-Stuffed Chicken with Cantaloupe Sauce

½	each large red and green bell pepper, seeded	½
4	boneless skinless chicken breasts (4 oz/125 g each)	4
	Salt and black pepper	
2 cups	water	500 mL
1	stalk celery, cut into ½-inch (1 cm) pieces	1
1	small onion, sliced	1
1	bay leaf	1
¼	large cantaloupe, peeled	¼
2 tsp	lemon juice	10 mL
	Chopped fresh parsley	

Roasted peppers add flavor and color to this unusual dish.

SERVES 4

Preheat broiler • Baking sheet

1. Roast peppers (see tip, below). Cut each into 4 long strips.
2. Place chicken between plastic wrap; flatten with mallet. Sprinkle with salt and pepper to taste. Place 1 green and 1 red pepper strip on each chicken breast; roll up tightly and secure with toothpick.
3. In a skillet, bring water, celery, onion, bay leaf and ¼ tsp (1 mL) each salt and pepper to a boil; add chicken rolls. Cover and simmer for 10 to 15 minutes or until chicken is no longer pink inside. Remove from liquid; drain.
4. In a food processor or blender, purée cantaloupe with lemon juice. Heat gently in small saucepan. Divide among 4 plates. Slice each chicken breast into 3 diagonal pieces. Place on cantaloupe purée. Sprinkle with parsley.

Tips

- To roast peppers: Heat barbecue or broiler; place peppers on grill or broiling pan and keep turning peppers until skins are blistered and black. Place roasted peppers in large pot with lid. Steam will make them sweat, and skin will be easier to peel off. Let peppers cool; remove stems, seeds and skin.
- Remove bay leaf before serving as it might cause someone to choke if eaten.
- The red pepper and cantaloupe boost the vitamin A and C content of this dish. Team it up with a spinach salad for a meal with eye appeal.

Nutritional Analysis (Per Serving)
- Calories: 169
- Protein: 28 g
- Fat: 2 g
- Carbohydrates: 10 g
- Fiber: 1 g
- Sodium: 98 mg
- Cholesterol: 64 mg

Citrus Grilled Chicken Breasts with Yogurt Sauce

1 tbsp	grated orange zest	15 mL
1 tbsp	grated lime zest	15 mL
¼ cup	fresh orange juice	50 mL
¼ cup	fresh lime juice	50 mL
2 tbsp	olive oil	25 mL
1	fresh jalapeño pepper, seeded and minced	1
4	chicken breasts, patted dry	4

YOGURT SAUCE

1 cup	plain yogurt	250 mL
1	shallot or small onion, finely diced	1
1 tsp	grated orange zest	5 mL
1 tsp	grated lime zest	5 mL
2 tbsp	fresh orange juice	25 mL
2 tbsp	chopped fresh coriander	25 mL
1 tbsp	fresh lime juice	15 mL
	Salt and pepper	

Make Ahead

The chicken breasts can be marinated up to 24 hours ahead in the refrigerator. Bring to room temperature 30 minutes before cooking.

The refreshing sauce is just right with this lively grilled chicken.

SERVES 4

Grease barbecue grill and preheat to medium-high

1. In a shallow dish or a sturdy plastic bag, combine orange and lime zest, orange juice, lime juice, olive oil and jalapeño pepper. Add chicken breasts and marinate for 30 minutes at room temperature.

2. Reserving the marinade, place chicken on grill and cook for 7 to 8 minutes a side, turning once and basting with the marinade, until the chicken is no longer pink inside.

3. *Yogurt Sauce:* Meanwhile, in a small bowl, stir together the yogurt, shallot, zest, orange juice, coriander, lime juice, and salt and pepper to taste. Cover and refrigerate. Serve the hot chicken with the cold sauce.

Nutritional Analysis (Per Serving)
- Calories: 408
- Protein: 39.6 g
- Fat: 22.7 g
- Carbohydrates: 9.3 g
- Fiber: 0.2 g
- Sodium: 157 mg
- Cholesterol: 109 mg

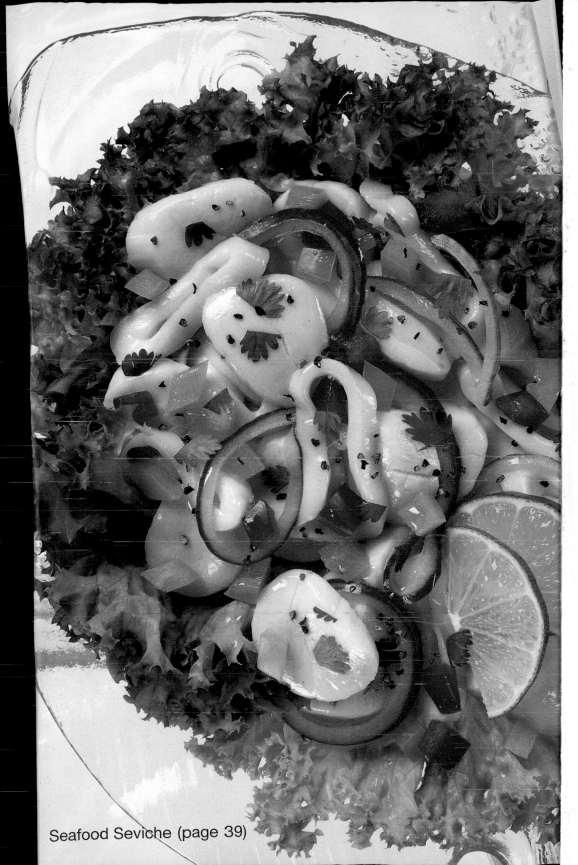

Seafood Seviche (page 39)

Garlic-Herb Chicken with Balsamic Glaze

6	bone-in, skin-on chicken breasts (about 4 lbs/2 kg)	6
1	package (5 oz/150 g) French soft cheese with garlic and herbs (such as Boursin), cut into 6 pieces	1
¼ cup	balsamic vinegar	50 mL
¼ cup	olive oil	50 mL
¾ tsp	salt	4 mL
¾ tsp	black pepper	4 mL
	Fresh herb sprigs (parsley, basil, thyme, oregano and/or tarragon)	

Make Ahead

Massage cheese into the chicken breasts then refrigerate, covered, for up to 24 hours.

This is one of those dishes that is very easy to prepare but somehow has that restaurant-dinner quality that will impress the you-know-what out of your guests.

SERVES 6

Preheat oven to 400°F (200°C) • Heavy baking sheet lined with lightly oiled foil

1. With your fingers, carefully lift skin from each chicken breast to form a pocket between skin and flesh. Place 1 piece of cheese under skin of each chicken breast; massage skin to spread cheese evenly. Place chicken breasts in a single layer on prepared baking sheet.

2. In a small bowl, whisk together balsamic vinegar and oil. Generously brush chicken breasts with half the vinegar mixture; sprinkle with salt and pepper.

3. Bake in preheated oven for 20 minutes. Whisk remaining vinegar mixture; brush generously over chicken breasts. Continue to bake for 20 to 30 minutes or until golden brown and juices that run out are no longer pink when thickest chicken breast is pierced with a skewer. Serve chicken on a bed of fresh herbs on a warm serving platter.

Tips

• For best flavor, look for air-chilled chicken breasts.

• Use a pastry brush when applying the vinegar glaze. Be sure to wash the brush well in hot, soapy water afterward.

Nutritional Analysis (Per Serving)
- Calories: 563
- Protein: 52.8 g
- Fat: 37.1 g
- Carbohydrates: 2.0 g
- Fiber: 0.4 g
- Sodium: 562 mg
- Cholesterol: 162 mg

Elizabeth Baird's Balsamic-Glazed Chicken Breasts

6	skinless boneless chicken breasts	6
1 tsp	dried thyme	5 mL
½ tsp	salt	2 mL
¼ tsp	pepper	1 mL
2 tsp	vegetable oil	10 mL
2 tbsp	balsamic or wine vinegar	25 mL
1 tsp	liquid honey	5 mL
1 tbsp	butter, cut into bits	15 mL

SERVES 6

1. Sprinkle both sides of chicken breasts with thyme, salt and pepper. In a large skillet, heat oil over medium-high heat. Add chicken, placing it smooth-side down; cook for 2 minutes or until browned. Turn and brown lightly on underside. Transfer to a plate.

2. Pour ⅓ cup (75 mL) water, balsamic vinegar and honey into the skillet; bring to a boil over high heat, stirring to scrape up any brown bits from the bottom of the pan. Boil for 2 minutes or until slightly syrupy and reduced by half. Add butter; stir until melted.

3. Reduce heat to medium-low. Return chicken, smooth-side down, to pan; cook, turning halfway through, for about 6 minutes or until glazed and no longer pink inside. Serve drizzled with glaze.

Nutritional Analysis (Per Serving)
- Calories: 221
- Protein: 39.4 g
- Fat: 5.5 g
- Carbohydrates: 1.5 g
- Fiber: 0.1 g
- Sodium: 322 mg
- Cholesterol: 101 mg

Creamy Mustard Chicken

2 lb	chicken pieces, skinned	1 kg
½ cup	lower-fat plain yogurt	125 mL
⅓ cup	light mayonnaise	75 mL
¼ cup	sliced green onions	50 mL
1 tbsp	Dijon mustard	15 mL
1 tbsp	Worcestershire sauce	15 mL
½ tsp	dried thyme	2 mL
½ tsp	salt	2 mL
¼ tsp	white pepper	1 mL
2 tbsp	grated Parmesan cheese	25 mL
	Chopped fresh parsley	

Yogurt, light mayonnaise, Dijon mustard and Worcestershire sauce combine to create this toothsome sauce, which is flavorful and light.

SERVES 6

Preheat oven to 350°F (180°C) • Lightly greased baking dish

1. Place chicken in single layer in lightly greased ovenproof casserole. Combine yogurt, mayonnaise, onions, mustard and seasonings. Spoon sauce over each chicken piece. Bake in preheated oven for about 45 minutes or until chicken is no longer pink inside. Sprinkle with Parmesan cheese and brown under the broiler. Serve garnished with chopped parsley.

Nutritional Analysis (Per Serving)
- Calories: 217
- Protein: 25 g
- Fat: 11 g
- Carbohydrates: 3 g
- Fiber: Trace
- Sodium: 599 mg
- Cholesterol: 98 mg

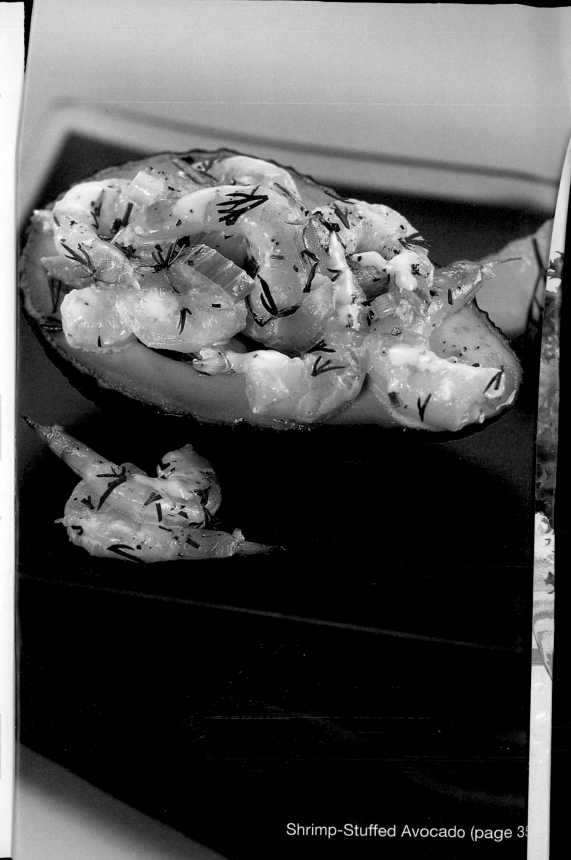

Shrimp-Stuffed Avocado (page 35)

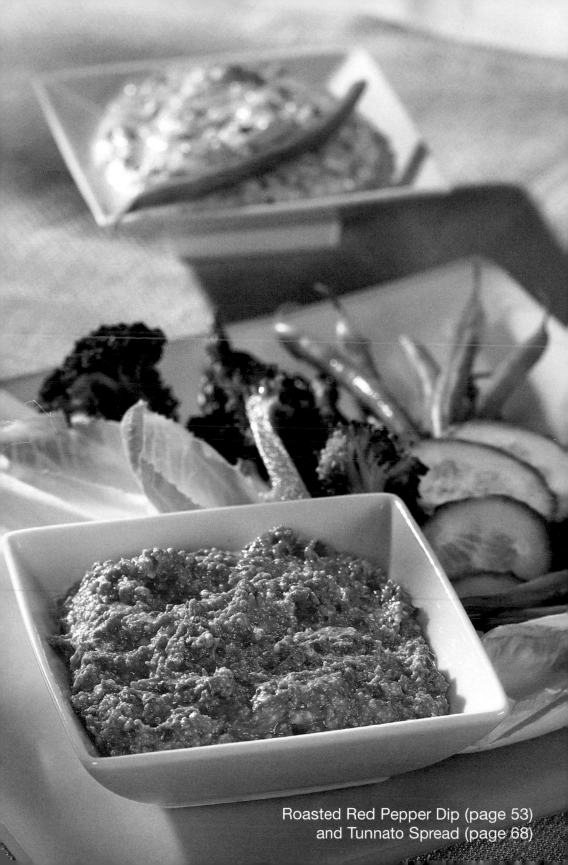

Roasted Red Pepper Dip (page 53)
and Tunnato Spread (page 68)

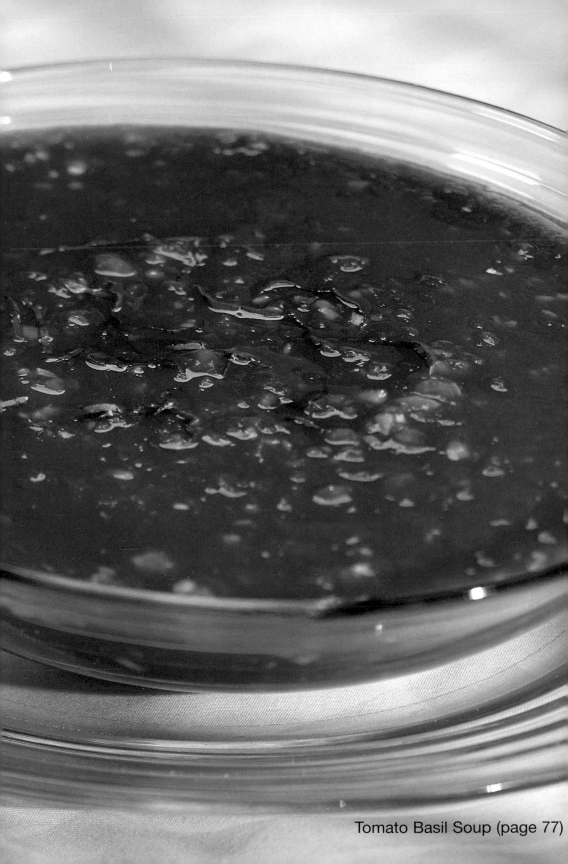
Tomato Basil Soup (page 77)

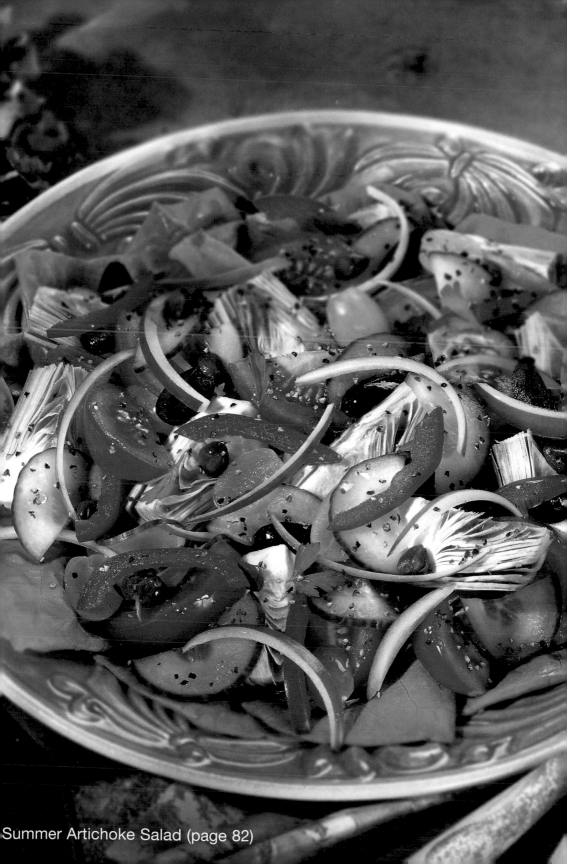

Summer Artichoke Salad (page 82)

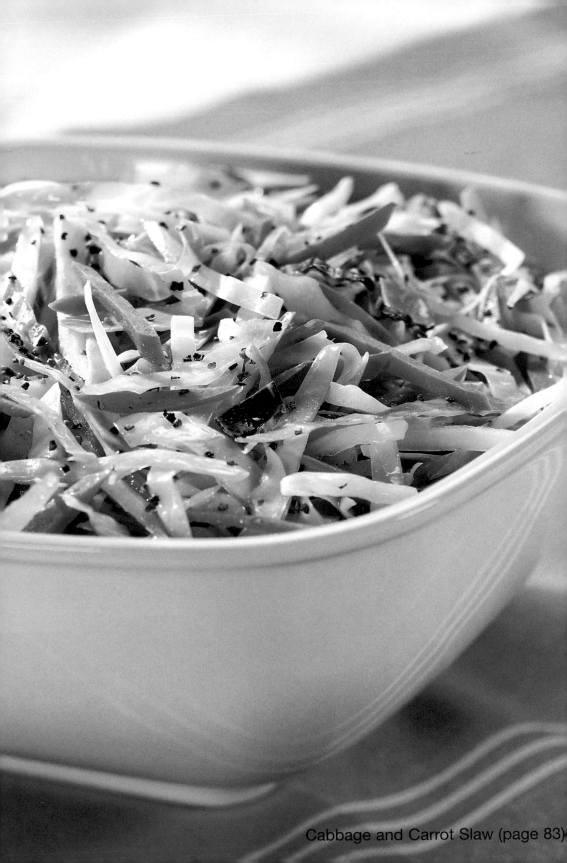

Cabbage and Carrot Slaw (page 83)

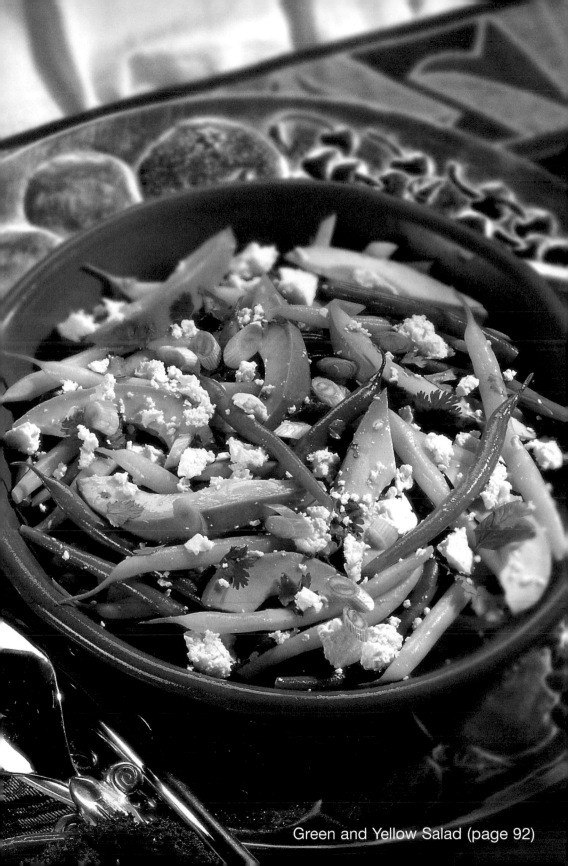

Green and Yellow Salad (page 92)

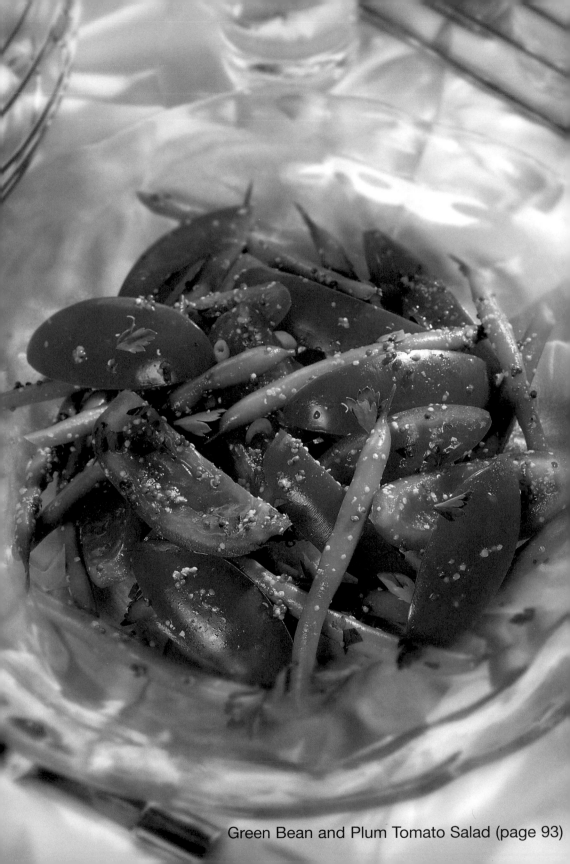

Green Bean and Plum Tomato Salad (page 93)

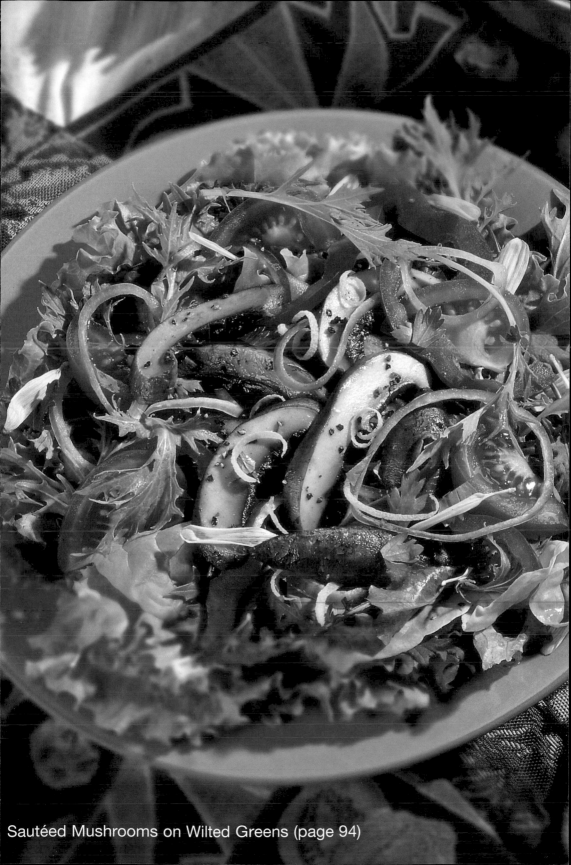

Sautéed Mushrooms on Wilted Greens (page 94)

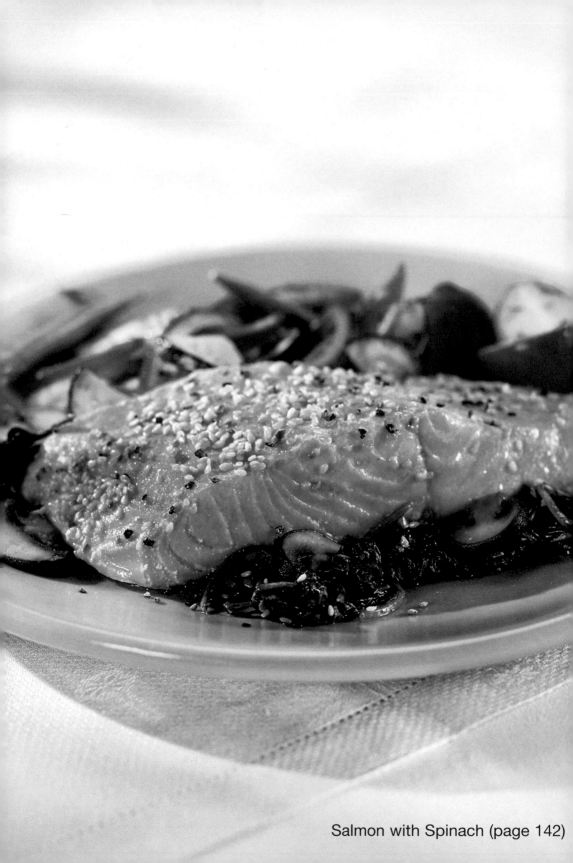

Salmon with Spinach (page 142)

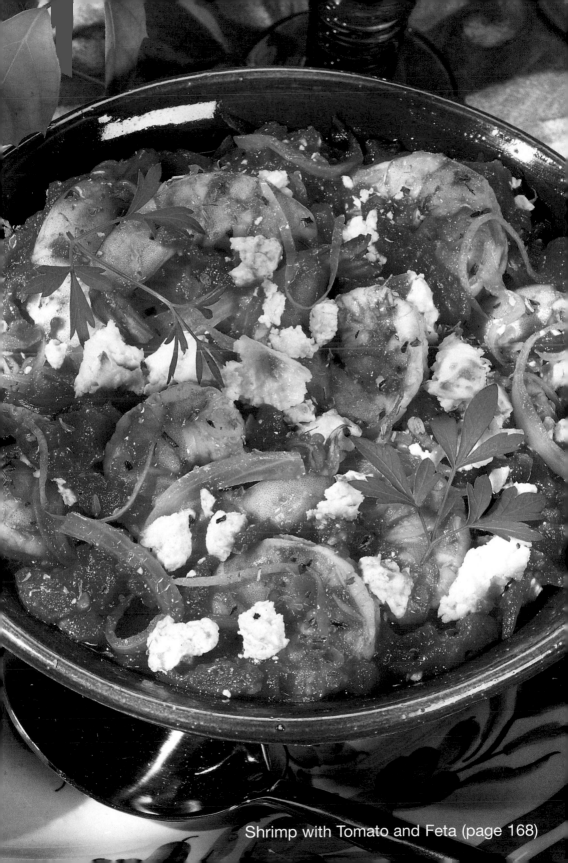

Shrimp with Tomato and Feta (page 168)

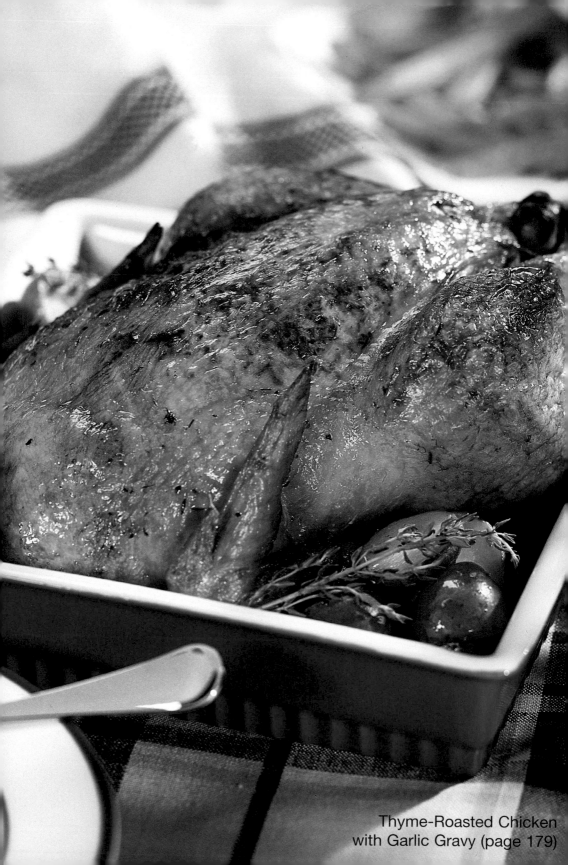

Thyme-Roasted Chicken
with Garlic Gravy (page 179)

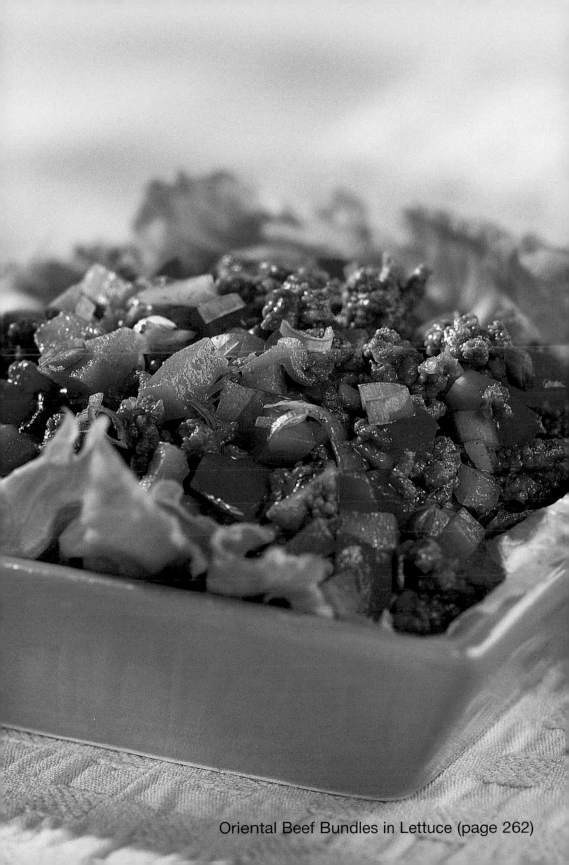

Oriental Beef Bundles in Lettuce (page 262)

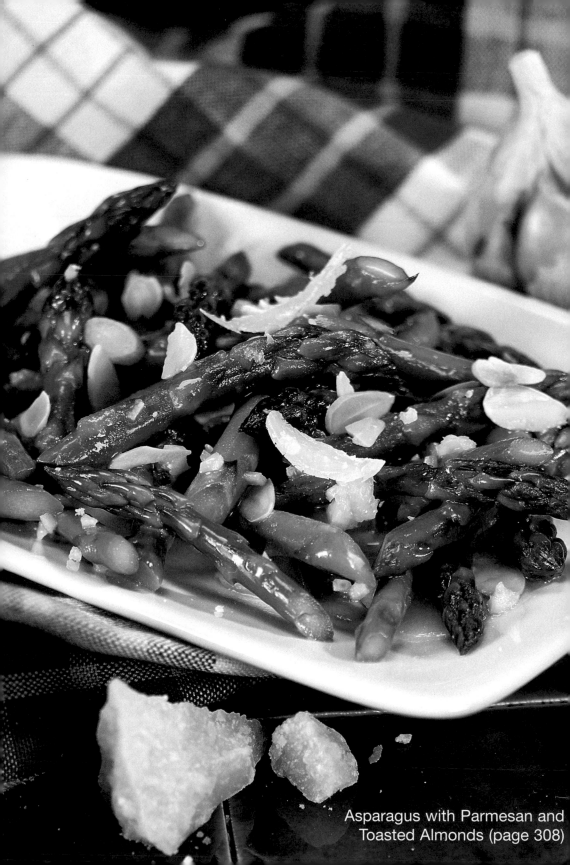

Asparagus with Parmesan and Toasted Almonds (page 308)

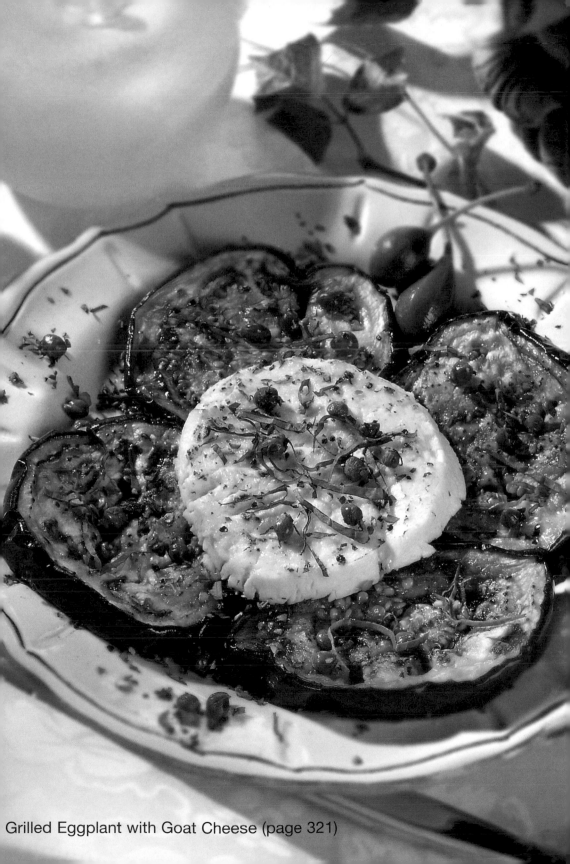

Grilled Eggplant with Goat Cheese (page 321)

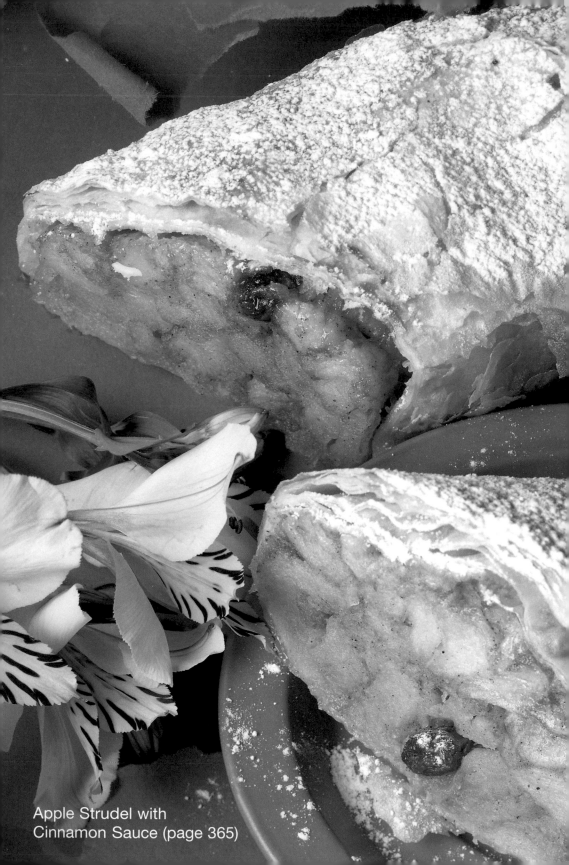

Apple Strudel with
Cinnamon Sauce (page 365)

Chicken Breasts with Wild Mushroom Sauce

4	boneless skinless chicken breasts	4
½ tsp	dried tarragon	2 mL
	Salt and pepper	
2 tbsp	all-purpose flour	25 mL
1 tbsp	butter	15 mL
2	cloves garlic, minced	2
8 oz	mushrooms, quartered or sliced	250 g
1½ cups	chicken stock	375 mL
1 tbsp	Dijon mustard	15 mL
½ cup	whipping (35%) cream	125 mL
	Chopped parsley	

SERVES 4

1. Sprinkle chicken with tarragon and a pinch of salt and pepper. Place flour on a piece of waxed paper and coat each breast with some. In a large skillet, heat butter over medium heat. Add chicken and cook for about 8 minutes a side or until no longer pink inside. Remove to a warm platter and keep warm.

2. Add garlic and mushrooms to skillet; cook, stirring for 3 minutes. Add chicken stock and mustard; increase heat to high and boil for 5 minutes. Stir in cream. Boil for 4 minutes or until thickened. Add salt and pepper to taste. Pour over chicken and garnish with parsley.

Nutritional Analysis (Per Serving)
- Calories: 156
- Protein: 3.7 g
- Fat: 14.3 g
- Carbohydrates: 4.9 g
- Fiber: 1.1 g
- Sodium: 299 mg
- Cholesterol: 49 mg

Chicken Curry with Red Peppers

1 cup	chicken stock	250 mL
2 tsp	cornstarch	10 mL
¼ tsp	salt	1 mL
4 tsp	vegetable oil, divided	20 mL
1 lb	skinless, boneless chicken breasts, cut into thin strips	500 g
2	cloves garlic, minced	2
1 tbsp	minced fresh gingerroot	15 mL
1 tbsp	mild curry paste or powder	15 mL
2	large red bell peppers, cut into thin strips	2
4	green onions, sliced	4

SERVES 4

1. In a liquid glass measure, combine stock, cornstarch and salt; set aside.

2. In a large nonstick skillet, heat 2 tsp (10 mL) oil over medium-high heat; cook chicken, stirring often, for 5 minutes or until no longer pink inside. Transfer to a plate.

3. Reduce heat to medium; add remaining oil; cook garlic, ginger and curry paste; cook, stirring, for 1 minute. Add peppers; cook, stirring, for 2 minutes. Stir reserved stock mixture and pour into skillet; bring to a boil. Cook, stirring, until thickened. Add chicken and green onions; cook, stirring, for 2 minutes or until heated through.

Nutritional Analysis (Per Serving)
- Calories: 206
- Protein: 28.1 g
- Fat: 6.3 g
- Carbohydrates: 9.2 g
- Fiber: 2.0 g
- Sodium: 365 mg
- Cholesterol: 64 mg

Grilled Chicken with Curry Sauce

CHICKEN

4	boneless skinless chicken breasts (about 1 lb/500 g)	4
2 tsp	grated lemon or lime zest	10 mL
1/3 cup	lemon or lime juice	75 mL
2 tbsp	chopped fresh basil (or 2 tsp/10 mL dried)	25 mL
4 tsp	Dijon mustard	20 mL
2 tsp	chopped fresh thyme (or 1/4 tsp/1 mL dried)	5 mL
	Black pepper	

CURRY SAUCE

1/4 cup	light mayonnaise	50 mL
1/4 cup	lower-fat plain yogurt	50 mL
1 tsp	grated lime zest	5 mL
1 tbsp	lime juice	15 mL
1/2 tsp	curry powder	2 mL

Here is an easy "fusion" recipe that combines a variety of toothsome flavors from around the world.

SERVES 4

1. *Chicken:* Place chicken in single layer in glass dish. Combine lemon zest and juice, basil, mustard, thyme, and pepper to taste; pour over chicken. Cover and refrigerate for 3 to 12 hours, turning chicken occasionally.

2. Preheat barbecue or grill. Remove chicken from marinade. Grill for 6 to 8 minutes per side or until no longer pink inside.

3. *Curry Sauce:* In a bowl, combine mayonnaise, yogurt, lime zest and juice, and curry powder. Serve with chicken.

Tip

• Sauce used to marinate raw meat, poultry or seafood should not be used on cooked foods as it may contain harmful bacteria. Boil leftover marinade or prepare extra for basting cooked food. Wash and sanitize your brush or use separate brushes when marinating raw and cooked foods.

Nutritional Analysis (Per Serving)
- Calories: 186
- Protein: 28 g
- Fat: 6 g
- Carbohydrates: 3 g
- Fiber: Trace
- Sodium: 264 mg
- Cholesterol: 64 mg

East Indian Chicken

4	skinless, boneless chicken breasts	4
3/4 cup	plain yogurt	175 mL
2 tsp	minced gingerroot	10 mL
1 tsp	cumin	5 mL
	Salt and freshly ground black pepper	

In keeping with Indian tradition, plain yogurt, grated gingerroot, some cumin or curry are added to flavor chicken. Yogurt helps to keep the chicken moist during baking.

SERVES 4
Pie plate, lined with foil

1. Rinse and wipe chicken with paper towel. Place chicken in a resealable plastic bag.

2. In a glass measuring cup, stir together yogurt, gingerroot, cumin, salt and pepper. Pour over chicken in bag and seal. Refrigerate for several hours or overnight.

3. Preheat oven to 350°F (180°C). Transfer chicken to prepared pan. Bake for 20 minutes or until meat is no longer pink inside.

Nutritional Analysis (Per Serving)
- Calories: 214
- Protein: 42.0 g
- Fat: 2.3 g
- Carbohydrates: 3.9 g
- Fiber: 0.1 g
- Sodium: 144 mg
- Cholesterol: 97 mg

Curried Red Pepper Chicken

2 tsp	vegetable oil	10 mL
1¼ lb	boneless skinless chicken breasts, cut into strips	625 g
1 cup	thinly sliced carrots	250 mL
2 cups	julienned red bell peppers	500 mL
3 tbsp	curry paste	45 mL
1 cup	chicken stock	250 mL
1 tsp	minced garlic	5 mL
¼ tsp	black pepper	1 mL
¼ cup	water	50 mL
1 tbsp	cornstarch	15 mL

Quick and colorful, this is a great meal to make when you suddenly find yourself with company for dinner!

SERVES 6

1. In a large nonstick skillet, heat 1 tsp (5 mL) of the oil over medium-high heat. Add chicken strips and cook for 4 to 5 minutes or until browned on all sides. Remove chicken and set aside.

2. In same skillet, heat remaining oil over medium-high heat. Add carrots and peppers; cook for 3 minutes. Add curry paste and cook, stirring, for 1 minute or until thoroughly combined.

3. Return chicken to skillet. Stir in stock, garlic and pepper; bring to a boil. Reduce heat and simmer for 5 to 6 minutes or until chicken is cooked through and vegetables are tender-crisp.

4. In a small bowl, whisk together water and cornstarch; add to skillet. Cook over medium heat for 1 to 2 minutes or until thickened.

Tips

- This dish is very spicy — so feel free to adjust the curry paste to suit your "fire" tolerance.

- Curry paste is available in Asian markets and in the specialty foods section of some supermarkets.

- Serve Raita Cucumber Salad (see recipe, page 87) on the side.

Nutritional Analysis (Per Serving)
- Calories: 188
- Protein: 23 g
- Fat: 7 g
- Carbohydrates: 6 g
- Fiber: 1 g
- Sodium: 165 mg
- Cholesterol: 53 mg

Chicken Tikka Masala

12	cooked tandoori chicken thighs (see recipe, page 199), divided	12
3	green chilies, preferably serranos	3
1	piece (1 inch/2.5 cm) peeled gingerroot	1
1	can (28 oz/796 mL) whole or diced tomatoes, including juice	1
½ cup	butter, divided	125 mL
2 tbsp	freshly ground toasted cumin seeds, divided (see tip, at right)	25 mL
2 tsp	paprika	10 mL
1 cup	whipping (35%) cream	250 mL
1½ tsp	salt or to taste	7 mL
2 tsp	garam masala	10 mL
¾ cup	cilantro, chopped	175 mL

This dish was called Chicken Makhanwalla (Butter Chicken) until the British adopted it as their favorite Indian dish and its name morphed into this one. Chicken Tikka means "bite-size boneless chicken."

SERVES 8

1. Carefully debone cooked chicken, taking care not to shred it.
2. In a food processor, process chilies and ginger. Add tomatoes with juice and purée until smooth.
3. In a large saucepan, melt ¼ cup (50 mL) of the butter over medium heat. Add one-third of the chicken and sauté until edges begin to brown, 3 to 4 minutes. Transfer with a slotted spoon to a bowl. Brown remaining 2 batches of chicken in the same manner, adding 2 tbsp (25 mL) of the remaining butter as needed to prevent sticking.
4. Melt remaining 2 tbsp (25 mL) of butter in saucepan. Reduce heat to medium-low. Cook, stirring and scraping up all browned bits. Stir in 4 tsp (20 mL) of the cumin seeds and paprika. Stir rapidly for 1 minute.
5. Pour in tomato mixture and return to a gentle boil. Cook, uncovered, stirring frequently to allow flavors to blend, about 10 minutes. Add cream, salt, chicken and accumulated juices. Simmer, uncovered, stirring gently a few times and scraping bottom to prevent burning, until chicken is heated through, 10 to 12 minutes.
6. Stir in garam masala and remaining cumin. Remove from heat and cover. Let stand for 10 minutes before serving. Serve garnished with cilantro.

Tips

- This dish is better prepared ahead. Let cool, cover and refrigerate for up to 4 days or freeze for up to 3 months. Reheat on very low heat or in microwave.

- To toast cumin seeds: Spread seeds in a single layer in a heavy dry skillet. Cook over medium heat, shaking skillet occasionally to toast evenly, until seeds are a little darker and aromatic, 3 to 4 minutes. Let cool. Grind to a powder in a spice grinder.

Nutritional Analysis (Per Serving)
- Calories: 545
- Protein: 50.2 g
- Fat: 32.0 g
- Carbohydrates: 14.7 g
- Fiber: 2.7 g
- Sodium: 1233 mg
- Cholesterol: 256 mg

Yogurt-Marinated Chicken

1¼ cups	lower-fat plain yogurt	300 mL
3	cloves garlic, minced	3
1 tbsp	minced gingerroot (or 2 tsp/10 mL ground ginger)	15 mL
1 tbsp	lemon juice	15 mL
1 tbsp	vegetable oil	15 mL
2 tsp	paprika	10 mL
1 tsp	chili powder	5 mL
1 tsp	crumbled dried rosemary	5 mL
1 tsp	black pepper	5 mL
½ tsp	turmeric	2 mL
8	boneless skinless chicken breasts (about 1½ lb/750 g)	8

Here's an interesting variation on Chicken Tandoori.

SERVES 8

Preheat oven to 350°F (180°C) • Baking pan

1. In a large bowl, combine yogurt, garlic, ginger root, lemon juice, oil, paprika, chili powder, rosemary, pepper and turmeric; whisk until smooth. Add chicken, turning to coat all over. Cover and refrigerate for 24 hours.

2. Place chicken in single layer in baking pan, reserving marinade. Bake in preheated oven for 20 to 25 minutes or until no longer pink inside, spooning additional marinade over chicken halfway through baking.

Tips

• Instead of using only chicken breasts, you can substitute one 3-lb (1.5 kg) chicken, cut into 8 pieces; bake for 45 to 60 minutes.

• Most marinated recipes call for vinegar, lemon juice or wine. This Indian-style recipe uses yogurt, which enhances the taste and tenderizes the texture. Serve with a green salad.

Nutritional Analysis (Per Serving)
• Calories: 129   • Protein: 21 g   • Fat: 3 g
• Carbohydrates: 3 g   • Fiber: Trace   • Sodium: 143 mg
• Cholesterol: 50 mg

Indian-Style Grilled Chicken Breasts

½ cup	plain low-fat yogurt	125 mL
1 tbsp	tomato paste	15 mL
2	green onions, coarsely chopped	2
2	cloves garlic, quartered	2
1	piece (1-inch/2.5 cm) peeled gingerroot, coarsely chopped (or 1 tsp/5 mL ground ginger)	1
½ tsp	ground cumin	2 mL
½ tsp	ground coriander	2 mL
½ tsp	salt	2 mL
¼ tsp	cayenne pepper	1 mL
4	chicken breasts (bone-in)	4
2 tbsp	chopped fresh coriander or parsley	25 mL

SERVES 4

Preheat barbecue grill or oven to 350°F (180°C)

1. In a food processor, combine yogurt, tomato paste, green onions, garlic, ginger, cumin, coriander, salt and cayenne pepper; purée until smooth.

2. Arrange chicken in a shallow dish; coat with yogurt mixture. Cover and refrigerate for 1 hour or up to 1 day ahead. Remove from refrigerator 30 minutes before cooking.

3. Place chicken skin-side down on greased grill over medium-high heat; cook for 15 minutes. Brush with marinade; turn and cook for 10 to 15 minutes longer or until golden and juices run clear. (Or place chicken on rack set on baking sheet; roast, basting after 30 minutes with marinade, for 50 to 55 minutes or until juices run clear.) Serve garnished with chopped coriander.

Tip

- If you have time, let the chicken marinate for several hours, or overnight, in the refrigerator to intensify the flavors. To avoid bacterial contamination, baste the chicken only once halfway through cooking, then discard any leftover marinade.

Nutritional Analysis (Per Serving)
- Calories: 133
- Protein: 24 g
- Fat: 2 g
- Carbohydrates: 4 g
- Fiber: 0 g
- Sodium: 300 mg
- Cholesterol: 59 mg

Tandoori Chicken

16	skinless bone-in chicken thighs, or thighs and drumsticks (about 5 lbs/2.5 kg)	16
1 cup	plain nonfat yogurt	250 mL
	Juice of 2 lemons	
1 tbsp	minced peeled gingerroot	15 mL
1 tbsp	minced garlic	15 mL
2 tsp	coriander powder	10 mL
2 tsp	cumin powder	10 mL
2 tsp	garam masala	10 mL
1 tsp	cayenne pepper	5 mL
1½ tsp	salt or to taste	7 mL
	Few drops red food coloring (optional)	
	Juice of 2 limes or additional lemons	
1	onion, cut into rings, for garnish	1
	Lemon wedges, for garnish	

A tandoor is a North Indian clay oven that is about three feet high, usually buried in the ground up to the neck. Live coals are placed in the bottom, and skewers with meat and poultry are angled at a suitable distance from the heat to cook them. It's the Indian version of a barbecue.

SERVES 8

Preheat oven to 375°F (190°C) • Shallow baking pan, lined with foil

1. Rinse chicken and pat dry. Cut long diagonal slits against the grain, almost to the bone.

2. In a shallow bowl, mix together yogurt, lemon juice, ginger, garlic, coriander, cumin, garam masala, cayenne pepper and salt. Add red food coloring, if using. Add chicken, turning to coat and making sure marinade goes into all slits. Cover and marinate in refrigerator for about 2 hours or for up to 12 hours.

3. Remove chicken from marinade and place in prepared shallow baking pan. Discard any remaining marinade. Bake in preheated oven until juices run clear when chicken is pierced, about 45 minutes.

4. Transfer pieces onto heated platter and squeeze lime juice on top while still warm. Discard accumulated juices. Garnish with sliced onion rings and lemon wedges.

Tips

• Tandoori chicken is best cooked on a charcoal grill. Buy split chickens or leg quarters if using this method. Grease barbecue grill and preheat to medium-high. Place chicken on grill and cook, covered, for 20 minutes. Turn and cook until juices run clear when chicken is pierced, 20 to 25 minutes.

• Ginger and garlic can be minced in a blender, grated on a ginger grater or purchased already prepared in jars.

Nutritional Analysis (Per Serving)
• Calories: 311 • Protein: 48.0 g • Fat: 8.9 g
• Carbohydrates: 7.7 g • Fiber: 0.9 g • Sodium: 654 mg
• Cholesterol: 185 mg

Easy Tandoori Chicken

2 tbsp	fresh lemon juice	25 mL
1 tbsp	minced ginger root	15 mL
3	cloves garlic, minced	3
¼ tsp	ground allspice	1 mL
¼ tsp	cinnamon	1 mL
¼ tsp	black pepper	1 mL
¼ tsp	cayenne pepper	1 mL
4	chicken legs with thighs attached	4

A spicy paste is rubbed on and under the skin, and the chicken is broiled close to the element or grilled over high heat to make it crisp and flavorful. Real tandoori chicken is marinated in yogurt and spices, then roasted in a tandoor, which reaches incredibly high temperatures.

SERVES 4

Preheat broiler • Broiler pan with greased rack

1. In a bowl combine lemon juice, ginger, garlic, allspice, cinnamon, black pepper and cayenne; mix to form a paste. Loosen skin of each thigh by slipping your fingers between the skin and the flesh and over the thigh-leg joint. Spread ¾ tsp (4 mL) of the paste on the flesh and squeeze to distribute evenly. Spread the remainder over the outside surfaces.

2. Place chicken skin-side down in prepared pan. Broil about 6 inches (15 cm) from the heat for 15 minutes. Turn the pieces over and broil 10 to 15 minutes longer or until meat near the thighbone is no longer pink inside, placing a piece of foil, shiny side up, on top if the chicken gets too brown. (Alternatively, place skin-side up on greased grill and barbecue, turning after 15 minutes.)

Nutritional Analysis (Per Serving)
- Calorie: 408
- Protein: 28.7 g
- Fat: 31.2 g
- Carbohydrates: 1.6 g
- Fiber: 0.3 g
- Sodium: 126 mg
- Cholesterol: 138 mg

Chinese Chicken with Garlic Ginger Sauce

3 lb	whole chicken	1.5 kg
SAUCE		
⅓ cup	chicken stock	75 mL
¼ cup	chopped green onions (about 2 medium)	50 mL
3 tbsp	vegetable oil	45 mL
4 tsp	soya sauce	20 mL
1 tsp	minced garlic	5 mL
1 tsp	minced ginger root	5 mL

Make Ahead

Prepare up to a day ahead and serve at room temperature.

SERVES 6

1. Remove neck and giblets from chicken and discard. Place chicken in large saucepan and add water to cover. Cover saucepan and bring to a boil over high heat. Reduce heat to low and simmer, covered, for 45 minutes, or until juices run clear from chicken leg when pierced.

2. Meanwhile, whisk together stock, green onions, oil, soya sauce, garlic and ginger in a small bowl.

3. Remove chicken from pot and let cool slightly. Remove skin; cut into serving pieces. Serve with dipping sauce.

Nutritional Analysis (Per Serving)
- Calories: 156
- Protein: 17 g
- Fat: 9 g
- Carbohydrates: 1 g
- Fiber: 0 g
- Sodium: 337 mg
- Cholesterol: 53 mg

Exotic Ginger Cumin Chicken

1 tbsp	vegetable oil, divided	15 mL
2 lb	boneless skinless chicken breasts, cut into bite-size pieces	1 kg
2 tsp	minced garlic	10 mL
1/2 cup	chopped onion	125 mL
1 tbsp	finely chopped gingerroot (or 1/2 tsp/2 mL ground ginger)	15 mL
1/4 to 1/2 tsp	cayenne pepper	1 to 2 mL
1 tsp	each ground coriander and cumin	5 mL
1 tsp	ground turmeric	5 mL
1/2 cup	chicken stock	125 mL
1	can (19 oz/540 mL) stewed tomatoes	1
2 tbsp	tomato paste	25 mL
2 tsp	granulated sugar	10 mL
1/2 tsp	salt	2 mL
3/4 cup	lower-fat plain yogurt	175 mL
2 tbsp	chopped fresh cilantro (optional)	25 mL

Here's another curry-style chicken dish you can make using ingredients you're likely to have on hand.

SERVES 8

1. In a large saucepan or Dutch oven, heat 2 tsp (10 mL) of the oil over medium high heat. Add half of the chicken and cook for 2 to 3 minutes or until brown. Remove from pan and set aside. Repeat with remaining chicken.

2. Add remaining oil to pan; add garlic, onion and ginger. Reduce heat to medium and cook, stirring constantly, for 4 to 5 minutes or until softened but not brown. Stir in cayenne, coriander, cumin and turmeric; sauté for 1 minute or until fragrant.

3. Stir in stock, tomatoes, tomato paste, sugar and salt; return chicken to pan. Bring to a boil; reduce heat and simmer for 5 minutes or until chicken is no longer pink inside.

4. Stir in yogurt and cilantro, if using; simmer over very low heat for 1 to 2 minutes.

Tips

- Try using canola oil in this and other recipes that call for vegetable oil. Canola oil is high in monounsaturated fat. It is inexpensive and widely available. And because of its neutral flavor, it is an excellent all-purpose oil for baking, cooking and salad dressings.

- Serve this flavorful chicken dish with a cool, creamy Raita Cucumber Salad (see recipe, page 87). Finish with a serving of fruit.

Nutritional Analysis (Per Serving)
- Calories: 193
- Protein: 28 g
- Fat: 4 g
- Carbohydrates: 10 g
- Fiber: 1 g
- Sodium: 277 mg
- Cholesterol: 64 mg

Ginger Chili Chicken

12	skinless bone-in chicken thighs	12
½ cup	freshly squeezed lime or lemon juice	125 mL
2½ tsp	freshly ground black pepper	12 mL
1½ tsp	mustard powder	7 mL
2 tsp	salt or to taste	10 mL
3 tbsp	vegetable oil	45 mL
½ cup	julienne peeled gingerroot	125 mL
6 to 8	green chilies, preferably serranos, julienned	6 to 8
	Lemon or lime slices, for garnish	
1	sprig cilantro, for garnish	1

The astonishing flavors of this simple dish will amaze you. Use the freshest ginger you can find, because the juice will greatly enhance the taste.

SERVES 8

1. Rinse chicken and pat dry.
2. In a large bowl, combine lime juice, pepper, mustard powder and salt. Add chicken and mix well. Marinate at room temperature for 30 minutes.
3. In a large skillet with a tight-fitting lid, heat oil over medium-high heat. Sauté ginger and chilies until almost crisp, about 2 minutes.
4. Add chicken with marinade. Reduce heat to medium and brown for 4 to 5 minutes per side. Add 2 tbsp (25 mL) water and cover. Reduce heat to medium-low and simmer, turning once, until chicken is no longer pink inside, about 30 minutes. Shake skillet periodically to prevent sticking, adding 1 or 2 tbsp (15 to 25 mL) water if necessary. Garnish with lime slices and cilantro.

Nutritional Analysis (Per Serving)
- Calories: 360
- Protein: 40.0g
- Fat: 13.0 g
- Carbohydrates: 23.8 g
- Fiber: 11.9 g
- Sodium: 769 mg
- Cholesterol: 138 mg

Tangy Glazed Chicken

1 lb	chicken breasts, skinned and boned	500 g
2 tbsp	sugar-reduced apricot jam or orange marmalade	25 mL
2 tbsp	unsweetened orange juice	25 mL
1	small clove garlic, minced	1
2 tsp	soy sauce	10 mL
½ tsp	ground ginger	2 mL
¼ tsp	dry mustard	1 mL

Apricot jam or orange marmalade and Asian flavors add flair to this easy-to-make dish.

SERVES 4

Preheat oven to 350°F (180°C) • Baking pan, lightly greased

1. Place chicken in pan. Combine remaining ingredients and spoon over chicken. Bake in preheated oven until chicken is glazed and no longer pink inside, about 45 minutes.

Tips

- Mustard is a versatile condiment and has many uses in cooking. Dry mustard, used here, is hot and pungent. It adds flavor without fat.
- Serve this tasty dish with steamed green beans. End the meal with sherbet sprinkled with fresh berries.

Nutritional Analysis (Per Serving)
- Calories: 151
- Protein: 26 g
- Fat: 3 g
- Carbohydrates: 3 g
- Fiber: 0 g
- Sodium: 161 mg
- Cholesterol: 64 mg

Coriander Chicken

12	skinless boneless chicken thighs, about 3 lbs (1.5 kg)	12
2 tbsp	minced peeled gingerroot	25 mL
2 tbsp	minced garlic	25 mL
2 tsp	salt or to taste	10 mL
	Juice of 1 lime or lemon	
3 tbsp	vegetable oil	45 mL
5 tbsp	coriander seeds, freshly toasted and powdered in spice grinder to yield about $1/4$ cup/50 mL powder (see tips, at right)	60 mL
1 tbsp	freshly ground black pepper	15 mL
2	green onions, finely sliced, with some green, for garnish	2

Coriander is one of the most popular seasonings in the Indian lexicon of spices and herbs. Its sweet, nutty flavor complements meats and vegetables alike. This simple but so delicious recipe showcases the highly aromatic spice.

SERVES 6

1. Rinse chicken and pat dry.
2. In a large bowl, combine ginger, garlic, salt and lime juice. Add chicken and toss to coat. Cover and marinate in refrigerator for 1 hour.
3. In a large saucepan, heat oil over medium-high heat. Add chicken with marinade and sauté until juices exuded from chicken cook down. When there is no more liquid, continue to brown chicken. The entire process will take 10 to 12 minutes.
4. Reduce heat to medium. Mix in coriander and pepper. Sauté for 2 minutes longer. If necessary, add water, 1 to 2 tbsp (15 to 25 mL) at a time, to prevent chicken from sticking to pan while browning.
5. Add $1/3$ cup (75 mL) water. Cover and simmer until chicken is no longer pink inside, 8 to 10 minutes. Shake pan periodically to prevent burning. There should be no liquid left in the pan and a thick gravy should coat the chicken.
6. Garnish with green onions.

Tips

- The key to success with this recipe lies in the freshly toasted and ground coriander seeds. The few extra minutes it takes to do this is well worth it. Do not use store-bought ground coriander.
- To toast coriander seeds: Spread in a dry heavy skillet. Cook over medium heat, shaking skillet occasionally to toast evenly, until seeds are a little darker and aromatic, 4 to 5 minutes. Let cool. Grind to a powder in a spice grinder.
- If doubling recipe, cook in 2 batches.

Nutritional Analysis (Per Serving)		
• Calories: 263	• Protein: 31.3 g	• Fat: 13.4 g
• Carbohydrates: 4.8 g	• Fiber: 2.6 g	• Sodium: 907 mg
• Cholesterol: 123 mg		

Pepper Chicken

12	skinless bone-in chicken thighs, or drumsticks and thighs (about 4 lbs/2 kg)	12
2 cups	plain nonfat yogurt	500 mL
2 tsp	cornstarch	10 mL
1 tbsp	minced peeled gingerroot	15 mL
1 tbsp	minced garlic	15 mL
2	minced green chilies, preferably serranos	2
2 tsp	salt or to taste	10 mL
1 cup	cilantro, chopped	250 mL
2 tbsp	vegetable oil	25 mL
1 tbsp	freshly cracked black peppercorns (see tip, at right)	15 mL

SERVES 8

1. Rinse chicken and pat dry.
2. In a large saucepan, stir together yogurt, cornstarch, ginger, garlic, chilies and salt. Add chicken and mix well. Marinate for 30 minutes at room temperature.
3. Cover and bring to a boil over medium heat. Reduce heat and simmer, shaking pan occasionally and turning pieces once to ensure even cooking, for 30 to 35 minutes. (Yogurt will curdle. Don't worry as it will be fine when dish is finished.) If there is too much liquid, increase heat and leave uncovered.
4. Reduce heat, shaking pan occasionally, until there is about 1 cup (250 mL) liquid and chicken is tender and no longer pink inside. Stir gently to loosen chicken from bottom of pan. Scatter cilantro over top.
5. In a small saucepan, heat oil over medium heat. Add peppercorns and cook until sizzling, about 1 minute. Pour over chicken and mix gently. Remove from heat. Cover and let stand for 5 minutes before serving.

Tips

- If planning to freeze, leave extra gravy to spoon over chicken to ensure it stays moist.
- To crack black peppercorns: Pound in a mortar and pestle or place in a heavy-duty resealable plastic bag and crack with a meat mallet or bottom of a saucepan until cracked. Do not grind.

Nutritional Analysis (Per Serving)
- Calories: 283
- Protein: 38.1 g
- Fat: 10.1 g
- Carbohydrates: 8.2 g
- Fiber: 0.8 g
- Sodium: 775 mg
- Cholesterol: 139 mg

Preeti's Brown Onion Chicken

12	skinless bone-in chicken thighs, about 4 lbs (2 kg)	12
1/4 cup	vegetable oil, divided	50 mL
2 cups	chopped onions (about 1 1/2)	500 mL
2 cups	plain nonfat yogurt, at room temperature	500 mL
2 tsp	cornstarch	10 mL
1 tsp	minced garlic	5 mL
1/2 tsp	minced peeled gingerroot	2 mL
3/4 tsp	black cumin (shah jeera)	4 mL
1/2 tsp	cumin seeds	2 mL
4	bay leaves	4
6	green cardamom pods, cracked open	6
5	whole cloves	5
1	stick cinnamon, about 1 inch (2.5 cm) long	1
3	whole dried red chilies, seeds removed if desired (see tip, at right)	3
2 tsp	salt or to taste	10 mL
1 cup	cilantro, chopped, divided	250 mL

SERVES 6 TO 8

1. Rinse chicken and pat dry.

2. In a large saucepan with a tight-fitting lid, heat 2 tbsp (25 mL) of the oil over medium-high heat. Sauté onions until beginning to color, 4 to 5 minutes. Reduce heat to medium and sauté until dark brown, 15 to 20 minutes longer.

3. Transfer onions to a blender. Stir yogurt to a creamy consistency and mix in cornstarch. Add 1 cup (250 mL) of the yogurt mixture to blender. Blend until smooth. Stir back into remaining yogurt. Set aside.

4. In the same saucepan, heat remaining oil over medium heat. Stir in garlic and ginger. Sauté for 30 seconds. Add black cumin, cumin seeds, bay leaves, cardamom pods, cloves, cinnamon and chilies. Sauté for 1 minute.

5. Increase heat to medium-high. Add chicken and salt and brown, 6 to 8 minutes per side.

6. Add yogurt mixture and half of the cilantro. Cover and bring to a boil. Reduce heat to low and simmer until chicken is no longer pink inside and gravy is thick, about 30 minutes. Discard bay leaves, cloves, cinnamon stick and chilies, if desired. Fold in remaining cilantro just before serving.

Tips

• Red chilies and whole spices should be removed before serving. They are used for flavor only, and the chilies are too fiery to eat.

• The key to success here is taking the time to caramelize the onions for the deep, rich flavor.

Nutritional Analysis (Per Serving)
• Calories: 371   • Protein: 43.8 g   • Fat: 15.5 g
• Carbohydrates: 12.4 g   • Fiber: 1.5 g   • Sodium: 886 mg
• Cholesterol: 159 mg

Chicken with Aromatic Puréed Spinach

12	skinless bone-in chicken thighs, about 4 lbs (2 kg)	12
1/4 cup	freshly squeezed lemon juice	50 mL
2 tbsp	vegetable oil	25 mL
2 cups	finely sliced onions (about 1 1/2)	500 mL
1 tbsp	minced green chilies, preferably serranos	15 mL
1 tsp	minced peeled gingerroot	5 mL
1 tsp	minced garlic	5 mL
2 tsp	coriander powder	10 mL
1 tsp	cumin powder	5 mL
1/2 tsp	turmeric	2 mL
1/2 tsp	cayenne pepper	2 mL
1 cup	chopped tomatoes	250 mL
2 tsp	salt or to taste	10 mL
2	packages (each 10 oz/300 g) frozen spinach, thawed	2
	Juice of 1 lime or lemon	

Chicken or lamb cooked with spinach is a north Indian favorite that appears on most restaurant menus. I like the flavor and texture of the creamy spinach complementing the chicken.

SERVES 8

1. Rinse chicken and pat dry. Marinate in lemon juice for 20 to 30 minutes.

2. Meanwhile, in a large saucepan, heat oil over medium-high heat. Sauté onions until beginning to color, 4 to 5 minutes. Reduce heat to medium and sauté until golden, 12 to 14 minutes longer. Stir in chilies, ginger and garlic. Sauté for 2 minutes.

3. Add coriander, cumin, turmeric and cayenne pepper. Reduce heat to low and sauté for 2 minutes.

4. Place chicken on top of masala. Scatter tomatoes over top of chicken. Sprinkle with salt. Cover and cook over low heat for 10 minutes.

5. Turn chicken over. Mix with masala, scraping bottom of pan. Add 2 tbsp (25 mL) water if necessary to deglaze. Cover and cook for 10 minutes longer.

6. Meanwhile, in a blender, purée spinach with 1 1/2 cups (375 mL) water. Pour into chicken and mix. Cover and simmer until gravy is thick and chicken is no longer pink inside, 10 to 15 minutes.

7. Remove from heat and stir in lime juice.

Nutritional Analysis (Per Serving)
- Calories: 287
- Protein: 37.9 g
- Fat: 10.3 g
- Carbohydrates: 11.1 g
- Fiber: 3.2 g
- Sodium: 810 mg
- Cholesterol: 138 mg

Chicken Kebabs with Ginger Lemon Marinade

8 oz	boneless skinless chicken breasts, cut into 2-inch (5 cm) cubes	250 g
16	squares sweet green pepper	16
16	pineapple chunks (fresh or canned)	16
16	cherry tomatoes	16

GINGER LEMON MARINADE

3 tbsp	lemon juice	45 mL
2 tbsp	water	25 mL
1 tbsp	vegetable oil	15 mL
2 tsp	sesame oil	10 mL
1½ tsp	red wine vinegar	7 mL
4 tsp	brown sugar	20 mL
1 tsp	minced gingerroot (or ¼ tsp/1 mL ground)	5 mL
½ tsp	ground coriander	2 mL
½ tsp	ground fennel seeds (optional)	2 mL

SERVES 4

1. *Ginger Lemon Marinade:* In small bowl, combine lemon juice, water, vegetable oil, sesame oil, vinegar, brown sugar, ginger, coriander and fennel seeds (if using); mix well. Add chicken and mix well; marinate for 20 minutes.

2. Alternately thread chicken cubes, green pepper, pineapple and tomatoes onto 4 long or 8 short barbecue skewers. Barbecue for 15 to 20 minutes or just until chicken is no longer pink inside, brushing often with marinade and rotating every 5 minutes.

Tips

- This tart yet sweet marinade also complements veal and firm white fish.

- For a change, try a combination of red and yellow peppers along with the green pepper.

Nutritional Analysis (Per Serving)
- Calories: 110
- Protein: 13 g
- Fat: 2
- Carbohydrates: 10 g
- Fiber: 2 g
- Sodium: 35 mg
- Cholesterol: 31 mg

Chicken with Teriyaki Vegetables

4	boneless skinless chicken breasts	4
1 tsp	vegetable oil	5 mL
1 tsp	crushed garlic	5 mL
1	large sweet red pepper, sliced thinly	1
1 cup	snow peas, trimmed	250 mL
MARINADE		
3 tbsp	sherry	45 mL
3 tbsp	brown sugar	45 mL
2 tbsp	water	25 mL
2 tbsp	soya sauce	25 mL
2 tbsp	vegetable oil	25 mL
1 1/2 tsp	minced gingerroot	7 mL

SERVES 4
Preheat oven to 425°F (220°C) • Baking dish sprayed with nonstick vegetable spray

1. *Marinade:* In medium bowl, combine sherry, sugar, water, soya sauce, oil and ginger. Set aside.

2. Place chicken between 2 sheets of waxed paper; pound until thin and flattened. Add to bowl and marinate for 30 minutes.

3. Remove chicken and place in baking dish. Pour marinade into saucepan; cook for 3 to 4 minutes or until thickened and syrupy. Set 2 tbsp (25 mL) aside; brush remainder over chicken. Cover and bake for 10 to 15 minutes or until no longer pink inside.

4. Meanwhile, in large nonstick skillet, heat oil; sauté garlic, red pepper and snow peas for 2 minutes. Add reserved marinade; cook for 2 minutes, stirring constantly. Serve over chicken.

Nutritional Analysis (Per Serving)
- Calories: 221
- Protein: 26 g
- Fat: 7 g
- Carbohydrates: 9 g
- Fiber: 1 g
- Sodium: 318 mg
- Cholesterol: 62 mg

Chicken with Peanut Sauce for One

1 tbsp	smooth peanut butter	15 mL
2 tsp	soya sauce	10 mL
2 tsp	rice or white wine vinegar	10 mL
Pinch	hot pepper flakes	Pinch
1 tsp	vegetable oil	5 mL
1	skinless boneless chicken breast, cut into (1/2-inch/1 cm) cubes	1
2 tsp	minced garlic	10 mL
1 tsp	minced gingerroot	5 mL

When you're home alone, this quick dish is very comforting. If someone comes along, it's easily doubled.

SERVES I

1. In a measuring cup, stir together 1/4 cup (50 mL) water, peanut butter, soya sauce, vinegar and hot pepper flakes.

2. In a nonstick skillet or wok, heat oil over medium-high heat. Add chicken, garlic and ginger; cook, stirring, 2 to 3 minutes or until the chicken is no longer pink inside.

3. Stir in peanut butter mixture; bring to a boil. Reduce heat to low; cook, stirring, for 3 minutes or until thickened.

Nutritional Analysis (Per Serving)
- Calories: 332
- Protein: 43.9 g
- Fat: 14.6 g
- Carbohydrates: 6.1 g
- Fiber: 1.2 g
- Sodium: 542 mg
- Cholesterol: 96 mg

Szechuan Chicken and Peanuts with Chili Peppers

2	whole chicken breasts,* cut into ¹/₂-inch (1 cm) pieces	2
1 tbsp	minced gingerroot	15 mL
2 tsp	light soya sauce	10 mL
¹/₄ tsp	salt	1 mL
1 tsp	cornstarch	5 mL
2 tbsp	peanut or vegetable oil	25 mL
¹/₂ cup	unsalted skinless peanuts	125 mL
4	small dried red chili peppers	4
1 tsp	rice vinegar	5 mL
¹/₂ tsp	granulated sugar	2 mL
	Boston or leaf lettuce leaves	

Chinese chefs usually bone the chicken breasts but leave the skin on before dicing. You can do the same or use 4 boneless skinless chicken breasts.

SERVES 4

1. In a bowl combine the chicken, ginger, soya sauce, salt and cornstarch; set aside.
2. In a wok, heat oil over medium-high heat. Add peanuts and stir-fry for 2 minutes. Remove with a slotted spoon; set aside. Add chili peppers; stir-fry for 30 seconds. Remove with a slotted spoon and set aside. Add chicken mixture and stir-fry for 2 minutes. Add vinegar, sugar, reserved peanuts and chilies; cook for another 1 to 2 minutes.
3. Serve immediately on a lettuce-lined platter.

Tips

- Szechuan vies with the Hunan province for the spiciest of Chinese regional cuisines. You can make this simple stir-fry hotter by adding more chili peppers if you wish; or reduce the heat by adding fewer.

- You can stir-fry vegetables like bok choy, mushrooms and red pepper strips in a bit of oil; add a small amount of water, cover and steam until tender. Or purchase a good frozen Oriental vegetable mix and cook according to the package instructions.

Nutritional Analysis (Per Serving)
- Calories: 507
- Protein: 41.6 g
- Fat: 34.0 g
- Carbohydrates: 9.2 g
- Fiber: 3.1 g
- Sodium: 527 mg
- Cholesterol: 108 mg

Spicy Peanut Chicken

1 tbsp	vegetable oil	15 mL
1 lb	skinless boneless chicken, cut into 1-inch (2.5 cm) cubes	500 g
1 cup	diced onion	250 mL
1 tbsp	minced garlic	15 mL
2 tsp	curry powder	10 mL
1 tsp	salt	5 mL
	Freshly ground black pepper	
1 cup	chopped red or green bell pepper or 1½ cups (375 mL) frozen mixed bell pepper strips	250 mL
1 tbsp	all-purpose flour	15 mL
2 cups	tomato juice	500 mL
¼ cup	peanut butter	50 mL

Surprise your family with this exotic stew, which is easily made with pantry ingredients. If you're a heat seeker, add Asian chili sauce.

SERVES 4

1. In a skillet, heat oil over medium heat. Add chicken and onion and cook, stirring, until onions are softened and chicken is no longer pink inside, about 8 minutes.
2. Add garlic, curry powder, salt, and black pepper to taste. Cook, stirring, for 1 minute. Add bell pepper and cook, stirring, for 1 minute. Add flour and cook, stirring, for 1 minute.
3. Add tomato juice. Bring to a boil. Cook, stirring, until thickened, about 5 minutes. Add peanut butter and stir until blended.

Tips

- If you prefer a spicier result, add 1 tsp (5 mL) Asian chili sauce along with the peanut butter.
- Maximize convenience by using frozen diced onion, bottled or frozen minced garlic and frozen mixed bell pepper strips.

Nutritional Analysis (Per Serving)
- Calories: 313
- Protein: 30.4 g
- Fat: 14.6 g
- Carbohydrates: 17.5 g
- Fiber: 3.4 g
- Sodium: 758 mg
- Cholesterol: 78 mg

Chicken with Chilies

1	roasting chicken (about 4 lbs/2 kg), fat trimmed and cut down the back, allowing it to lie flat	1
3 tbsp	extra virgin olive oil	45 mL
½ tsp	salt	2 mL
¼ tsp	freshly cracked black peppercorns	1 mL
2 tsp	red pepper flakes	10 mL
	Juice of 1 large lemon	

There is something so good about this roast chicken — with its rub-down of olive oil, dried chilies, coarse salt, lots of cracked pepper and squirt of lemon — that it's completely addictive. The only cure is to make it again.

SERVES 4 TO 6

1. Place chicken skin-side up in an ovenproof dish, preferably terra cotta. Rub all over with olive oil, salt and cracked peppercorns; sprinkle with pepper flakes. Pour lemon juice over chicken, cover with plastic wrap and leave it to sit for at least 1 hour.

2. Preheat oven to 400°F (200°C). Roast chicken for about 60 to 65 minutes or until golden brown and crispy. If the skin begins to brown too quickly, reduce heat. Serve while very hot.

Tips

- Use a kitchen mallet to crack the bones of the chicken. This encourages them to release their flavorful marrow; it also helps to flatten the chicken somewhat, making for a quicker cooking time.

- Take care not to overcook the chicken or the white meat will become dry.

- This dish is even more phenomenal when grilled over charcoal.

Nutritional Analysis (Per Serving)
- Calories: 424
- Protein: 32.1 g
- Fat: 31.6 g
- Carbohydrates: 1.0 g
- Fiber: 0.3 g
- Sodium: 350 mg
- Cholesterol: 123 mg

Shrimp-Stuffed Chicken

25	medium raw shrimp, peeled and deveined	25
1/2 cup	firm tofu	125 mL
1/4 cup	chopped onion	50 mL
2	cloves garlic, minced	2
1 tbsp	grated gingerroot	15 mL
1 tbsp	lime juice	15 mL
1 tbsp	chopped fresh cilantro	15 mL
2 tsp	soy sauce	10 mL
1/4 tsp	each salt and white pepper	1 mL
6	boneless skinless chicken breasts (about 1 1/2 lb/750 g)	6
1	egg white, lightly beaten	1
	Grated lime zest	

YOGURT LIME SAUCE

1 cup	strong chicken broth	250 mL
1 tbsp	chopped shallots	15 mL
2 tbsp	cornstarch	25 mL
2 tbsp	lime juice	25 mL
1 tbsp	Dijon mustard	15 mL
1/4 cup	lower-fat plain yogurt	50 mL

Tofu, cilantro, ginger and lime give this tasty chicken an Asian flair. The unusual Yogurt Lime Sauce, which is flavored with Dijon mustard, adds a "fusion" element to the dish.

SERVES 6
Preheat oven to 350°F (180°C) • 9-inch (2.5 L) square baking pan • Roasting pan

1. In a food processor, chop shrimp very finely. Add tofu, onion, garlic, ginger root, lime juice, cilantro, soy sauce, salt and pepper; process to form paste.

2. With meat mallet, pound chicken between plastic wrap to flatten. Divide shrimp mixture among breasts. Brush edges with egg white; fold chicken around filling to seal. Wrap individually in plastic wrap; place in 9-inch (2.5 L) square baking pan. Place in roasting pan (or broiler pan). Add boiling water to come three-quarters of the way up sides of square pan. Cover and bake in preheated oven for 25 to 30 minutes or until firm and moist.

3. *Yogurt Lime Sauce:* In a saucepan, bring broth and shallots to a boil. Combine cornstarch, lime juice and mustard; stir into broth until boiling and thickened. Over low heat, add yogurt and heat through. Serve with chicken. Garnish with lime zest.

Tips

• When mincing ginger root, peel off the skin and chop finely, or use a fine grater. If you have leftover chopped ginger root, cover it with sherry and refrigerate in a sealed jar. Use the drained ginger to flavor oil before sautéing meat.

• Poaching the chicken, rather than frying, and using a lower-fat yogurt for the sauce make this tangy entrée lower in calories and fat. Serve with Orange Broccoli (see recipe, page 311).

Nutritional Analysis (Per Serving)
• Calories: 210 • Protein: 35 g • Fat: 4 g
• Carbohydrates: 7 g • Fiber: 1 g • Sodium: 473 mg
• Cholesterol: 179 mg

Baked Chicken Parmesan

2 tsp	vegetable oil	10 mL
4	boneless skinless chicken breasts	4
1 cup	diced zucchini	250 mL
1/2 cup	sliced onions	125 mL
1 1/2 cups	tomato pasta sauce	375 mL
1 tsp	dried basil or dried Italian seasoning	5 mL
1 cup	shredded part-skim mozzarella cheese	250 mL
1/2 cup	grated Parmesan cheese	125 mL

Here's another kid-friendly dinner that can be made using ingredients you're likely to have on hand.

SERVES 4

Preheat oven to 350°F (180°C) • 11- by 7-inch (2 L) baking dish, greased

1. In a large nonstick skillet, heat 1 tsp (5 mL) of the oil over medium-high heat. Add chicken breasts and sear for 1 to 2 minutes per side or until golden brown. Transfer to greased 11- by 7-inch (2 L) baking dish.

2. Heat remaining oil in skillet. Add zucchini and onions; sauté for 3 to 5 minutes or until lightly browned. Remove from pan and place on top of chicken.

3. In a small bowl, blend together Piquant Tomato Sauce and basil; pour over chicken and vegetables. Sprinkle with mozzarella and Parmesan cheese. Bake in preheated oven for 25 to 30 minutes or until juices run clear when chicken is pierced with a fork.

Tips

• After preparing uncooked meat and poultry, be sure to clean cutting boards and utensils in hot, soapy water and sanitize by rinsing in hot water that has a capful of bleach added to it. Having two cutting boards — one for raw meat and the other for everything else — helps reduce chances of bacterial contamination.

• Using commercially prepared pasta sauce can increase salt intake; if this is a concern, make your own.

Nutritional Analysis (Per Serving)
- Calories: 372
- Protein: 47 g
- Fat: 15 g
- Carbohydrates: 12 g
- Fiber: 2 g
- Sodium: 468 mg
- Cholesterol: 125 mg

Crisp Parmesan Chicken

2	skinless boneless chicken breasts	2
	Salt and pepper	
¼ cup	all-purpose flour	50 mL
1	egg	1
½ cup	freshly grated Parmesan cheese	125 mL
¼ tsp	dried oregano	1 mL
¼ tsp	dried basil	1 mL
1 tbsp	olive oil	15 mL

Make Ahead

Recipe can be prepared to the end of step 3, covered and refrigerated for up to 8 hours.

This flavorful chicken has a lovely texture that will go well with any number of crisply cooked vegetables.

SERVES 2

1. Place chicken between 2 pieces of plastic wrap and pound with a mallet or rolling pin to an even thickness of about ¼ inch (5 mm). Pat dry and sprinkle with salt and pepper.

2. Place flour on waxed paper. In a shallow bowl, beat egg with 1 tbsp (15 mL) cold water. In another shallow bowl, mix cheese with oregano and basil.

3. Dust each breast with flour, dip in egg and coat with cheese. Place on a plate and refrigerate if making ahead.

4. In a large skillet, heat oil over medium-high heat. Add chicken and cook 3 minutes. Using a wide spatula to get all the crust, turn and cook 1 to 2 minutes longer or until no longer pink inside.

Nutritional Analysis (Per Serving)
- Calories: 435
- Protein: 52.4 g
- Fat: 17.6 g
- Carbohydrates: 13.6 g
- Fiber: 0.7 g
- Sodium: 1675 mg
- Cholesterol: 219 mg

Chicken Breasts in Pizzaiola Sauce

¼ cup	olive oil	50 mL
4	garlic cloves, minced	4
4	anchovy fillets, rinsed, drained, patted dry and finely chopped	4
2 tbsp	finely chopped flat-leaf parsley	25 mL
2 tsp	finely chopped oregano	10 mL
2½ cups	canned, peeled plum tomatoes, chopped, plus ¼ cup (50 mL) of their juice or, in season, 2½ lbs (1.25 kg) fresh, ripe plum tomatoes, chopped or *passata* (puréed, sieved tomatoes)	625 mL
½ tsp	salt	2 mL
¼ tsp	freshly ground black pepper	1 mL
3 tbsp	olive oil	45 mL
6	boneless, skinless chicken breasts, pounded flat	6

Pizzaiola is Naples' classic tomato sauce, so named because the ingredients for this fresh-tasting, simple sauce are the same as those used to dress pizzas. This preparation is simplicity itself.

SERVES 4 TO 6

1. In a skillet heat the olive oil over medium-high heat. Add garlic and cook for 1 minute or until softened. Stir in chopped anchovies, parsley, and oregano.

2. Using the back of a fork, mash the anchovies into a paste. Cook, stirring, for another 2 or 3 minutes. Add tomatoes, salt and pepper; stir until well combined. Cook until thickened, about 15 minutes.

3. In another skillet, heat remaining olive oil. Add chicken breasts and cook for about 8 minutes on each side, until cooked through.

4. Season thickened tomato sauce to taste. Pour some of the sauce to pool in the center of each warmed plate. Place a chicken breast on top of the sauce and serve immediately.

Tips

- Try to use fresh oregano; there is no comparison between it and the dried version.

- You can omit the anchovies if you prefer. If using anchovies, you may need less salt.

- The sauce is equally good with mild-tasting white fish, shrimp or seared scallops.

Nutritional Analysis (Per Serving)
- Calories: 391
- Protein: 41.8 g
- Fat: 21.6 g
- Carbohydrates: 6.6 g
- Fiber: 1.6 g
- Sodium: 493 mg
- Cholesterol: 99 mg

Chicken Cacciatore with Thick Tomato Sauce

4	chicken drumsticks, skinned	4
4	chicken thighs, skinned	4
	All-purpose flour for dusting	
1 tbsp	vegetable oil	15 mL
2 tsp	crushed garlic	10 mL
1 cup	chopped onion	250 mL
½ cup	chopped sweet green pepper	125 mL
1 cup	sliced mushrooms	250 mL
1	can (19 oz/540 mL) tomatoes, crushed	1
2 tbsp	tomato paste	25 mL
1 tsp	dried basil	5 mL
1 tsp	dried oregano	5 mL
¼ cup	red wine	50 mL
1 tbsp	grated Parmesan cheese	15 mL
¼ cup	chopped fresh parsley	50 mL

SERVES 4

1. Dust chicken with flour. In large nonstick skillet, heat oil; sauté chicken just until browned on all sides. Remove and set aside.
2. To skillet, add garlic, onion, green pepper and mushrooms; sauté for 5 minutes or until softened. Add tomatoes, tomato paste, basil, oregano and wine; stir to mix well.
3. Return chicken to skillet; cover and simmer for 20 to 30 minutes or until juices run clear when chicken is pierced, stirring occasionally and turning pieces over. Serve sprinkled with cheese and parsley.

Tip
- You can use vegetables such as zucchini or eggplant to replace the peppers and mushrooms.

Nutritional Analysis (Per Serving)
- Calories: 192
- Protein: 17 g
- Fat: 7 g
- Carbohydrates: 13 g
- Fiber: 3 g
- Sodium: 341 mg
- Cholesterol: 4 mg

Chicken Tuscan Hunter Style

¼ cup	olive oil	50 mL
4	garlic cloves, finely chopped	4
1	branch rosemary, leaves only, finely chopped	1
12	sage leaves, finely chopped	12
4½ lbs	chicken thighs, skin removed	2.25 kg
½ tsp	salt	2 mL
¼ tsp	freshly ground black pepper	1 mL
1 cup	dry red wine	250 mL
2 tbsp	tomato paste	25 mL
1½ cups	chicken stock	375 mL

SERVES 4 TO 6

1. In a large skillet, heat olive oil over medium heat. Add garlic, rosemary and sage; cook for 1 or 2 minutes. Add chicken, in batches if necessary, and sear on both sides; continue cooking until chicken is golden brown, about 15 minutes.

2. Season chicken with salt and pepper. Splash in the red wine. Bring to a gentle boil and cook for about 5 minutes.

3. Blend the tomato paste into the stock and pour over chicken. Cover and let simmer 30 to 35 minutes or until chicken is cooked through and sauce is thickened. Serve immediately.

Nutritional Analysis (Per Serving)
- Calories: 359
- Protein: 35.5 g
- Fat: 17.8 g
- Carbohydrates: 6.1 g
- Fiber: 1.9 g
- Sodium: 556 mg
- Cholesterol: 138 mg

This Tuscan version of chicken cacciatore eases up on the tomatoes and relies more on the qualities of a good Italian red wine (don't stint!) — with outstanding results.

Greek-Style Baked Chicken

4	small skinless boneless chicken breasts	4
	Black pepper	
2	small tomatoes (preferably plum), diced	2
2 tbsp	diced red or yellow bell pepper	25 mL
2 tbsp	chopped fresh parsley	25 mL
½ tsp	dried oregano	2 mL
2	cloves garlic, minced	2
1 cup	crumbled feta cheese	250 mL
1 tbsp	olive oil	15 mL

SERVES 4

Preheat oven to 400°F (200°C) • Baking dish, greased

1. Arrange chicken breasts in a greased baking dish just big enough to hold them in a single layer. Sprinkle with pepper and set aside.

2. In a bowl, toss together tomatoes, bell pepper, parsley, oregano, garlic and feta cheese. Spoon over chicken, drizzle with olive oil and bake in preheated oven for 25 to 30 minutes or until chicken is no longer pink inside.

Nutritional Analysis (Per Serving)
- Calories: 337
- Protein: 45.7 g
- Fat: 13.7 g
- Carbohydrates: 6.3 g
- Fiber: 1.4 g
- Sodium: 532 mg
- Cholesterol: 130 mg

This dish is so colorful and delicious, no one will know how easy and quick it is to prepare. Garnish it with some black olives if you wish.

Chicken with Sage

2 tbsp	butter	25 mL
¼ cup	olive oil	50 mL
1	chicken (about 4 to 5 lbs/2 to 2.5 kg), cut into parts or equivalent weight of pre-cut chicken pieces	1
1½ cups	dry white wine	375 mL
24	sage leaves, chopped	24
1 tsp	salt	5 mL
¼ tsp	freshly ground black pepper	1 mL

The Italians are fond of preparing chicken in a simple braise — first browning in a little oil then cooking in liquid — and have devised many variations on this theme. Here is one of the best and easiest.

SERVES 4 TO 6

1. In a large skillet, melt butter over medium-high heat. Add olive oil and stir to blend. Add chicken pieces, in batches if necessary, and cook until they are golden on all sides. Drain all but ¼ cup (50 mL) of fat.

2. Return all chicken pieces to the pan, nestling them together in a single layer. Pour wine over chicken; increase heat and bring to a gentle boil. Cook for about 5 minutes.

3. Add sage, salt and pepper. Turn chicken pieces over to cover them with the sage, shaking the pan a little to help them to nestle down. Reduce heat to low, cover loosely and let it gently bubble away until chicken is cooked through and very tender, about 45 minutes. (Turn the pieces over periodically and check to make sure the liquid is not evaporating too quickly; if it is, add a little water.) Serve immediately.

Tip

- Try to use chicken pieces that are all more or less the same size. Serve with a salad of peppery greens.

Nutritional Analysis (Per Serving)
- Calories: 327
- Protein: 12.4 g
- Fat: 24.6 g
- Carbohydrates: 3.5 g
- Fiber: 2.0 g
- Sodium: 558 mg
- Cholesterol: 58 mg

Chicken with Lemon

1	chicken (about 4 lbs/2 kg), cut lengthwise down back or breastbone, allowing it to lie flat	1
2 tbsp	olive oil	25 mL
3	small lemons, halved and juiced (about 3/4 cup/175 mL juice)	3
6	cloves garlic, smashed	6
Half	bunch flat-leaf parsley, washed, dried and roughly chopped	Half
1/3 cup	chicken stock, cooled	75 mL
1/2 tsp	salt	2 mL
1/4 tsp	freshly ground black pepper	1 mL

SERVES 4 TO 6

1. Trim chicken of any excess fat and transfer to a terra cotta or casserole dish. (It should be large enough to accommodate the chicken comfortably.) Drizzle with olive oil; pour lemon juice over. Add garlic and parsley, nestling it in and around the chicken.

2. Pour stock over the chicken; season with salt and pepper. Cover loosely with plastic wrap and marinate at room temperature for about 1 hour, turning it over periodically. (If kitchen is hot, marinate in refrigerator.)

3. Preheat oven to 400°F (200°C). Remove plastic wrap. Make sure chicken is skin side up and roast in preheated oven for about 55 to 65 minutes, until chicken is cooked through, basting occasionally with the marinade. Be careful not to overcook. Remove from oven and let stand for about 5 minutes before serving.

Tips

- Cutting open a whole chicken and flattening it speeds up cooking time. This works well for oven roasting or grilling.

- Be sure to use lemons of the same size — too much fresh lemon juice will overpower all the other flavors and make the sauce bitter.

Nutritional Analysis (Per Serving)
- Calories: 416
- Protein: 32.9 g
- Fat: 29.0 g
- Carbohydrates: 4.3 g
- Fiber: 0.7 g
- Sodium: 395 mg
- Cholesterol: 123 mg

Chicken with Olives

3 tbsp	olive oil	45 mL
4	cloves garlic, peeled and smashed	4
1	chicken (about 4$\frac{1}{2}$ lbs/ 2.25 kg), cut into parts or equivalent weight of pre-cut chicken pieces	1
1 cup	dry white wine	250 mL
2 tbsp	balsamic vinegar	25 mL
1 cup	whole black olives, pitted	250 mL
1 cup	finely chopped black olives	250 mL
$\frac{1}{2}$ cup	chopped flat-leaf parsley	125 mL
$\frac{1}{2}$ tsp	salt	2 mL
$\frac{1}{4}$ tsp	freshly ground black pepper	1 mL
	Fresh lemon wedges (optional)	

SERVES 4 TO 6

1. In a large skillet, heat olive oil over medium heat. Add garlic and cook for 1 minute or until softened. Do not allow to brown. Add chicken pieces; cook until browned on all sides.

2. Add wine and vinegar; increase heat slightly and bring to a gentle boil. Cook for about 5 minutes. Add whole and chopped olives, parsley, salt and pepper. Stir until well mixed.

3. Reduce heat, cover and simmer for 20 to 30 minutes, periodically turning chicken to make sure it cooks thoroughly. Add a splash of water or wine if chicken looks too dry.

4. Arrange chicken pieces on a warm serving platter and pour sauce over. Serve with fresh lemon wedges if desired.

Tip

• Canned, pitted olives tend to have an unpleasant metallic taste, as well as an unappealing texture. Far better are the olives sold at delis and Italian markets. If you have a cherry pitter, use it to remove olive pits.

Nutritional Analysis (Per Serving)
• Calories: 483   • Protein: 32.6 g   • Fat: 34.0 g
• Carbohydrates: 3.4 g   • Fiber: 0.8 g   • Sodium: 545 mg
• Cholesterol: 123 mg

Chicken and Swiss Chard

3 tbsp	olive oil	45 mL
1	onion, chopped	1
2	carrots, scraped and finely chopped	2
1	stalk celery, chopped	1
4	cloves garlic, peeled and smashed	4
1	chicken, (about 4½ lbs /2.25 kg), cut into pieces or equivalent weight of pre-cut chicken pieces	1
1 cup	dry white wine	250 mL
½ cup	chicken stock	125 mL
½ tsp	salt	2 mL
¼ tsp	freshly ground black pepper	1 mL
2 lbs	Swiss chard, washed, trimmed and chopped	1 kg
1 cup	whipping (35%) cream	250 mL

SERVES 4 TO 6

1. In a large skillet or Dutch oven, heat olive oil over medium heat. Add onion, carrot and celery; cook 5 minutes or until softened. Add garlic and cook until softened but not brown.

2. Add chicken, in batches if necessary, and brown on all sides. With all chicken in skillet, add wine and stock; increase heat slightly, bring to a gentle boil and cook for about 5 minutes. Add salt and pepper; mix well.

3. Reduce heat, cover and simmer for 20 to 30 minutes, turning chicken occasionally to make sure it cooks thoroughly. If it gets too dry, add a little more water or wine.

4. Add Swiss chard, nestling it beneath and around chicken pieces. Cook for 5 minutes or until Swiss chard is wilted. Add cream and bring to a boil; cook for about 5 minutes or until sauce thickens. Serve chicken with sauce poured over.

Tips

- Use spinach, turnip tops or kale instead of Swiss chard.

- Don't omit the heavy cream — it adds a wonderfully rich dimension to the sauce.

Nutritional Analysis (Per Serving)
- Calories: 689
- Protein: 37.4 g
- Fat: 49.7 g
- Carbohydrates: 17.1 g
- Fiber: 5.0 g
- Sodium: 840 mg
- Cholesterol: 188 mg

Chicken with Eggplant and Tomato

2 lbs	eggplant, trimmed, cut into 1-inch (2.5 cm) cubes	1 kg
2 tbsp	salt	25 mL
¼ cup	olive oil	50 mL
4	cloves garlic, chopped	4
2	stalks celery, chopped	2
2 tbsp	chopped flat-leaf parsley	25 mL
1	chicken (about 4 to 5 lbs/ 2 to 2.5 kg) cut into parts or equivalent weight of pre-cut chicken pieces	1
1 tbsp	red pepper flakes	15 mL
½ tsp	salt	2 mL
¼ tsp	freshly ground black pepper	1 mL
1½ cups	dry white wine	375 mL
2 cups	canned plum tomatoes, peeled, with juice or, in season, 2 lbs (1 kg) fresh, ripe plum tomatoes, chopped or *passata* (puréed, sieved tomatoes)	500 mL
	Flat-leaf parsley, chopped	

Here's a very popular dish from Sicily, where eggplant is the winner and undefeated champion of vegetables.

SERVES 4 TO 6

Preheat oven to 375°F (190°C) • Baking sheet, lightly oiled

1. Place the eggplant in a colander set in the sink and sprinkle with salt. Leave to drain for about 1 hour. Rinse and pat dry with paper towels.

2. Put eggplant on prepared baking sheet. Roast in preheated oven for about 20 to 25 minutes or until soft and brown.

3. Meanwhile, in a large skillet, heat olive oil over medium-high heat. Add garlic, celery and parsley; cook for a few minutes or until slightly softened. In batches, add chicken pieces, sprinkling them with red pepper flakes, salt and pepper; cook, turning often, until golden brown on all sides.

4. Add white wine and bring to a gentle boil; cook for about 5 minutes. Add tomatoes, shaking the pan a little to settle them down between the chicken pieces; return to the boil. Reduce heat to low; cover loosely and simmer for about 35 minutes, stirring occasionally, until chicken is cooked through. Add a little water if sauce becomes too dry.

5. Gently combine eggplant with chicken. Transfer everything to a warmed serving platter and serve sprinkled with plenty of chopped flat-leaf parsley.

Tip

- Any variety of eggplant may be used for this dish: the regular elongated variety, the smaller, rounder Italian type, or the long, slender Asian eggplant.

Nutritional Analysis (Per Serving)
- Calories: 570
- Protein: 35.4 g
- Fat: 34.8 g
- Carbohydrates: 18.9 g
- Fiber: 6.7 g
- Sodium: 1341 mg
- Cholesterol: 123 mg

Chicken with Sun-Dried Tomatoes

4	boneless skinless chicken breasts (4 oz/125 g each)	4
4	large basil leaves (or 1 tsp/5 mL dried)	4
4	sun-dried tomatoes, softened (see tip, page 327)	4
2 oz	fontina or mozzarella cheese, cut in 4 long strips	60 g
1 cup	chicken broth	250 mL
SAUCE		
8	sun-dried tomatoes, softened	8
1 tbsp	chopped fresh basil (or 1 tsp/5 mL dried)	15 mL

Here's a yummy Italian-inspired recipe for chicken breasts stuffed with cheese, basil and flavor-packed sun-dried tomatoes.

SERVES 4

1. Cut slit in underside of thickest part of chicken breast. Insert 1 basil leaf (or sprinkle with dried basil), 1 sun-dried tomato and 1 strip of cheese into each breast; seal with toothpick.

2. In a skillet, bring chicken broth to a boil; add chicken and return to boil. Cover and reduce heat to simmer for 10 to 15 minutes or until chicken is no longer pink inside. Remove chicken from pan and keep warm.

3. *Sauce:* Add sun-dried tomatoes and dried basil, if using, to stock in skillet; bring to a boil and cook until reduced to ½ cup (125 mL). In a food processor or blender, purée until smooth. Add fresh basil, if using. Serve over chicken.

Nutritional Analysis (Per Serving)
- Calories: 206
- Protein: 32 g
- Fat: 6 g
- Carbohydrates: 4 g
- Fiber: 1 g
- Sodium: 332 mg
- Cholesterol: 80 mg

Moroccan Baked Chicken

½ cup	packed parsley	125 mL
½ cup	fresh coriander leaves	125 mL
¼ cup	fresh lemon juice	50 mL
2 tsp	paprika	10 mL
2 tsp	ground cumin	10 mL
¼ tsp	hot pepper flakes	1 mL
¼ tsp	cinnamon	1 mL
2	cloves garlic	2
¼ cup	olive oil	50 mL
	Salt and pepper	
4	skinless boneless chicken breasts, 4 diagonal slits (each ½ inch/1 cm) cut on smooth side of each breast	4

Chicken is often on the menus in Morocco — but always enlivened with wonderful spice combinations.

SERVES 4
Preheat oven to 425°F (220°C) • Foil-lined baking sheet

1. In a food processor, chop parsley and coriander. Add lemon juice, paprika, cumin, hot pepper flakes and cinnamon; with the motor running, drop garlic through the feed tube; process until finely chopped. Transfer to a bowl; whisk in the oil. Set aside 1 tbsp (15 mL) of parsley mixture.

2. Sprinkle each breast with salt and pepper; coat with the parsley mixture and place in a single layer on prepared baking sheet. Bake in preheated oven for 20 to 25 minutes or until chicken is no longer pink inside.

3. Top with reserved parsley mixture.

Nutritional Analysis (Per Serving)
- Calories: 385
- Protein: 53.2 g
- Fat: 16.7 g
- Carbohydrates: 3.4 g
- Fiber: 1.0 g
- Sodium: 443 mg
- Cholesterol: 128 mg

Chicken Breasts with Goat Cheese and Sun-Dried Tomatoes

1/3 cup	sun-dried tomatoes	75 mL
1 1/2 oz	goat cheese	40 g
1/2 tsp	dried basil	2 mL
1 lb	skinless, boneless chicken breasts (about 4)	500 g
2 tsp	vegetable oil	10 mL
2 tbsp	all-purpose flour	25 mL

Make Ahead

Prepare rolled breasts early in the day, sauté, then refrigerate and bake just before serving. Add 5 minutes to baking time.

SERVES 4

Preheat oven to 425°F (220°C) • Baking sheet sprayed with nonstick vegetable spray

1. Pour boiling water over sun-dried tomatoes. Let rest for 15 minutes. Drain and chop.

2. In a small bowl, mix sun-dried tomatoes, goat cheese and basil; set aside.

3. Between sheets of waxed paper, pound each chicken breast to 1/4 -inch (5-mm) thickness. Put 1 1/2 tbsp (20 mL) of sun-dried tomato filling at the short end of each flattened breast. Roll up tightly; secure edge with a toothpick.

4. Heat oil in large nonstick skillet sprayed with nonstick vegetable spray over high heat. Roll breasts in the flour; cook for 4 minutes, turning often, or until browned on all sides. Put on prepared baking sheet. Bake for 10 minutes, or until chicken is just done at center. Remove toothpicks before serving.

Tips

• Instead of serving each breast whole, slice each crosswise into medallions and fan out on plates.

• Veal or turkey scaloppine can replace chicken.

• Feta cheese can replace goat cheese.

Nutritional Analysis (Per Serving)
- Calories: 191
- Protein: 28 g
- Fat: 6 g
- Carbohydrates: 5 g
- Fiber: 13 g
- Sodium: 203 mg
- Cholesterol: 66 mg

Chicken Breasts Stuffed with Goat Cheese and Pecans in Leek Sauce

4	boneless skinless chicken breasts	4
2 oz	goat cheese	50 g
1 tbsp	chopped pecans	15 mL
1	egg white	1
1/3 cup	dry bread crumbs	75 mL
1 tbsp	vegetable oil	15 mL
1 1/2 tsp	margarine	7 mL
1	medium leek, thinly sliced	1
1/2 tsp	crushed garlic	2 mL
1 tbsp	all-purpose flour	15 mL
3/4 cup	chicken stock	175 mL
1/3 cup	2% milk	75 mL

Make Ahead

Assemble and refrigerate breasts early in day; brown and bake just before serving. Prepare and refrigerate sauce, adding more stock if too thick when reheating.

SERVES 4

Preheat oven to 400°F (200°C) • Baking dish sprayed with nonstick vegetable spray

1. Place chicken between 2 sheets of waxed paper; pound until flattened and thin.

2. Combine cheese and pecans until mixed; divide among breasts and roll up to enclose. Fasten with toothpicks. Dip into egg white, then into bread crumbs until well coated.

3. In nonstick skillet, heat oil; brown breasts all over, approximately 5 minutes. Place in baking dish; cover and bake for approximately 10 minutes or until chicken is no longer pink inside. Place on serving plate.

4. Meanwhile, add margarine to skillet; sauté leeks and garlic until softened, approximately 10 minutes. Add flour and cook, stirring, for 1 minute. Gradually stir in stock and milk; cook, stirring, until thickened, approximately 3 minutes. Pour over chicken.

Tip

• To wash leeks properly, separate leaves and rinse under running water to remove all dirt trapped between leaves.

Nutritional Analysis (Per Serving)
- Calories: 304
- Protein: 32 g
- Fat: 13 g
- Carbohydrates: 11 g
- Fiber: 1 g
- Sodium: 472 mg
- Cholesterol: 81 mg

Stuffed Chicken Breasts with Goat Cheese and Red Pepper Sauce

RED PEPPER SAUCE

4	red bell peppers	4
¾ cup	chicken stock	175 mL
1 tbsp	olive oil	15 mL
¼ tsp	salt	1 mL
¼ tsp	black pepper	1 mL

STUFFED CHICKEN BREASTS

¾ cup	crumbled goat cheese (about 4 oz/125 g)	175 mL
2 tbsp	olive oil, divided	25 mL
½ tsp	herbes de Provence (see tip, page 250) or dried thyme leaves	2 mL
6	boneless, skinless chicken breasts (about 6 oz/175 g each)	6
¼ tsp	salt	1 mL
¼ tsp	black pepper	1 mL
⅓ cup	finely shredded fresh basil	6

Make Ahead

Stuff chicken up to six hours ahead, cover and refrigerate. Red pepper sauce can be prepared, covered and refrigerated up to a day ahead.

This is a special dish for entertaining, but requires just a little last-minute cooking.

SERVES 6

1. To prepare sauce, arrange red peppers on a baking sheet. Place about 3 inches (7.5 cm) from preheated broiler. Convection broil for 10 to 15 minutes, or until skin is charred, turning peppers about three times during broiling time. Let stand at room temperature until cool enough to handle.

2. Peel peppers and discard seeds and core. (Dip fingers in cold water when peeling peppers to help remove any clinging seeds and skins. Do not rinse peppers.)

3. Cut peppers into large pieces and puree in a food processor or blender until smooth. Add chicken stock, olive oil, salt and pepper. Blend to combine thoroughly. (An immersion blender can also be used.) Refrigerate if not serving immediately. (Just before serving, heat sauce in saucepan.)

4. To prepare chicken, in a small bowl, combine goat cheese, 1 tbsp (15 mL) olive oil and herbes de Provence. Stir until softened.

5. Make a 3-inch (7.5 cm) slit lengthwise in thickest part of chicken breast. Spoon in cheese filling. Close opening with toothpick or skewer. Repeat with remaining chicken breasts. Refrigerate for 1½ hours.

6. Heat remaining 1 tbsp (15 mL) olive oil in a large nonstick skillet over medium-high heat (if you don't have a nonstick skillet, you may need more oil). Sprinkle chicken with salt and pepper. Brown chicken breasts for about 2 minutes per side, or until golden. Place on a parchment-lined baking sheet.

7. Convection bake chicken in a preheated 350°F (180°C) oven for 25 minutes, or until juices run clear and chicken is no longer pink inside. Remove skewers. Serve with sauce. Garnish with shredded basil.

Nutritional Analysis (Per Serving)
- Calories: 407
- Protein: 57.6 g
- Fat: 15.4 g
- Carbohydrates: 7.4 g
- Fiber: 2.1 g
- Sodium: 509 mg
- Cholesterol: 143 mg

Chicken Souvlaki with Tzatziki

CHICKEN

2 tbsp	olive oil	25 mL
2 tbsp	dry white wine or chicken stock	25 mL
2 tbsp	lemon juice	25 mL
1	clove garlic, minced	1
1 tsp	dried oregano leaves	5 mL
1 tsp	grated lemon zest	5 mL
1/4 tsp	salt	1 mL
1/4 tsp	black pepper	1 mL
3	bay leaves	3
1 lb	boneless, skinless chicken breasts, cut in 1-inch (2.5 cm) pieces	500 g

TZATZIKI

1 cup	unflavored yogurt	250 mL
1/2	English cucumber, grated	1/2
1/2 tsp	salt	2 mL
2	cloves garlic, minced	2
1 tbsp	chopped fresh dillweed	15 mL
1 tbsp	chopped fresh mint	15 mL
1 tbsp	lemon juice	15 mL
	Salt and black pepper to taste	

Make Ahead

Tzatziki can be made and refrigerated, covered, up to six hours ahead.

Anyone who has visited Greece and spent leisurely hours in the open-air taverns and restaurants may be transported back with this recipe. Traditionally grilled over charcoal cookers, souvlaki can also be cooked quickly under the broiler.

SERVES 4

1. To prepare chicken, combine olive oil, wine, lemon juice, garlic, oregano, lemon zest, salt, pepper, bay leaves and chicken in a large bowl. Stir thoroughly. Cover and refrigerate for 1 to 8 hours.

2. To prepare tzatziki, line a sieve or strainer with cheesecloth or a clean dish towel. Spoon yogurt into sieve. Let drain, refrigerated, for 1 hour.

3. Meanwhile, combine cucumber with salt and place in a strainer. Drain for 30 minutes. Pat cucumber dry.

4. Combine drained yogurt, cucumber, garlic, dill, mint and lemon juice. Taste and season with salt and pepper.

5. To cook souvlaki, thread chicken onto skewers. Arrange on a lightly greased broiler rack. Place 4 inches (10 cm) from heat and convection broil under preheated broiler for 4 minutes. Turn and broil for 4 to 6 minutes longer, or until pinkness disappears. Serve with tzatziki.

Tip

- Slice fresh tomatoes and lemon wedges to serve alongside.

Nutritional Analysis (Per Serving)

- Calories: 236
- Protein: 30.2 g
- Fat: 8.4 g
- Carbohydrates: 7.6 g
- Fiber: 0.5 g
- Sodium: 556 mg
- Cholesterol: 65 mg

Chicken Breast Tapenade Bob Dees

8 oz	skinless boneless chicken breast cut into ½-inch (1 cm) strips	250 g
2 tbsp	all-purpose flour	25 mL
2 tbsp	olive oil	25 mL
¼ tsp	freshly ground black pepper	1 mL
1 tbsp	finely chopped garlic	15 mL
2	anchovies, minced	2
1 tbsp	lemon zest, cut into ribbons	15 mL
2 tbsp	lemon juice	25 mL
1 cup	chicken stock	250 mL
½ tsp	dried thyme	5 mL
8	black olives, pitted and finely chopped	8
1	small tomato, finely diced, with juices	1
	Few sprigs fresh basil or parsley, chopped	

SERVES 2 OR 3

1. Lightly dredge chicken in the flour and set aside.

2. In a large nonstick frying pan, heat oil with black pepper over high heat for 1 minute. Add garlic, anchovies and lemon zest; stir-fry for 10 seconds. Add chicken and stir-fry actively for 2 to 3 minutes or until browned on all sides.

3. Immediately add lemon juice; cook, stirring, for 30 seconds or until sizzling. Add chicken stock and thyme; bring to a boil. Add olives and cook, stirring, for 2 minutes or until the sauce is syrupy. Remove from heat.

4. Transfer to plates and apportion sauce equally. Garnish with tomatoes and chopped parsley. Serve immediately.

Nutritional Analysis (Per Serving)
- Calories: 335
- Protein: 30.6 g
- Fat: 17.6 g
- Carbohydrates: 13.2 g
- Fiber: 2.1 g
- Sodium: 690 mg
- Cholesterol: 68 mg

This recipe is dedicated to Robert Rose president Bob Dees. Traditionally, such a dish would have a tapenade simply spread over grilled chicken, but this recipe features a sauce that contains all of the essential ingredients of tapenade and acts as a simmering agent for the chicken itself. The combination is, as you will see, explosive. The various complementary flavors and tastes weave in and out of the sauce, anchored by the sweetness of quickly sautéed chicken.

Mediterranean Sautéed Chicken and Vegetables

4	skinless boneless chicken breasts	4
½ tsp	dried oregano	2 mL
	Salt and pepper	
4 tbsp	olive oil	50 mL
1	small eggplant, diced	1
1	red bell pepper, cut into strips	1
2	small zucchini, sliced	2
2	cloves garlic, minced	2
1 tsp	dried thyme	5 mL
¼ tsp	cayenne	1 mL
1	tomato, unpeeled and diced	1
4 oz	goat cheese or feta cheese, crumbled	125 g

SERVES 4

1. Sprinkle chicken breasts on both sides with oregano and ¼ tsp (1 mL) each salt and pepper. In a large skillet, heat half the oil over medium-high heat; brown chicken 2 minutes a side. Reduce heat to medium and cook chicken for about 10 minutes, turning once, until no longer pink inside.

2. Meanwhile, in another large skillet, heat remaining oil over medium heat. Add eggplant, sprinkle with salt and pepper to taste; cook for 5 minutes. Add red pepper and cook for 3 minutes. Add zucchini and garlic; cook for 2 minutes. Stir in thyme, cayenne and tomato. Cover and set aside.

3. Remove cooked chicken to a warm platter and keep warm. Add 2 tbsp (25 mL) water to chicken skillet and bring to a boil, stirring up any brown bits from the bottom. Stir into vegetables and reheat if necessary. Arrange around chicken and sprinkle with cheese to serve.

Nutritional Analysis (Per Serving)
- Calories: 475
- Protein: 48.4 g
- Fat: 24.6 g
- Carbohydrates: 15.9 g
- Fiber: 5.7 g
- Sodium: 554 mg
- Cholesterol: 118 mg

Skillet Chicken Stroganoff

1 tbsp	butter	15 mL
1 tbsp	vegetable oil	15 mL
1 lb	skinless boneless chicken breasts or thighs, cut into thin strips	500 g
	Salt and pepper	
2 cups	tiny whole mushrooms or sliced large mushrooms	500 mL
1	red bell pepper, cut into strips	1
2	cloves garlic, minced	2
4 tsp	Dijon mustard	20 mL
1 tbsp	Worcestershire sauce	15 mL
2/3 cup	light sour cream	150 mL
	Chopped parsley (optional)	

Anyone who likes mushrooms with chicken in a creamy sauce will love this quick and easy skillet supper. Serve on top of hot buttered egg noodles.

SERVES 4

1. In a large skillet, melt butter with oil over medium-high heat. Add chicken and cook, stirring often, for 5 minutes or until it changes color. Sprinkle with salt and pepper.
2. Add mushrooms, red pepper and garlic; cook, stirring often, for 4 minutes. Reduce heat to low; stir in mustard, Worcestershire sauce and sour cream. Taste and adjust seasoning. Heat through but do not boil. Sprinkle with parsley if desired.

Tip
- To save time, look for chicken already cut into stir-fry strips. Also look for prepackaged sliced mushrooms.

Nutritional Analysis (Per Serving)
- Calories: 255
- Protein: 29.3 g
- Fat: 10.3 g
- Carbohydrates: 7.1 g
- Fiber: 1.6 g
- Sodium: 192 mg
- Cholesterol: 88 mg

Mushroom Chicken Stroganoff

4 cups	thickly sliced mushrooms	1 L
2/3 cup	sour cream	150 mL
2 tsp	all-purpose flour	10 mL
	Salt, freshly ground black pepper and paprika	
4	skinless, boneless chicken breasts	4

Sour cream and mushrooms combined with sautéed chicken make a stroganoff reminiscent of Eastern Europe.

SERVES 4
Nonstick cooking spray

1. In a large nonstick skillet lightly sprayed with cooking spray, sauté mushrooms, turning often, on medium-high for 6 minutes or until golden brown. Remove and set aside.
2. In a small bowl, whisk together sour cream, flour, salt, pepper and paprika. Set aside.
3. Meanwhile, rinse and wipe chicken with paper towel. Spray same skillet again and sauté chicken on medium-high for 5 minutes or until browned on each side. Add mushrooms and sour cream mixture. Cover, reduce heat to medium-low and cook slowly for 10 minutes or until meat is no longer pink inside.

Nutritional Analysis (Per Serving)
- Calories: 284
- Protein: 43.2 g
- Fat: 9.2 g
- Carbohydrates: 6.4 g
- Fiber: 1.3 g
- Sodium: 201 mg
- Cholesterol: 109 mg

Slow-Cooked Creole Chicken

2 lb	boneless skinless chicken thighs	1 kg
2 cups	diced green bell peppers	500 mL
½ cup	chopped green onions or cooking onions	125 mL
1	can (19 oz/540 mL) stewed tomatoes	1
1	can (5.5 oz/155 g) tomato paste	1
2 tsp	minced garlic	10 mL
1 tsp	hot pepper sauce	5 mL
1	bay leaf	1
2 tsp	dried thyme leaves	10 mL
8 oz	spicy smoked Polish sausage, sliced	250 g

Children love the succulent chicken and sausage in this recipe — they'll be sure to ask for more.

SERVES 8

Electric slow cooker

1. Place chicken thighs in bottom of slow cooker. Add peppers, onions, tomatoes, tomato paste, garlic, hot pepper sauce, bay leaf and dried thyme. Cook, covered, on Low heat setting for 4 to 5 hours. Increase heat setting to High; add sausage and cook for 20 to 30 minutes. Remove bay leaf.

Tips

- If you prefer a less-pronounced tomato flavor, substitute 1 can (10 oz/285 mL) condensed tomato soup for the tomato paste.

- This recipe provides 1 serving of meat and 2 servings of vegetables.

Nutritional Analysis (Per Serving)
- Calories: 284
- Protein: 27 g
- Fat: 14 g
- Carbohydrates: 12 g
- Fiber: 2 g
- Sodium: 363 mg
- Cholesterol: 112 mg

Cajun Chicken "Ribs" with Garlic and Shallots

2 tsp	salt	10 mL
1½ tsp	ground black pepper	7 mL
1 tsp	ground white pepper	5 mL
1 tsp	cayenne pepper	5 mL
1½ tsp	sweet paprika	7 mL
3 tsp	dried thyme	15 mL
2 tsp	dried basil	10 mL
5	skinless chicken breasts, bone-in, cut into pieces ½-inch (1 cm) thick	5
10	cloves garlic, minced	10
14	shallots, finely chopped	14
2 tbsp	olive oil	25 mL

SERVES 4

Preheat barbecue or grill

1. In a plastic bag, combine salt, black pepper, white pepper, cayenne, paprika, thyme and basil; shake until well mixed. Add chicken pieces, in batches if necessary, and shake until thoroughly coated.

2. In a bowl mix garlic and shallots with olive oil; coat chicken pieces with mixture.

3. Grill chicken over medium-low heat until cooked, about 15 minutes. (Or bake for about 30 minutes in 350°F/180°C oven.)

Nutritional Analysis (Per Serving)
- Calories: 362
- Protein: 54.8 g
- Fat: 9.7 g
- Carbohydrates: 13.5 g
- Fiber: 1.4 g
- Sodium: 1314 mg
- Cholesterol: 128 mg

Quick-Roasted Lemon Thighs

6	chicken thighs	6
2	cloves garlic	2
3 tbsp	fresh lemon juice	45 mL
1 tbsp	Worcestershire sauce	15 mL
1/2 tsp	salt	2 mL

*If you wish, you can substitute
3 bone-in breasts for the thighs in this
simple and easy recipe that creates a
wonderfully crisp skin and moist meat.*

SERVES 3
Preheat oven to 425°F (220°C) • Foil-lined roasting pan

1. Place chicken thighs in a glass dish just big enough to hold them in a single layer.
2. In a blender or mini chopper, combine garlic, lemon juice and Worcestershire sauce; purée until smooth. Coat chicken with mixture and leave at room temperature for 15 minutes.
3. Arrange chicken on a rack in prepared roasting pan; sprinkle with salt. Roast in preheated oven for about 30 minutes or until chicken is no longer pink inside.

Nutritional Analysis (Per Serving)
- Calories: 544
- Protein: 38.1 g
- Fat: 41.6 g
- Carbohydrates: 1.9 g
- Fiber: 0.1 g
- Sodium: 577 mg
- Cholesterol: 184 mg

Lemon Roast Chicken Thighs

1/4 cup	fresh lemon juice	50 mL
2 tbsp	olive oil	25 mL
2 tbsp	balsamic vinegar	25 mL
2	cloves garlic, minced	2
2 tsp	grated lemon zest	10 mL
6 to 12	chicken thighs, trimmed of excess fat	6 to 12
1/2 tsp	salt	2 mL
1/2 tsp	black pepper	2 mL
	Chopped fresh parsley	

Make Ahead

Chicken thighs must be marinated in the refrigerator for at least 1 hour or up to 24 hours.

*Sometimes it takes only the simplest of
marinades to add flavor to a dish. In
this case, the magic comes from lemon,
olive oil, balsamic vinegar and garlic.*

SERVES 6
Large shallow nonreactive baking dish

1. In the baking dish, whisk together lemon juice, olive oil, vinegar, garlic and lemon zest. Add chicken thighs; turn to coat well. Refrigerate, covered, for at least 1 hour or up to 24 hours, turning occasionally.
2. When ready to cook, preheat oven to 425°F (220°C). Remove chicken thighs from marinade, shaking off excess. Arrange thighs on oiled rack in a shallow roasting pan (line roasting pan with foil for easy clean up); sprinkle with salt and pepper. Bake for 25 to 35 minutes or until skin is crisp and golden, and juices that run out are no longer pink when thickest thigh is pierced with a skewer. Transfer to a warm platter; serve garnished with parsley.

Nutritional Analysis (Per Serving)
- Calories: 447
- Protein: 28.6 g
- Fat: 35.7 g
- Carbohydrates: 1.3 g
- Fiber: 0.1 g
- Sodium: 320 mg
- Cholesterol: 138 mg

Broiled Rosemary Thighs

8	chicken thighs	8
3 tbsp	fresh lemon juice	45 mL
3 tbsp	olive oil	45 mL
1 tbsp	chopped fresh rosemary (or 1 tsp/5 mL crumbled dried)	15 mL
½ tsp	grated lemon zest	2 mL
	Salt and pepper	

Make Ahead

The chicken can be marinated, covered and refrigerated, for up to 4 hours. Bring to room temperature for 30 minutes before cooking.

This very simple recipe creates wonderfully moist and delicious chicken.

SERVES 4
Preheat Broiler • Foil-lined broiling pan

1. Place chicken thighs in a glass dish just big enough to hold them in a single layer. In a bowl whisk together the lemon juice, olive oil, rosemary and lemon zest. Pour over chicken and turn to coat well. Cover and let stand at room temperature for 30 minutes.

2. Reserving the marinade, arrange chicken thighs skin-side down on prepared pan; sprinkle with salt and pepper. Broil 4 inches (10 cm) from heat for 7 minutes, basting occasionally.

3. Turn, baste and broil 5 to 8 minutes longer, or until chicken is no longer pink inside.

Nutritional Analysis (Per Serving)
- Calories: 498
- Protein: 28.5 g
- Fat: 10.4 g
- Carbohydrates: 1.2 g
- Fiber: 0.4 g
- Sodium: 127 mg
- Cholesterol: 138 mg

Gremolata Grilled Chicken

2	cloves garlic, minced	2
2 tbsp	minced fresh parsley	25 mL
1 tbsp	chopped lemon zest	15 mL
2 tbsp	fresh lemon juice	25 mL
1 tbsp	vegetable oil	15 mL
4	boneless chicken thighs	4

The gremolata mixture is usually a final garnish for veal stew, but it makes a delicious addition to grilled chicken as well. It also works well for boneless chicken breasts.

SERVES 2
Grease barbecue grill and preheat to medium-high

1. In a small bowl, combine garlic, parsley and lemon zest. Set aside 1 tbsp (15 mL) of the mixture and combine remainder of the mixture with lemon juice and oil. Press mixture into both sides of the thighs.

2. Grill for about 12 minutes, turning once, until the chicken is no longer pink inside. Sprinkle with the reserved gremolata and serve.

Nutritional Analysis (Per Serving)
- Calories: 471
- Protein: 28.8 g
- Fat: 38.0 g
- Carbohydrates: 2.1 g
- Fiber: 0.3 g
- Sodium: 128 mg
- Cholesterol: 138 mg

Yummy Parmesan Chicken Fingers

½ cup	finely crushed soda cracker crumbs (about 16 crackers)	125 mL
⅓ cup	freshly grated Parmesan cheese	75 mL
½ tsp	dried basil leaves	2 mL
½ tsp	dried marjoram leaves	2 mL
½ tsp	paprika	2 mL
½ tsp	salt, optional	2 mL
¼ tsp	freshly ground black pepper	1 mL
4	skinless, boneless chicken breasts	4
1	egg	1
2 tbsp	margarine or butter	25 mL
1	clove garlic, minced	1

SERVES 4

Preheat oven to 400°F (200°C) • Baking sheet, with greased rack

1. In a food processor, combine cracker crumbs, Parmesan cheese, basil, marjoram, paprika, optional salt and pepper. Process to make fine crumbs. Place in a shallow bowl.

2. Cut chicken breasts into four strips each. In a bowl, beat egg; add chicken strips. Using a fork, dip chicken strips in crumb mixture until evenly coated. Arrange on greased rack set on baking sheet. In small bowl, microwave butter and garlic at High for 45 seconds or until melted. Brush chicken strips with melted butter.

3. Bake in preheated oven for 15 minutes or until no longer pink in center. (If frozen, bake for up to 25 minutes.)

Tips

- You can also make extra batches of the crumb mixture and store in the freezer.

- Instead of boneless chicken breasts, prepare skinless chicken drumsticks in the same way but bake in a 375°F (190°C) oven for 35 to 40 minutes or until tender.

- Adding salt brings the sodium to 674 mg.

Nutritional Analysis (Per Serving)
- Calories: 236
- Protein: 22 g
- Fat: 12 g
- Carbohydrates: 10 g
- Fiber: 1 g
- Sodium: 400 mg
- Cholesterol: 114 mg

Crunchy Cheese and Herb Drumsticks

1½ cups	bran or corn flakes cereal	375 mL
1½ tbsp	fresh chopped parsley	20 mL
2½ tbsp	grated Parmesan cheese	35 mL
1 tsp	minced garlic	5 mL
¾ tsp	dried basil (or ½ tsp/2 mL dried)	4 mL
½ tsp	chili powder	2 mL
⅛ tsp	ground black pepper	0.5 mL
1	egg	1
2 tbsp	milk or water	25 mL
8	skinless chicken drumsticks	8

Make Ahead

Coat the drumsticks up to 1 day ahead. They can be baked a few hours in advance and then gently reheated. Great for leftovers.

SERVES 4

Preheat oven to 400°F (200°C) • Baking sheet sprayed with vegetable spray

1. In a food processor combine bran flakes, parsley, Parmesan, garlic, basil, chili powder and pepper; process into fine crumbs. Set aside.
2. In a bowl whisk together egg and milk. Dip each drumstick into egg wash, then roll in crumbs; place on prepared baking sheet. Bake, turning halfway, for 35 minutes or until browned and chicken is cooked through.

Tip

• Use bran flakes instead of natural bran; it has a sweetness that children love.

Nutritional Analysis (Per Serving)
• Calories: 238   • Protein: 28 g   • Fat: 9 g
• Carbohydrates: 11 g   • Fiber: 2 g   • Sodium: 186 mg
• Cholesterol: 151 mg

Spicy Roasted Drumsticks or Wings

¼ cup	Dijon mustard	50 mL
4	cloves garlic, crushed	4
2 tbsp	Worcestershire sauce	25 mL
1 tbsp	vegetable oil	15 mL
2 tsp	Tabasco sauce	10 mL
2 tsp	paprika	10 mL
½ tsp	black pepper	2 mL
8	chicken drumsticks, skin scored through (or 3 lbs/1.5 kg divided wings)	8

Make Ahead

Drumsticks can be coated with mustard mixture, covered and refrigerated for up to 24 hours. Bring to room temperature for 30 minutes before cooking.

SERVES 4

Preheat oven to 425°F (220°C) • Foil-lined baking sheet

1. In a shallow bowl, stir together the mustard, garlic, Worcestershire sauce, oil, Tabasco, paprika and pepper.
2. Dip each drumstick in the mixture and arrange in a single layer on a rack on prepared baking sheet. Cover and let sit for 30 minutes at room temperature.
3. Roast in preheated oven for about 30 minutes or until chicken is no longer pink inside, turning once.

Nutritional Analysis (Per Serving)
• Calories: 453   • Protein: 29.4 g   • Fat: 35.1 g
• Carbohydrates: 3.6 g   • Fiber: 1.0 g   • Sodium: 450 mg
• Cholesterol: 138 mg

Tex-Mex Wings

2 lbs	chicken wings, patted dry, separated at the joints, tips removed	1 kg
1 tbsp	vegetable oil	15 mL
2	jalapeño peppers, minced	2
1¾ cups	bottled salsa, preferably chunky	425 mL
1 tbsp	vinegar	15 mL
1 tbsp	Worcestershire sauce	15 mL
1 tsp	chili powder	5 mL
½ tsp	paprika	2 mL
½ tsp	ground cumin	2 mL
½ tsp	dried oregano	2 mL
	Salt and pepper	

Bottled salsa makes a quick and easy glaze for these zesty wings.

SERVES 3

Preheat oven to 450°F (230°C) • Foil-lined baking sheet, greased

1. Arrange wings meaty-side down in a single layer on prepared baking sheet. Bake in preheated oven for 15 minutes, turning once.
2. Meanwhile, in a small saucepan, heat oil over medium-high heat. Add jalapeños and cook for 2 minutes. Stir in salsa, vinegar, Worcestershire sauce, chili powder, paprika, cumin, oregano, and salt and pepper to taste. Bring to a boil; reduce heat and simmer, uncovered, for 5 minutes.
3. Brush jalapeño mixture liberally over browned wings, reserving remaining sauce over low heat. Bake the wings, uncovered, in preheated oven for about 15 to 20 minutes or until tender and glazed, turning once and brushing again with the sauce. Arrange on a heated platter and serve with remaining hot sauce in a bowl.

Nutritional Analysis (Per Serving)
- Calories: 469
- Protein: 33.4 g
- Fat: 32.0 g
- Carbohydrates: 11.3 g
- Fiber: 2.9 g
- Sodium: 805 mg
- Cholesterol: 132 mg

Feta Cheese Burgers

1½ lbs	lean ground chicken	750 g
½ tsp	salt	2 mL
¼ tsp	pepper	1 mL
¼ tsp	ground cumin	1 mL
2 oz	feta cheese	50 g
2 tbsp	chopped fresh mint (or 2 tsp/10 mL dried)	25 mL

SERVES 4

Grease barbecue grill and preheat to medium-high

1. In a bowl combine chicken, salt, pepper and cumin. Divide mixture into 4 portions. Cut cheese into 4 cubes; flatten the cubes and sprinkle with mint. Form 4 chicken patties with the cheese and mint buried in the center of each patty.
2. Place patties on grill; cook, turning once, for 12 to 14 minutes or until patties are no longer pink inside.

Nutritional Analysis (Per Serving)
- Calories: 233
- Protein: 38.8 g
- Fat: 7.3 g
- Carbohydrates: 0.7 g
- Fiber: 0.1 g
- Sodium: 575 mg
- Cholesterol: 130 mg

Spinach and Cheese Stuffed Turkey Breasts

4	skinless, boneless turkey scallopini	4
1½ tsp	vegetable oil	7 mL
1 tsp	crushed garlic	5 mL
¼ cup	finely chopped red onions	50 mL
¼ cup	drained, cooked, chopped spinach	50 mL
¼ cup	diced red peppers	50 mL
¼ cup	shredded Swiss cheese	50 mL
¼ cup	chicken stock	50 mL
SAUCE		
1½ tsp	margarine or butter	7 mL
1 tsp	crushed garlic	5 mL
1½ cups	diced plum tomatoes	375 mL
⅓ cup	chicken stock	75 mL
3 tbsp	chopped fresh basil	45 mL

Make Ahead

Assemble and refrigerate stuffed breasts early in day, but bake just before eating. Prepare sauce early in the day. Reheat gently.

SERVES 4

Preheat oven to 400°F (200°C) • Baking dish sprayed with nonstick vegetable spray

1. Place turkey between 2 sheets of waxed paper; pound until flattened. Set aside.

2. In nonstick skillet, heat oil; sauté garlic, onions, spinach and red peppers until softened, approximately 3 minutes. Spoon evenly over breasts; sprinkle with cheese. Roll up and fasten with toothpicks.

3. Place turkey in baking dish; pour in ¼ cup (50 mL) stock. Cover and bake for 12 to 15 minutes or until turkey is no longer pink. Remove turkey to serving dish and keep warm.

4. *Sauce:* Meanwhile, in small saucepan, melt margarine; sauté garlic for 1 minute. Stir in tomatoes and chicken stock; cook for 3 minutes or until heated through. Add basil and serve over turkey.

Tips

• Substitute boneless chicken breasts, or use veal or pork scaloppine.

• If using fresh spinach, use 1½ cups (375 mL). Cook, drain well and chop.

• A milder cheese can replace Swiss.

Nutritional Analysis (Per Serving)
- Calories: 225
- Protein: 30 g
- Fat: 10 g
- Carbohydrates: 4 g
- Fiber: 1 g
- Sodium: 247 mg
- Cholesterol: 80 mg

Cider-Glazed Turkey Breast

¼ cup	cider vinegar	50 mL
2 tbsp	coarse-grain mustard	25 mL
2 tbsp	soy sauce	25 mL
2	cloves garlic, finely chopped	2
½ tsp	dried sage or savory leaves	2 mL
½ tsp	salt	2 mL
¼ tsp	black pepper	1 mL
1	3-lb (1.5 kg) turkey breast, bone in	1

For people who like white meat only. For a smaller family, this will also provide extra for lunches. Garnish with orange sections and sage leaves.

SERVES 6 TO 8

1. In a small bowl, whisk together vinegar, mustard, soy sauce, garlic, sage, salt and pepper.
2. Place turkey breast skin side up on a rack over broiler pan. Spread half of vinegar mixture over turkey.
3. Convection roast in a preheated 325°F (160°C) oven for 50 minutes. Baste with vinegar mixture. Continue to roast for 30 to 40 minutes, basting every 15 minutes, until meat thermometer registers 170°F (75°C) when inserted into thickest part. Remove turkey to a platter. Cover loosely with foil and let stand for 10 minutes before carving.

Variation

- **Mediterranean Glazed Turkey Breast:** For the basting mixture, in a small bowl, whisk together 3 tbsp (45 mL) orange juice, 3 tbsp (45 mL) balsamic vinegar, 2 tbsp (25 mL) pesto, 1½ tsp (7 mL) dried thyme leaves, 1 tsp (5 mL) grated orange zest and ½ tsp (2 mL) salt.

Nutritional Analysis (Per Serving)
- Calories: 132
- Protein: 28.4 g
- Fat: 0.9 g
- Carbohydrates: 1.6 g
- Fiber: 0.2 g
- Sodium: 422 mg
- Cholesterol: 72 mg

Turkey Scaloppine with Pesto Cream Sauce

SAUCE

1/3 cup	pesto	75 mL
1 1/2 tbsp	light sour cream	22 mL
1 1/2 tbsp	grated Parmesan cheese	22 mL
1 lb	turkey scaloppine	500 g
1/4 cup	all-purpose flour	50 mL
1 tbsp	vegetable oil	15 mL

Make Ahead

Prepare pesto sauce up to a day ahead, or freeze for up to 3 weeks. Cook just before serving.

SERVES 4

1. In small bowl combine pesto, sour cream and Parmesan; set aside.
2. Between sheets of waxed paper, pound turkey to 1/4 -inch (5-mm) thickness. Dust with flour.
3. In nonstick skillet sprayed with vegetable spray, heat oil over medium-high heat. Cook 2 minutes per side, or until just done at center. Serve with a dollop of pesto sauce on top.

Tips

- If you can't find turkey scaloppine, get your butcher to cut thin crosswise slices from a turkey breast for you. You can also substitute chicken or veal scaloppine.

- If you use store-bought pesto, calories and fat will be higher.

Nutritional Analysis (Per Serving)
- Calories: 283
- Protein: 31 g
- Fat: 15 g
- Carbohydrates: 7 g
- Fiber: 1 g
- Sodium: 200 mg
- Cholesterol: 74 mg

Cajun-Style Turkey Cutlet with Citrus

2 tbsp	paprika	25 mL
1 tbsp	dried sage	15 mL
1 tsp	black pepper	5 mL
1/2 tsp	each salt, garlic powder and cayenne pepper	2 mL
6	turkey cutlets (3 oz/90 g each)	6
1 tbsp	vegetable oil	15 mL
1	large orange, peeled and sectioned	1
1	medium grapefruit, peeled and sectioned	1

Turkey cutlets are available fresh and frozen in most supermarkets and are a convenient way of enjoying turkey — without the leftovers!

SERVES 6

1. Mix together paprika, sage, pepper, salt, garlic powder and cayenne; place on waxed paper. With meat mallet, pound turkey between 2 pieces of plastic wrap to 3/8-inch (9 mm) thickness. Coat cutlets well with seasoning mixture.
2. In a large skillet, heat oil over high heat; quickly brown turkey on both sides. Reduce heat and add orange and grapefruit; cook until turkey is no longer pink inside.

Tip

- In this recipe, spices reduce the need for fat. Serve this quick and easy dinner with broccoli florets.

Nutritional Analysis (Per Serving)
- Calories: 153
- Protein: 21 g
- Fat: 4 g
- Carbohydrates: 8 g
- Fiber: 2 g
- Sodium: 42 mg
- Cholesterol: 54 mg

Turkey Hazelnut Roll

1/2	turkey breast, boned and halved lengthwise	1/2
1	turkey thigh, boned	1
1/2 cup	whole hazelnuts	125 mL
1/2 cup	wheat germ	125 mL
1 tbsp	brandy or cognac	15 mL
1	egg, beaten	1
1 tsp	salt	5 mL
1 tsp	dried thyme	5 mL
1/2 tsp	black pepper	2 mL
	Cranberry sauce	

Serve this tasty dish instead of a big bird for an easy-to-manage Thanksgiving or holiday meal.

SERVES 6

Preheat oven to 350°F (180°C) • Baking pan

1. Flatten boned turkey breast pieces by pounding between 2 sheets of heavy plastic wrap. Cut one-third of turkey thigh into 1/2-inch (1 cm) cubes. Grind remaining two-thirds of turkey thigh to the consistency of minced meat.

2. In a bowl, combine ground turkey with turkey cubes, hazelnuts, wheat germ, brandy, egg and seasonings. Spread mixture over 1 flattened turkey breast and cover with the other to form a sandwich. Sew the edges of the sandwich closed with needle and thread. Roll up; tie with string like a roast. Wrap in aluminum foil (dull side on the outside) to form an airtight seal.

3. Place turkey roll in baking pan containing 1 inch (2.5 cm) of boiling water. Bake, uncovered, in preheated oven for 1 1/2 hours. Slice and serve with cranberry sauce.

Tips

- Pounding the boned turkey helps to tenderize the meat and produces a piece of breast that is even and thin enough to work in this recipe. If you don't have a wooden mallet, use a wooden rolling pin or a heavy saucepan.

- To obtain firm slices of this roll, cook the night before and refrigerate. The next day, slice the chilled roll and reheat slices in the oven, or microwave on Low, making sure they are well covered with either aluminum foil or plastic wrap, depending upon the method used.

Nutritional Analysis (Per Serving)
- Calories: 208
- Protein: 23 g
- Fat: 10 g
- Carbohydrates: 7 g
- Fiber: 2 g
- Sodium: 493 mg
- Cholesterol: 149 mg

Turkiaki Fiesta

2 tsp	vegetable oil	10 mL
1 lb	ground or slivered turkey or chicken	500 g
2 tbsp	teriyaki sauce	25 mL
Pinch	each salt and black pepper	Pinch
1 cup	diagonally sliced celery	250 mL
¾ cup	chopped green onions	175 mL
1	large red bell pepper, cubed	1
2 cups	snow peas, trimmed	500 mL
1	can (10 oz/284 mL) water chestnuts, drained	1
1 tbsp	sesame seeds (optional)	15 mL

SERVES 5

1. In a wok or nonstick skillet, heat oil over high heat. Add turkey and stir-fry for about 4 minutes or until lightly browned and no longer pink inside. Add teriyaki sauce, salt, pepper, celery and onion. Cover and steam for 4 minutes. Add red pepper, snow peas and water chestnuts; cover and cook for 6 minutes, stirring occasionally. Serve sprinkled with sesame seeds, if using.

Tips

- If using ground turkey or chicken, ensure that the meat is cooked through and no longer pink. Ground meat is considered a high-risk food as bacteria can spread during the grinding process.

- If you don't have any sesame seeds in your cupboard, stir ½ tsp (2 mL) sesame oil into the dish just before serving.

Nutritional Analysis (Per Serving)
- Calories: 175
- Protein: 23 g
- Fat: 4 g
- Carbohydrates: 12 g
- Fiber: 4 g
- Sodium: 145 mg
- Cholesterol: 115 mg

Herbed Roast Turkey Roll

1	turkey roll (about 4 lbs/2 kg)	1
10	large cloves garlic, minced	10
3 tbsp	chopped fresh rosemary or 1 tbsp (15 mL) dried	45 mL
1 tsp	salt	5 mL
¼ tsp	freshly ground black pepper	1 mL
2 tbsp	olive oil	25 mL

Turkey adapts readily to added flavorings, especially to herbs, spices and garlic. The finished roast carves into neat slices to enjoy hot or cold.

SERVES 10
Preheat oven to 325°F (160°C)

1. Place turkey roll on a cutting board and unroll as flat as possible.

2. In a small bowl, combine garlic, rosemary, salt, pepper and oil. Spread half of mixture over inside of turkey. Reroll and tie firmly with string. Spread remaining mixture over outside of roll.

3. Roast on a rack in preheated oven for 1½ hours or until a meat thermometer registers 180°F (82°C). Remove from oven and let stand for 10 minutes before carving.

Nutritional Analysis (Per Serving)
- Calories: 300
- Protein: 33.1 g
- Fat: 15.5 g
- Carbohydrates: 5.5 g
- Fiber: 0.5 g
- Sodium: 1296 mg
- Cholesterol: 102 mg

Quail Roasted with Pancetta

10	quail	10
10	sprigs sage	10
10	cloves garlic, peeled and left whole	10
4 oz	butter, softened	125 g
½ tsp	salt	2 mL
¼ tsp	freshly ground black pepper to taste	1 mL
10	slices pancetta (Italian bacon), unrolled	10
	Wedges of lemon	

SERVES 4 TO 6

Preheat oven to 400°F (200°C)

1. Wipe clean each quail, inside and out. Pat dry with paper towel. Place a sprig of sage and a clove of garlic inside the cavity of each quail, along with a small knob of the butter.

2. Spread the remaining butter over each quail's breast and legs. Season with salt and pepper. Wrap each one with a strip of pancetta. (You may wish to secure the pancetta with a toothpick.)

3. Place birds in a roasting pan and roast in preheated oven for about 15 minutes. Remove from oven and let rest for 5 minutes. Serve with a squeeze of fresh lemon.

Tip

- Look for good-sized plump quail with broad breasts — well, as broad as a quail's breast can be. Serve with a green vegetable.

Nutritional Analysis (Per Serving)
- Calories: 1827
- Protein: 174.2 g
- Fat: 119.7 g
- Carbohydrates: 4.5 g
- Fiber: 1.8 g
- Sodium: 1660 mg
- Cholesterol: 698 mg

Beef, Pork and Lamb

Beef Stroganoff

1 tbsp	vegetable oil	15 mL
2 tbsp	butter, divided	25 mL
8 oz	sliced mushrooms	250 g
1 lb	sirloin steak, cut into ½-inch (1 cm) slices	500 g
¼ tsp	salt	1 mL
	Freshly ground black pepper	
2 tbsp	minced shallots or finely chopped green onion (white part only)	25 mL
1 tbsp	all-purpose flour	15 mL
1 cup	beef stock	250 mL
1 tbsp	Dijon mustard	15 mL
½ cup	sour cream	125 mL
1	dill pickle, finely chopped	1

Here's a dish that is quick to make, yet elegant enough for special occasions. Just add a bottle of robust red wine and a crisp green salad.

SERVES 4

Preheat oven to 250°F (120°C)

1. In a skillet, heat oil and 1 tbsp (15 mL) of the butter over medium-high heat. Add mushrooms and cook, stirring, until they begin to lose their liquid, about 7 minutes. Using a slotted spoon, transfer to a plate and keep warm in preheated oven.

2. Add remaining butter to pan. Add steak slices and sauté until desired degree of doneness, about 1½ minutes per side for medium. Season with salt, and black pepper to taste. Transfer to a warm platter and keep warm in oven.

3. Reduce heat to medium. Add shallots to pan and cook, stirring, for 1 minute. Add flour and cook, stirring, for 1 minute. Add stock. Bring to a boil. Cook, stirring, until thickened, about 3 minutes. Stir in mustard.

4. Return mushrooms to pan. Add sour cream and chopped dill pickle and cook, stirring, just until cream is heated through, about 1 minute. (Do not let mixture boil or it will curdle.) Pour over steak.

Nutritional Analysis (Per Serving)
- Calories: 276
- Protein: 27.3 g
- Fat: 15.5 g
- Carbohydrates: 6.0 g
- Fiber: 1.4 g
- Sodium: 414 mg
- Cholesterol: 84 mg

Beef with Broccoli

1 lb	sirloin steak, cut into thin strips	500 g
1/4 cup	soy sauce	50 mL
2 tbsp	cornstarch, divided	25 mL
1	clove garlic, minced	1
1	thin slice ginger root, minced	1
2 tbsp	safflower oil, divided	25 mL
2	medium onions, cut into wedges	2
3	large carrots, sliced into coins	3
1	head broccoli, cut into florets	1
1 1/4 cups	water, divided	300 mL
1 tbsp	oyster sauce	15 mL
1 tsp	granulated sugar	5 mL

This classic stir-fry marries Asian flavors with beef and vegetables and is perfect for a busy weeknight.

SERVES 4 TO 6

1. Place steak in a medium bowl. In a separate bowl, combine soy sauce, 1 tbsp (15 mL) of the cornstarch, garlic and ginger root; pour over steak.

2. In a wok or nonstick skillet, heat 1 tbsp (15 mL) of the oil over high heat. Add beef and stir-fry until browned. Set aside.

3. In wok, heat remaining oil over high heat. Add onions and stir-fry for 1 minute. Add carrots, broccoli and 1 cup (250 mL) of the water; cover and steam for 4 minutes.

4. Combine remaining water, oyster sauce, remaining cornstarch and sugar. Stir sauce into wok; cook until smooth and thickened. Return meat to wok. Reheat to serving temperature.

Tips

- When preparing food for stir-frying, cut into small pieces of approximately equal size so that they will cook through rapidly and in the same period of time. Have sauce and ingredients prepared and easily accessible before starting to cook.

- For a quick and easy dessert that continues the Asian theme, serve sliced melon, such as cantaloupe, sprinkled with gingered sugar (granulated sugar mixed with ground ginger to taste).

Nutritional Analysis (Per Serving)
- Calories: 189
- Protein: 15 g
- Fat: 10 g
- Carbohydrates: 11 g
- Fiber: 2 g
- Sodium: 600 mg
- Cholesterol: 109 mg

Hoisin Beef and Broccoli Stir-Fry

2 tsp	vegetable oil	10 mL
12 oz	sirloin or inside round steak, cut into 3- by 1/2-inch (7.5 by 1 cm) strips	375 g
1 tbsp	chopped ginger root	15 mL
1 tsp	minced garlic	5 mL
3 cups	small broccoli florets	750 mL
1/3 cup	sliced water chestnuts	75 mL
1/2 tsp	cornstarch	2 mL
1/3 cup	orange juice or beef stock	75 mL
2 tbsp	hoisin sauce	25 mL
1/2 tsp	sesame oil (optional)	2 mL
	Black pepper	
1 tbsp	toasted sesame seeds (optional)	15 mL

There are endless variations on the theme of stir-fried beef and broccoli. This one highlights flavorful hoisin sauce, a spicy-sweet condiment made from fermented soybeans.

SERVES 4

1. In a large nonstick skillet, heat oil over medium-high heat; add beef strips and stir-fry for 1 to 2 minutes or until browned. Add ginger, garlic, broccoli and water chestnuts; stir-fry for another 2 to 3 minutes or until broccoli is tender-crisp.

2. In a small bowl or glass measuring cup, whisk together cornstarch, orange juice, hoisin sauce and, if using, sesame oil. Add to skillet; cook, stirring, for 1 to 2 minutes or until thickened and heated through. Season with pepper to taste. If desired, sprinkle with sesame seeds.

Tips

- Hoisin sauce also makes a great glaze for fish fillets or chicken breasts. Look for it in the Asian food section of most supermarkets. Refrigerate after opening.

- Using a nonstick skillet helps you cook with very small amounts of oil — and makes cleanup a breeze. Adding a tiny amount of flavored oil, such as sesame oil, provides taste without adding too much fat.

Nutritional Analysis (Per Serving)
- Calories: 178
- Protein: 20 g
- Fat: 6 g
- Carbohydrates: 11 g
- Fiber: 2 g
- Sodium: 196 mg
- Cholesterol: 51 mg

Flank Steak Stir-Fry

1 lb	flank steak	500 g
¼ cup	soy sauce	50 mL
1 tbsp	water	15 mL
2 tsp	cornstarch	10 mL
1 tsp	dry sherry	5 mL
1	clove garlic, minced	1
1 tbsp	vegetable oil	15 mL
2½ cups	cubed green bell pepper	625 mL
2	large tomatoes, cut into wedges	2
¼ tsp	black pepper	1 mL

Finding recipes the whole family will like that can be made in less than 20 minutes is a challenge. This tasty stir-fry, made with green peppers and tomatoes, fits the bill on both counts!

SERVES 6

1. Trim steak and thinly slice across the grain; cut into bite-size pieces. In a medium bowl, combine soy sauce, water, cornstarch, sherry and garlic. Stir in steak and let stand for 10 minutes.

2. In a nonstick skillet, heat oil over medium heat; cook green peppers, stirring, until almost tender. Add beef; cook to desired doneness, about 2 minutes. Stir in tomatoes and pepper; cook just until heated through.

Tip

- For variety, replace the green pepper in this recipe with shredded cabbage, chopped napa cabbage or broccoli florets.

Nutritional Analysis (Per Serving)
- Calories: 174
- Protein: 18 g
- Fat: 8 g
- Carbohydrates: 7 g
- Fiber: 2 g
- Sodium: 414 mg
- Cholesterol: 53 mg

Thai Beef Satay

1 lb	fast fry or sirloin steak	500 g
¼ cup	peanut butter	50 mL
2 tbsp	soy sauce	25 mL
2 tbsp	freshly squeezed lime or lemon juice	25 mL
	Salt and freshly ground black pepper	

This is a very traditional recipe for a very traditional Thai dish. It can be served on small skewers for appetizers or on larger skewers for the main course. The Canadian Beef Information Center is the source of this recipe, with only a modest change.

SERVES 4

Preheat broiler or barbecue • Skewers

1. Cut beef into long strips about ½ inch (1 cm) wide. Set aside.

2. In a medium bowl, whisk together peanut butter, soy sauce, juice, 2 tbsp (25 mL) water, salt and pepper until smooth. Add beef strips and stir to coat. Let stand at room temperature for 15 minutes or refrigerate for several hours.

3. If using wooden skewers, soak them in cold water for at least 10 minutes to prevent charring during cooking.

4. Remove beef from peanut butter mixture. Thread strips loosely on skewers. Broil or grill for 4 minutes per side or until desired doneness and slightly pink inside. Serve at once.

Nutritional Analysis (Per Serving)
- Calories: 257
- Protein: 28.4 g
- Fat: 13.7 g
- Carbohydrates: 4.8 g
- Fiber: 1.1 g
- Sodium: 408 mg
- Cholesterol: 68 mg

Sautéed Beef with Asparagus in Oyster Sauce

½ tsp	black peppercorns	2 mL
½ tsp	Szechuan peppercorns or green or red peppercorns	2 mL
SAUCE		
2 tbsp	oyster sauce	25 mL
1 tbsp	soya sauce	15 mL
1 tbsp	chicken stock or water	15 mL
2 tsp	cornstarch	10 mL
2 tbsp	vegetable oil	25 mL
2 tsp	minced ginger root	10 mL
2 tsp	minced garlic	10 mL
1	small onion, sliced	1
12 oz	flank steak, thinly sliced across the grain	375 g
1 lb	asparagus, cut into 2-inch (5 cm) segments	500 g

Flank steak is juicy and flavorful, and it's great in stir-fry dishes. Slice it across the grain, and it will be tender when cooked.

SERVES 4

1. Combine peppercorns. Coarsely grind in a pepper grinder, mortar and pestle, or by crushing with a wine bottle between two sheets of waxed paper.

2. In a small bowl, combine ingredients for sauce; mix well and set aside.

3. In a nonstick wok or skillet, heat oil over medium-high heat for 30 seconds. Add ginger root, garlic and onion; stir-fry 1 minute or until fragrant. Add beef; cook, stirring to separate pieces, about 2 minutes. Season with mixed peppercorns. Add asparagus; toss to mix and cook 2 minutes. Add sauce mixture; stir and cook until thickened. Transfer to a serving platter and serve immediately.

Nutritional Analysis (Per Serving)
- Calories: 318
- Protein: 26.3 g
- Fat: 18.8 g
- Carbohydrates: 10.9 g
- Fiber: 2.1 g
- Sodium: 338 mg
- Cholesterol: 60 mg

Bistecca alla Florentine

1	T-bone steak (3 to 3½ lbs/1.5 to 1.75 kg)	1
	Salt and freshly ground black pepper, to taste	
	Extra virgin olive oil	

Simplicity itself — since its only partners are salt, pepper and very good olive oil — the T-bone must be of the absolute best quality, preferably prime, and as thick as 3 inches (7.5 cm). Traditionally, this steak is served rare.

SERVES 4 TO 6
Preheat grill to high

1. Coat entire steak with salt and pepper. Place on grill. Cook undisturbed for about 5 minutes on first side.

2. Using tongs, flip steak; cook undisturbed for another 5 minutes, then continue to cook, turning every 5 minutes, for 10 to 12 minutes or according to taste.

3. Remove steak to a cutting board. Let rest for 5 minutes before carving. Arrange on serving platter; drizzle with olive oil. Serve immediately.

Nutritional Analysis (Per Serving)
- Calories: 282
- Protein: 36.1 g
- Fat: 13.9 g
- Carbohydrates: 0 g
- Fiber: 0 g
- Sodium: 96 mg
- Cholesterol: 102 mg

Anticuchos

3	cloves garlic	3
1 tbsp	ground cumin	15 mL
	Salt and freshly ground black pepper, to taste	
1 to 2	fresh chilies, seeded and chopped	1 to 2
1/2 tsp	red pepper flakes	2 mL
2/3 cup	red wine vinegar	150 mL
1/3 cup	annatto-flavored oil (see tip, at right)	75 mL
2 lbs	sirloin, cut into 1-inch (2.5 cm) cubes	1 kg

> *Anticuchos is the name of Peru's national dish, which used to consist of skewered barbecued llama hearts. Today, this recipe is more likely to include beef hearts or chunks of tender beef.*

SERVES 4 TO 6

1. With a mortar and pestle or in a food processor, combine garlic, cumin, salt, pepper, chilies and red pepper flakes until a chunky paste forms. Scrape mixture into a large bowl. Add vinegar and flavored oil, stirring to combine well.

2. Add sirloin; toss to coat well. Marinate, covered, in refrigerator overnight or at room temperature for at least 4 hours.

3. Preheat grill to high. Remove sirloin from marinade. Transfer remaining marinade to a small saucepan. Place over medium heat; boil for 3 minutes. Set aside.

4. Thread cubes of beef onto skewers (if using wooden skewers, soak in water for 1 hour before using). Place skewers of beef on grill; cook, brushing with reserved marinade, for 4 to 6 minutes or according to taste, turning once or twice. Serve immediately.

Tip

- Available in Latin and South American supermarkets, annatto seeds are used to make a spicy, colorful cooking oil to brush over the beef while grilling. To make this oil, combine 1 cup (250 mL) vegetable oil, 1/2 cup (125 mL) annatto seeds (or 1/4 cup/50 mL paprika and 1 tsp/5 mL ground turmeric), a dried chili and 1 bay leaf. After sitting for about 30 minutes, place over gentle heat and simmer for 30 minutes, stirring occasionally. Cool and strain through a cheesecloth-lined sieve. Store in a jar with a tight-fitting lid in the refrigerator.

Nutritional Analysis (Per Serving)
- Calories: 382
- Protein: 39.0 g
- Fat: 22.9 g
- Carbohydrates: 3.0 g
- Fiber: 0.4 g
- Sodium: 105 mg
- Cholesterol: 109 mg

Quick Bistro-Style Steak

4	boneless striploin steaks, each 6 oz (175 g)	4
½ tsp	coarsely ground black pepper	2 mL
2 tsp	olive oil	10 mL
2 tsp	butter	10 mL
	Salt	
¼ cup	finely chopped shallots	50 mL
1	large clove garlic, finely chopped	1
¼ tsp	dried herbes de Provence (see tip, at right)	1 mL
⅓ cup	red wine or additional beef stock	75 mL
½ cup	beef stock	125 mL
1 tbsp	Dijon mustard	15 mL
2 tbsp	chopped fresh parsley	25 mL

Dressed up with wine, garlic and herbs, this steak recipe becomes a special dish when you're entertaining friends.

SERVES 4

1. Remove steaks from refrigerator 30 minutes before cooking. Season with pepper.

2. Heat a large heavy skillet over medium heat until hot; add oil and butter. Increase heat to high; brown steaks about 1 minute on each side. Reduce heat to medium; cook to desired degree of doneness. Transfer to a heated serving platter; season with salt and keep warm.

3. Add shallots, garlic and herbes to skillet; cook, stirring, for 1 minute. Stir in red wine; cook, scraping up any brown bits from bottom of pan, until liquid has almost evaporated.

4. Stir in stock, mustard and parsley; season with salt and pepper to taste. Cook, stirring, until slightly reduced. Spoon sauce over steaks. Serve immediately.

Tip

- Herbes de Provence is a blend of French herbs that often includes thyme, rosemary, basil and sage. If you can't find this blend in your supermarket, substitute a generous pinch of each of these herbs.

Nutritional Analysis (Per Serving)
- Calories: 296
- Protein: 36.8 g
- Fat: 12.8
- Carbohydrates: 2.4 g
- Fiber: 0.3 g
- Sodium: 231 m
- Cholesterol: 107 mg

Sesame Steak

¼ cup	light soy sauce	50 mL
1	clove garlic, minced	1
1	small onion, finely chopped	1
1 tbsp	liquid honey	15 mL
1 tbsp	sesame seeds	15 mL
1 tsp	grated ginger root	5 mL
1 tsp	black pepper	5 mL
1 lb	flank steak	500 g

Flank steak is a popular cut of beef because it is versatile and extremely flavorful. In this recipe, the steak is marinated in a soy, garlic, ginger and honey sauce. The result is both tender and packed with flavor.

SERVES 4

1. In a shallow nonaluminum pan, mix together soy sauce, garlic, onion, honey, sesame seeds, ginger and pepper. Add steak, turning to coat. Cover and marinate in refrigerator for at least 4 to 6 hours or preferably overnight.

2. Preheat barbecue or broiler; place steak on greased grill or under broiler; cook for 4 to 5 minutes per side for medium-rare. Slice across the grain to serve.

Tips

- Flank steak is a lean cut of meat that can be quite elegant when grilled and cut across the grain. Serve this delicious steak with stir-fried vegetables or Sautéed Spinach with Pine Nuts (see recipe, page 335).

- Marinade adds flavor while it tenderizes. For convenience, marinate meat in a resealable plastic freezer bag.

Nutritional Analysis (Per Serving)
- Calories: 200
- Protein: 26 g
- Fat: 9 g
- Carbohydrates: 2 g
- Fiber: Trace
- Sodium: 701 mg
- Cholesterol: 160 mg

Saucy Swiss Steak

1 tbsp	vegetable oil	15 mL
2 lbs	round steak or "simmering" steak	1 kg
2	medium onions, finely chopped	2
1/4 cup	thinly sliced carrots	50 mL
1	small carrot, thinly sliced, about 1/4 cup (50 mL)	1
1	small stalk celery, thinly sliced, about 1/4 cup (50 mL)	1
1/2 tsp	salt	2 mL
1/4 tsp	black pepper	1 mL
2 tbsp	all-purpose flour	25 mL
1	can (28 oz/796 mL) plum tomatoes, drained and chopped, 1/2 cup (125 mL) juice reserved	1
1 tbsp	Worcestershire sauce	15 mL
1	bay leaf	1

Make Ahead

This dish can be partially prepared the night before it is cooked. Complete Step 2, heating 1 tbsp (15 mL) oil in pan before softening onions, carrots and celery. Cover and refrigerate mixture overnight. The next morning, brown steak (Step 1), or skip this step and place steak directly in stoneware. Continue cooking as directed. Alternatively, cook steak overnight and refrigerate. When ready to serve, bring to a boil in a large skillet and simmer for 10 minutes, until meat is heated through and sauce is hot and bubbling.

SERVES 8
Slow cooker

1. In a skillet, heat oil over medium-high heat. Add steak, in pieces, if necessary, and brown on both sides. Transfer to slow cooker stoneware.

2. Reduce heat to medium-low. Add onion, carrots, celery, salt and pepper to pan. Cover and cook until vegetables are softened, about 8 minutes. Sprinkle flour over vegetables and cook for 1 minute, stirring. Add tomatoes, reserved juice and Worcestershire sauce. Bring to a boil, stirring until slightly thickened. Add bay leaf.

3. Pour tomato mixture over steak and cook on Low for 8 to 10 hours or on High for 4 to 5 hours, until meat is tender. Discard bay leaf.

Nutritional Analysis (Per Serving)
- Calories: 196
- Protein: 28 g
- Fat: 4 g
- Carbohydrates: 11 g
- Fiber: 2 g
- Sodium: 330 mg
- Cholesterol: 49 mg

Salisbury Steak in Wine Sauce

2 tbsp	vegetable oil, divided	25 mL
6	4-oz (125 g) tenderized round steaks (see tip, at right), pounded to $1/2$-inch (1 cm) thickness and patted dry	6
1 cup	sliced onions	250 mL
2 cups	sliced mushrooms	500 mL
3 tbsp	all-purpose flour	45 mL
1	beef bouillon cube	1
$1^1/2$ cups	hot water	375 mL
$1/2$ cup	dry red wine	125 mL
2 tsp	Worcestershire sauce	10 mL
$1/2$ tsp	each garlic powder and paprika	2 mL
1	bay leaf	1
$1/8$ tsp	black pepper	0.5 mL
1 tbsp	chopped fresh parsley (optional)	15 mL

This recipe is a delicious way to cook a less tender cut of beef.

SERVES 6

Preheat oven to 350°F (180°C) • 11- by 7-inch (2 L) baking dish, greased

1. In a nonstick skillet, heat 1 tsp (5 mL) of the oil over medium-high heat; cook steaks in 2 batches, turning once, until brown on both sides. Transfer to prepared dish.

2. Heat another 1 tsp (5 mL) of the oil in skillet. Add onions and mushrooms; cook until softened. Transfer to baking dish, placing vegetables on top of steaks. Remove skillet from heat and add remaining oil; blend in flour.

3. In a small bowl, dissolve bouillon cube in hot water. Slowly add bouillon to flour mixture, whisking constantly until well combined. Return skillet to medium heat; stir in wine, Worcestershire sauce, garlic powder, paprika, bay leaf and pepper. Whisk constantly until sauce is thickened and smooth. Pour sauce over steaks.

4. Cook, covered, in preheated oven for 45 to 50 minutes or until meat is fork-tender. Remove bay leaf before serving. Sprinkle with parsley, if desired.

Tips

- To tenderize steaks, place meat between 2 pieces of plastic wrap and pound with a flat wooden or rubber mallet until flattened slightly. This process helps to break down the tough fibers in the meat.

- If desired, replace the red wine in this recipe with beef stock.

Nutritional Analysis (Per Serving)
- Calories: 212
- Protein: 28 g
- Fat: 7 g
- Carbohydrates: 7 g
- Fiber: 1 g
- Sodium: 164 mg
- Cholesterol: 11 mg

Peppered Beef Steaks with Tuna Caper Sauce

1	can (6.5 oz/184 g) water-packed tuna, drained	1
½ cup	chicken stock	125 mL
2 tbsp	light mayonnaise	25 mL
2 tbsp	olive oil	25 mL
1 tbsp	drained capers	15 mL
1½ tsp	minced garlic	7 mL
3 lb	beef tenderloin steaks, about 8, each approx. 6 oz (150 g)	1.5 kg
3 tbsp	coarsely ground black pepper	45 mL

Make Ahead

Prepare sauce up to a day ahead.

SERVES 8
Preheat broiler or start barbecue

1. Put tuna, stock, mayonnaise, olive oil, capers and garlic in food processor; purée until smooth.
2. Rub approximately 1 tsp (5 mL) pepper onto each steak, covering all sides. Barbecue or cook under broiler for 5 minutes; turn and cook for 3 minutes longer for medium-rare. Warm sauce slightly and serve over top.

Tip

- Use any other good quality steaks, such as sirloin, rib eye or porterhouse, totaling 3 lbs (1.5 kg).

Nutritional Analysis (Per Serving)
- Calories: 320
- Protein: 40 g
- Fat: 16 g
- Carbohydrates: 1 g
- Fiber: 0 g
- Sodium: 268 mg
- Cholesterol: 89 mg

Beef Tenderloin

1 lb	beef tenderloin (see tip, at right)	500 g
2 tsp	olive oil	10 mL
2	cloves garlic, sliced	2
1 tbsp	balsamic vinegar	15 mL
	Salt and freshly ground black pepper	

This simple recipe is all it takes to make a gourmet treat of this succulent cut of beef.

SERVES 4

1. Cut beef into four thick slices. Set aside.
2. In a heavy nonstick skillet, heat oil on medium-high heat. Cook garlic for 30 seconds. Add beef and sauté on each side until brown and beef is still pink inside.
3. Add vinegar and salt and pepper to taste.

Tip

- Beef suitable for this recipe is often described as "grilling steak," indicating that the beef will be tender when prepared using this fast grilling method. You can also use rib, rib eye, strip loin, T-bone or top sirloin.

Nutritional Analysis (Per Serving)
- Calories: 211
- Protein: 23.7 g
- Fat: 12.0 g
- Carbohydrates: 0.7 g
- Fiber: 0.1 g
- Sodium: 60 mg
- Cholesterol: 72 mg

Poached Beef Tenderloin

1	can (10 oz/284 mL) beef consommé	1
1½ lb	beef tenderloin	750 g
1	can (5½ oz/156 mL) tomato paste	1
1 tbsp	butter, melted	15 mL
1 tbsp	all-purpose flour	15 mL
2 tbsp	Madeira	25 mL
¼ tsp	black pepper	1 mL
	Watercress	

This variation of a classic pot-au-feu is sophisticated enough for even the most elegant dinner.

SERVES 8

1. In a covered skillet, bring consommé and 1 soup can of water to a boil. Add beef; cover and simmer for 25 to 30 minutes or until desired doneness. Remove beef and keep warm.

2. Reserve 1 cup (250 mL) of the cooking liquid in skillet; stir in tomato paste. Combine butter and flour; stir into skillet and cook, stirring, until thickened and bubbly. Add Madeira and pepper; heat through.

3. To serve, slice beef. Serve sauce on the side. Garnish with watercress.

Variation

- Use this recipe as the basis for a superb beef fondue. Cut the beef into ³⁄₄-inch (2 cm) cubes. Bring the consommé and soup can of water to a boil, then pour all but 1 cup (250 mL) of the liquid into fondue pot and maintain at a simmer. Proceed with Step 2, using reserved liquid (beef will not have been cooked in it) and serve sauce as a dipping sauce. (Or skip this step and serve cooked beef with Dijon mustard, horseradish or other dipping sauce of your choice.) Spear beef pieces with a fondue fork and cook until desired doneness (about 3 minutes).

Tip

- Although beef tenderloin, a lean meat option, is more likely to be grilled than poached, poaching produces a moist, flavorful result. Balance this meal with abundant vegetables.

Nutritional Analysis (Per Serving)
- Calories: 158
- Protein: 18 g
- Fat: 7 g
- Carbohydrates: 6 g
- Fiber: 1 g
- Sodium: 126 mg
- Cholesterol: 58 mg

Beef Tenderloin with Blue Cheese Herb Crust

SAUCE

1 cup	beef broth	250 mL
1 tbsp	cornstarch	15 mL
¼ tsp	crushed dried thyme	1 mL

BEEF

⅓ cup	crumbled blue cheese	75 mL
¼ cup	fresh white bread crumbs	50 mL
2 tbsp	chopped fresh parsley	25 mL
2 tbsp	chopped fresh chives or green onions	25 mL
1	clove garlic	1
4	beef tenderloin medallions (3 oz/90 g each)	4

Although it is costly, beef tenderloin is both lean and tender, and there is no waste as there is with some less expensive cuts of meat. This elegant recipe improves on the higher-fat approach of serving steak with Roquefort butter.

SERVES 4

Preheat oven to 350°F (180°C) • Baking sheet

1. *Sauce:* In a small saucepan, bring broth, cornstarch and thyme to a boil, stirring; simmer for 1 minute. Keep warm.

2. *Beef:* In a food processor, process cheese, crumbs, parsley, chives and garlic until in fine crumbs.

3. In a nonstick skillet, brown medallions quickly on each side. Remove from skillet and place on baking sheet. Pack cheese mixture evenly on top of each. Bake in preheated oven for about 20 minutes for medium doneness or as desired. Spoon sauce onto plates and top with beef.

Tips

- If fresh thyme is available, use 1 tsp (5 mL) leaves in the sauce instead of the dried thyme.

- There are many different types of blue cheese, ranging in flavor from very mild to very strong. You may want to sample some at the cheese counter before deciding which is for you.

- In this recipe, the strong tastes of the blue cheese and the garlic complement the lower-fat preparation. Complete this rich-tasting meal with a steamed green vegetable.

Nutritional Analysis (Per Serving)
- Calories: 171
- Protein: 19 g
- Fat: 8 g
- Carbohydrates: 4 g
- Fiber: Trace
- Sodium: 567 mg
- Cholesterol: 68 mg

Beef Tenderloin with Mustard Horseradish Sauce

2 tbsp	soy sauce	25 mL
1 tbsp	Dijon mustard	15 mL
1 tbsp	olive oil	15 mL
1 tsp	grated lemon zest	5 mL
1	1½-lb (750 g) piece beef tenderloin	1

MUSTARD HORSERADISH SAUCE

½ cup	mayonnaise	125 mL
3 tbsp	prepared horseradish	45 mL
2 tbsp	Russian-style mustard	25 mL

SERVES 4

1. In a small bowl, combine soy sauce, mustard, oil and lemon zest.

2. Place beef in a shallow dish. Rub soy sauce marinade over beef. Let stand at room temperature for 30 minutes.

3. Place beef on broiler rack set over oven pan. Roast in preheated 500°F (260°C) toaster oven for 20 minutes.

4. Reduce heat to 350°F (180°C) and continue to roast for 25 to 30 minutes, or until a meat thermometer registers 140°F (60°C) for medium-rare. Let stand for 10 minutes.

5. Meanwhile, to prepare sauce, in a bowl, stir together mayonnaise, horseradish and mustard. Carve beef and serve with sauce.

Variation

- *Beef Tenderloin with Wasabi Sauce:* Combine ½ cup (125 mL) mayonnaise, 2 tbsp (25 mL) chopped pickled ginger and ½ tsp (2 mL) prepared wasabi (or more to taste). Serve with beef.

Tip

- As there is little waste and no bone, beef tenderloin is easy to carve. Ask for a section that is about 3 inches (7.5 cm) thick. (If your tenderloin is thicker than this, it may be necessary to lengthen the cooking time by 10 minutes, but use a meat thermometer to be sure.) Serve with sautéed wild mushrooms.

Nutritional Analysis (Per Serving)
- Calories: 527
- Protein: 36.6 g
- Fat: 40.4 g
- Carbohydrates: 3.6 g
- Fiber: 0.8 g
- Sodium: 525 mg
- Cholesterol: 124 mg

Faheem's Beef and Tomato Curry

1	medium onion, coarsely chopped	1
4	cloves garlic, coarsely chopped	4
1	1-inch (2.5 cm) piece gingerroot, coarsely chopped	1
¼ cup	canola oil or vegetable oil	50 mL
1 tbsp	hot curry powder	15 mL
1	can (28 oz/796 mL) diced tomatoes	1
2 tsp	granulated sugar	10 mL
½ tsp	salt	2 mL
2 lbs	stew beef, trimmed of excess fat and cut into 1-inch (2.5 cm) cubes	1 kg
1	hot banana pepper, washed	1
¼ tsp	cayenne pepper (or to taste)	1 mL
¼ cup	chopped fresh coriander	50 mL

Make Ahead

This is a perfect make-ahead dish as it tastes even better after 24 hours. The curry can be cooked, cooled then refrigerated for up to 2 days. Reheat over medium heat, stirring occasionally, until piping hot and bubbly.

When this beef curry is on the table, it's usually the first thing to disappear. It's spicy without being fiery — a great introduction for anyone unfamiliar with Pakistani or Indian food.

SERVES 4 TO 6
12-cup (3 L) Dutch oven or flameproof casserole

1. In a food processor or mini chopper, combine onion, garlic and ginger; process until finely ground. In Dutch oven, heat oil over medium-high heat. Add onion mixture; cook, stirring, for 3 to 5 minutes or until just beginning to brown. Add curry powder; cook, stirring, for 1 minute.

2. Stir in tomatoes, sugar and salt. Increase heat to high; bring to a boil, stirring to scrape up any brown bits from bottom of Dutch oven. Add beef and whole banana pepper. Reduce heat to medium-low; simmer, covered, for 1½ hours or until beef is tender.

3. If sauce seems a little thin, increase heat to high. Boil, stirring occasionally, for 8 to 10 minutes or until sauce is reduced and slightly thickened. Discard banana pepper; stir in cayenne pepper. Spoon curry into a warm shallow serving dish. Sprinkle with coriander; serve at once.

Tip
- Hot banana peppers resemble bell peppers but are longer and slimmer. They're fairly hot without being too fiery.

Nutritional Analysis (Per Serving)
- Calories: 616
- Protein: 35.5 g
- Fat: 46.5 g
- Carbohydrates: 13.8 g
- Fiber: 2.4 g
- Sodium: 359 mg
- Cholesterol: 128 mg

Foolproof Roast Beef

RUB

1	prime-rib roast, about 6 lbs (3 kg)	1
1	clove garlic, crushed with the flat blade of a large knife	1
1	onion, thickly sliced	1
1/2 tsp	black pepper	2 mL
1/4 cup	grainy Dijon mustard	50 mL
2 tsp	fresh thyme leaves (or 1 tsp/5 mL dried)	10 mL

GRAVY

2 tbsp	all-purpose flour	25 mL
2 cups	beef stock	500 mL
1/4 tsp	salt	1 mL
	Fresh thyme sprigs	

Make Ahead

The roast can be rubbed with garlic and pepper, covered with the mustard mixture then refrigerated, covered, for up to 24 hours. Let the beef stand at room temperature for 30 minutes before roasting.

> *It's hard to beat a really good roast beef — and even harder to mess it up when you use this wonderfully simple recipe.*

SERVES 8

Preheat oven to 475°F (250°C) • Shallow roasting pan

1. *Rub:* Rub roast all over with garlic; place garlic in roasting pan, along with onion. Sprinkle roast with black pepper. In a small bowl, stir together mustard and thyme leaves; spread over roast. Place roast bone-side down on top of onion and garlic. Roast in preheated oven, uncovered, for 20 minutes. Reduce oven temperature to 325°F (160°C); cook for 2 1/2 to 3 hours or until a meat thermometer inserted in roast (but not the touching the bones) registers 140°F (60°C) for rare or 160°F (70°C) for medium. Remove roast to a cutting board; tent loosely with foil and let stand in a warm place for 20 minutes before carving.

2. *Gravy:* Drain off all but 2 tbsp (25 mL) fat from roasting pan; reserve onion and garlic in pan. Sprinkle flour evenly over fat remaining in pan; stir until no lumps of flour remain. Place roasting pan on stovetop; cook over medium-high heat for 1 minute, stirring constantly. Gradually whisk in stock; bring to a boil, stirring constantly. Reduce heat to low; simmer for 5 minutes or until gravy has thickened and is smooth. If desired, season to taste with salt and additional pepper. Strain gravy through a sieve into a pitcher.

3. If your butcher has separated the meat from the bones, snip strings on roast, remove bones and slice meat thinly. Arrange meat on a warm serving platter; garnish with thyme. Serve with gravy.

Tip

• Using a meat thermometer is the most accurate way to establish whether a roast is done to your taste. For an accurate reading with a bone-in roast, be sure the shaft of the thermometer does not touch any bones.

Nutritional Analysis (Per Serving)
• Calories: 659   • Protein: 26.3 g   • Fat: 59.9 g
• Carbohydrates: 1.0 g   • Fiber: 0.3 g   • Sodium: 111 mg
• Cholesterol: 126 mg

Pot Roast of Beef with Wild Mushrooms

1 cup	boiling water	250 mL
1/2 oz	dried porcini mushrooms	15 g
1 tbsp	olive oil	15 mL
1	cross-rib, blade or short-rib beef roast (about 3 lbs/1.5 kg)	1
1/2 tsp	salt	2 mL
1/2 tsp	black pepper	2 mL
8 oz	shallots, peeled but left whole	250 g
1 cup	red wine	250 mL
1 tsp	dried thyme	5 mL
1	bay leaf	1
3 cups	sliced mixed mushrooms (button, shiitake, portobello; about 8 oz/250 g)	750 mL
1 tbsp	cornstarch	15 mL
1 tbsp	cold water	15 mL
	Fresh thyme or parsley sprigs	

A pot roast like this one needs very little in the way of preparation, after which it happily looks after itself for 2 or 3 hours in the oven. The result is moist and tender meat in an intensely flavored gravy.

SERVES 6

Preheat oven to 325°F (160°C) • 12-cup (3 L) Dutch oven or flameproof casserole

1. In a small heatproof bowl, combine boiling water and porcini mushrooms; let stand for 20 minutes. Line a sieve with paper towels; drain porcini mushrooms through sieve, reserving soaking liquid. Rinse porcini mushrooms under running water; pat dry on paper towels. Set aside.

2. In the Dutch oven, heat oil over medium-high heat. Sprinkle roast with salt and pepper; place in Dutch oven. Cook, turning often, for 3 to 5 minutes or until browned on all sides. Remove roast to a plate.

3. Add shallots to the fat remaining in Dutch oven; cook, stirring, for 3 to 5 minutes or until golden brown. Add porcini mushrooms, reserved soaking liquid, red wine, thyme and bay leaf. Bring to a boil, stirring to scrape up any browned bits from bottom of Dutch oven. Return beef to Dutch oven; cover with lid. Transfer to preheated oven; cook for 2 1/2 hours. Remove from oven; add sliced mushrooms, stirring to combine with cooking juices. Return to oven; cook, covered, for 30 minutes or until beef is very tender and mushrooms are cooked. Remove beef to a large plate. Cover loosely with foil; keep warm.

4. In a small bowl, whisk together cornstarch and cold water until smooth; add to cooking juices in Dutch oven. Bring to a boil over medium-high heat, stirring constantly. Reduce heat to medium-low; simmer, stirring often, for 2 to 3 minutes or until mushroom gravy has thickened and is smooth. If desired, season to taste with additional salt and pepper; discard bay leaf.

5. Cut beef into thick slices; arrange on a warm serving platter. Drizzle some mushroom gravy evenly over beef; pour remaining gravy into a warm serving bowl. Garnish beef with thyme. Serve at once.

Nutritional Analysis (Per Serving)
- Calories: 658
- Protein: 43.9 g
- Fat: 46.5 g
- Carbohydrates: 8.2 g
- Fiber: 0.9 g
- Sodium: 337 mg
- Cholesterol: 160 mg

Roast Prime Rib of Beef

¼ cup	Dijon mustard	50 mL
3	cloves garlic, finely chopped	3
1 tbsp	chopped fresh thyme, or 1 tsp (5 mL) dried	15 mL
1 tbsp	Worcestershire sauce	15 mL
¾ tsp	salt	4 mL
½ tsp	black pepper	2 mL
1	prime rib roast of beef (about 4 lbs/2 kg)	1

SAUCE

1 tbsp	all-purpose flour	15 mL
¾ cup	water	175 mL
½ cup	dry red wine	125 mL
½ tsp	salt	2 mL
¼ tsp	black pepper	1 mL

For a special and truly delicious meal, few can resist a prime roast beef dinner. Serve with pan juices, horseradish and your favorite mustard.

SERVES 6

1. In a small bowl, combine mustard, garlic, thyme, Worcestershire, salt and pepper.

2. Place roast, fat side up, on a rack over broiler pan. Rub paste mixture over top and sides of meat.

3. Convection roast in a preheated 325°F (160°C) oven for 1¾ hours, or until meat is cooked to desired doneness: 140°F (60°C) for rare to medium-rare or 160°F (70°C) for medium. Remove roast to a carving board and cover loosely with foil. Let stand for 10 to 15 minutes before carving.

4. Meanwhile, to prepare sauce, pour fat from roasting pan and place pan on stovetop on medium-high heat. Sprinkle flour over remaining meat juices and cook, stirring, for 2 minutes. Add water and wine. Bring to a boil over medium-high heat, stirring and scraping any caramelized bits from bottom of pan. Reduce heat to medium and cook for 5 minutes. Add any accumulated juices from carving board to sauce. Strain sauce if desired and season with salt and pepper. Serve with sliced roast beef.

Nutritional Analysis (Per Serving)
- Calories: 685
- Protein: 26.9 g
- Fat: 60.2 g
- Carbohydrates: 3.6 g
- Fiber: 0.7 g
- Sodium: 699 mg
- Cholesterol: 126 mg

Oriental Beef Bundles in Lettuce

12 oz	lean ground beef	375 g

SAUCE

2 tbsp	hoisin sauce	25 mL
1 tbsp	rice wine vinegar	15 mL
2 tsp	minced garlic	10 mL
1½ tsp	minced gingerroot	7 mL
1 tsp	sesame oil	5 mL
1 tsp	vegetable oil	5 mL
⅓ cup	finely chopped carrots	75 mL
¾ cup	finely chopped red or green peppers	175 mL
¾ cup	finely chopped mushrooms	175 mL
½ cup	chopped water chestnuts	125 mL
2	green onions, chopped	2
2 tbsp	hoisin sauce	25 mL
1 tbsp	water	15 mL
8	large iceberg lettuce leaves	8

Make Ahead

Prepare entire beef mixture earlier in the day. Reheat gently before placing in lettuce leaves.

SERVES 4

1. *Sauce:* In small bowl, whisk together hoisin, vinegar, garlic, ginger and sesame oil; set aside.

2. In nonstick skillet sprayed with vegetable spray, cook beef over medium heat for 5 minutes, or until browned; remove from skillet. Drain any excess liquid.

3. In same nonstick skillet, heat oil over medium heat. Add carrots and cook for 3 minutes. Add red peppers and mushrooms and cook for 3 minutes or until softened. Return beef to pan along with water chestnuts and green onions. Add sauce and cook for 2 minutes.

4. Combine hoisin sauce and water in small bowl. Place a little over leaves. Divide beef mixture among lettuce leaves. Serve open or rolled up.

Tips

- Look for a large iceberg lettuce to get the best quality leaves.
- Use other vegetables, such as celery and oyster mushrooms, as substitutes.

Nutritional Analysis (Per Serving)
- Calories: 252
- Protein: 17 g
- Fat: 15 g
- Carbohydrates: 12 g
- Fiber: 1 g
- Sodium: 236 mg
- Cholesterol: 45 mg

Italian Pizza Egg Rolls

1 tsp	vegetable oil	5 mL
1 tsp	minced garlic	5 mL
¼ cup	finely chopped carrots	50 mL
¼ cup	finely chopped onions	50 mL
¼ cup	finely chopped green peppers	50 mL
3 oz	lean ground beef	75 g
½ cup	tomato pasta sauce	125 mL
½ cup	grated mozzarella cheese (1½ oz/40g)	125 mL
1 tbsp	grated Parmesan cheese	15 mL
9	egg roll wrappers (5½ inches/13 cm square)	9

Make Ahead

Prepare these up to a day ahead and keep refrigerated. Bake an extra 5 minutes. These can also be prepared and frozen for up to a month.

Roll the wrappers any way that's easy. Wetting the edges of the wrappers with water may help secure roll.

MAKES 9

Preheat oven to 425°F (220°C) • Baking sheet sprayed with vegetable spray

1. In nonstick skillet sprayed with vegetable spray, heat oil over medium heat. Add garlic, carrots and onions; cook for 8 minutes, or until softened and browned. Add peppers and cook 2 minutes longer. Add beef and cook for 2 minutes, stirring to break it up, or until it is no longer pink. Remove from heat and stir in tomato sauce, mozzarella and Parmesan cheeses.

2. Keeping rest of wrappers covered with a cloth to prevent drying out, put one wrapper on work surface with a corner pointing towards you. Put 2 tbsp (25 mL) of the filling in the center. Fold the lower corner up over the filling, fold the 2 side corners in over the filling, and roll the bundle away from you. Put on prepared pan and repeat until all wrappers are filled. Bake for 14 minutes, until browned, turning the pizza rolls at the halfway mark.

Tips

• Children devour these tasty egg rolls. Double the recipe if necessary.

• Ground chicken or veal can replace beef.

• Cheddar cheese can replace mozzarella for a more intense flavor.

Nutritional Analysis (Per Serving)
• Calories: 87   • Protein: 4 g   • Fat: 4 g
• Carbohydrates: 8 g   • Fiber: 0 g   • Sodium: 138 mg
• Cholesterol: 9 mg

Meatloaf Topped with Sautéed Vegetables and Tomato Sauce

1½ tsp	vegetable oil	7 mL
1 tsp	crushed garlic	5 mL
½ cup	finely diced onions	125 mL
½ cup	finely diced sweet red pepper	125 mL
½ cup	thinly sliced mushrooms	125 mL
½ cup	tomato sauce, heated	125 mL

MEATLOAF

1 lb	lean ground beef	500 g
1	green onion, finely chopped	1
2 tsp	crushed garlic	10 mL
1	egg	1
⅓ cup	dry bread crumbs	75 mL
1 tbsp	grated Parmesan cheese	15 mL
2 tbsp	chili sauce or ketchup	25 mL
½ tsp	dried basil	2 mL
½ tsp	dried oregano	2 mL
½ cup	tomato sauce	125 mL

SERVES 6

Preheat oven to 375°F (190°C) • 9- by 5-inch (2 L) loaf pan sprayed with nonstick vegetable spray

1. *Meatloaf:* In bowl, mix together beef, onion, garlic, egg, bread crumbs, cheese, chili sauce, basil, oregano and tomato sauce until well combined. Pat into loaf pan.

2. In small nonstick skillet, heat oil; sauté garlic, onions, red pepper and mushrooms until softened, about 5 minutes. Spoon over meatloaf. Bake, uncovered, for 40 to 50 minutes or until meat thermometer registers 170°F (75°C). Cover and let stand for 20 minutes before serving. Serve with tomato sauce.

Nutritional Analysis (Per Serving)
- Calories: 219
- Protein: 18 g
- Fat: 11 g
- Carbohydrates: 11 g
- Fiber: 2 g
- Sodium: 411 mg
- Cholesterol: 82 mg

Hoisin Garlic Burgers

1 lb	lean ground beef	500 g
¼ cup	bread crumbs	50 mL
¼ cup	chopped green onions (about 2 medium)	50 mL
3 tbsp	chopped coriander or parsley	45 mL
2 tbsp	hoisin sauce	25 mL
2 tsp	minced garlic	10 mL
1 tsp	minced gingerroot	5 mL
1	egg	1
2 tbsp	water	25 mL
2 tbsp	hoisin sauce	25 mL
1 tsp	sesame oil	5 mL

SERVES 4 TO 5

Start barbecue or preheat oven to 450°F (230°C)

1. In bowl combine beef, bread crumbs, green onions, coriander, hoisin sauce, garlic, gingerroot and egg; mix well. Make 4 to 5 burgers.

2. In small bowl whisk together water, hoisin sauce and sesame oil. Brush half of the sauce over top of burgers.

3. Place on greased grill and barbecue, or place on rack on baking sheet and bake for 10 to 15 minutes (or until no longer pink inside). Turn patties once and brush with remaining sauce.

Make Ahead

Prepare beef mixture up to a day ahead and form into burgers. Freeze up to 6 weeks.

Nutritional Analysis (Per Serving)
- Calories: 292
- Protein: 21 g
- Fat: 18 g
- Carbohydrates: 10 g
- Fiber: 1 g
- Sodium: 305 mg
- Cholesterol: 100 mg

Hamburgers Stuffed with Cheese and Onions

1 lb	lean ground beef	500 g
2 tsp	crushed garlic	10 mL
¼ cup	finely chopped green onion	50 mL
2 tbsp	ketchup	25 mL
	Salt and pepper	
1	egg	1
2 tbsp	dry bread crumbs	25 mL
½ cup	finely chopped onions	125 mL
1 tsp	vegetable oil	5 mL
¼ cup	shredded Cheddar cheese	50 mL

Make Ahead

Make patties in advance and freeze. Thaw and barbecue just prior to serving.

SERVES 4 TO 5

Barbecue or preheat oven to 450°F (230°C)

1. In bowl, mix together beef, garlic, green onion, ketchup, salt and pepper to taste, egg and bread crumbs until well combined. Form into 4 or 5 hamburgers.

2. In small nonstick skillet, sauté onions in oil until softened. Make pocket in each hamburger and evenly stuff with onions and cheese. Press meat mixture around opening to seal.

3. Place on greased grill and barbecue, or place on rack on baking sheet and bake for 10 to 15 minutes or until no longer pink inside, turning patties once.

Tips

- Try ground veal or chicken for a change.
- Substitute other cheeses, such as Swiss or mozzarella.

Nutritional Analysis (Per Serving)
- Calories: 240
- Protein: 21 g
- Fat: 13 g
- Carbohydrates: 5 g
- Fiber: 1 g
- Sodium: 181 mg
- Cholesterol: 102 mg

Mixed Meat Burgers with Cheese and Mushroom Pockets

8 oz	lean ground beef	250 g
8 oz	lean ground veal or chicken	250 g
2 tsp	crushed garlic	10 mL
1/4 cup	finely chopped red onions	50 mL
2 tbsp	barbecue sauce	25 mL
1	egg	1
2 tbsp	seasoned bread crumbs	25 mL

STUFFING

1 tsp	vegetable oil	5 mL
1/2 cup	finely chopped mushrooms	125 mL
1/4 cup	shredded mozzarella cheese	50 mL

Make Ahead

Make patties in advance and freeze. Thaw and barbecue just prior to serving.

SERVES 4 TO 5

Start barbecue or preheat oven to 450°F (230°C)

1. In bowl, mix together both meats, garlic, red onions, barbecue sauce, egg and bread crumbs until well combined. Form into 4 or 5 hamburgers.

2. *Stuffing:* In small nonstick skillet, heat oil and sauté mushrooms until softened. Make pocket in each hamburger and evenly stuff with mushrooms and cheese. Press meat mixture around opening to seal.

3. Place on greased grill and barbecue, or place on rack on baking sheet and bake for 10 to 15 minutes or until no longer pink inside, turning patties once.

Tips

- Other combinations of ground meat can be used.
- Substitute another cheese for the mozzarella.
- Try wild mushrooms, such as oyster mushrooms.

Nutritional Analysis (Per Serving)
- Calories: 231
- Protein: 21 g
- Fat: 12 g
- Carbohydrates: 5 g
- Fiber: 1 g
- Sodium: 200 mg
- Cholesterol: 102 mg

Veal Stuffed with Cheese in Mushroom Sauce

1 lb	veal cutlets	500 g
1 tsp	vegetable oil	5 mL
1/2 cup	finely diced mushrooms	125 mL
1/4 cup	finely diced onions	50 mL
1 tsp	crushed garlic	5 mL
1/3 cup	shredded mozzarella cheese	75 mL
1/4 cup	beef stock	50 mL
	Chopped fresh parsley	

SAUCE

1 tbsp	margarine	15 mL
1 1/2 cups	sliced mushrooms	375 mL
2 tbsp	all-purpose flour	25 mL
1 cup	beef stock	250 mL
1 tbsp	sherry (optional)	15 mL
2 tbsp	light sour cream	25 mL

Make Ahead

Assemble and refrigerate veal rolls early in the day. Make sauce ahead of time but add sour cream after reheating.

SERVES 4
Preheat oven to 400°F (200°C)

1. Pound veal until flat and divide into 4 serving pieces.
2. In small nonstick skillet, heat oil; sauté mushrooms, onions and garlic until softened, approximately 3 minutes. Remove from heat.
3. Divide vegetable mixture among cutlets. Sprinkle cheese over top. Roll up and secure with toothpick. Place in baking dish and add stock. Cover and bake for 8 to 10 minutes or just until veal is tender. Remove rolls to serving platter. Keep warm.
4. *Sauce:* In small nonstick skillet, melt margarine; sauté mushrooms until softened and liquid is released. Add flour and cook, stirring, for 1 minute. Add stock, and sherry (if using); cook until thickened, approximately 2 minutes, stirring constantly. If too thick, add more stock. Remove from heat and stir in sour cream; pour over veal. Garnish with parsley.

Tips

- If the veal seems tough, marinate it in milk for 2 hours before using. Be sure not to overcook the veal, which will make it tough.
- You can substitute boneless chicken breasts for the veal.

Nutritional Analysis (Per Serving)
- Calories: 222
- Protein: 24 g
- Fat: 10 g
- Carbohydrates: 7 g
- Fiber: 1 g
- Sodium: 360 mg
- Cholesterol: 82 mg

Spiced Veal Stir-Fry

1 tsp	ground ginger	5 mL
½ tsp	garlic powder	2 mL
¼ tsp	red pepper flakes	1 mL
Pinch	ground cinnamon	Pinch
Pinch	each allspice and ground cloves	Pinch
1¼ lb	veal scaloppine, cut into thin strips	625 g
1 cup	chicken broth	250 mL
¼ cup	dry white wine (optional)	50 mL
3 tbsp	soy sauce	45 mL
2 tbsp	cornstarch	25 mL
2 tbsp	vegetable oil, divided	25 mL
1	medium onion, chopped	1
2 cups	mushrooms, quartered	500 mL
3	medium carrots, sliced	3
3	stalks celery, diagonally sliced	3
1	medium green bell pepper, chopped	1

This delicious stir-fry recipe uses veal seasoned with ginger, garlic, red pepper flakes — and cinnamon!

SERVES 6

1. Combine ginger, garlic powder, red pepper flakes, cinnamon, allspice and cloves. Transfer one-third of the spice mixture to bowl; add veal and toss to coat. Chill for 1 to 2 hours.

2. Combine remaining spice mixture, chicken broth, wine, if using, soy sauce and cornstarch; set sauce aside.

3. In a large skillet, heat 1 tbsp (15 mL) of the oil over medium-high heat; sauté onion, mushrooms, carrots, celery and green pepper for 5 minutes or until tender. Remove from pan. Add remaining oil to skillet; brown veal for about 2 minutes. Add sauce and bring to a boil; cook, stirring, until thickened. Return vegetables to skillet and heat through.

Tips

- Stir-frying and sautéing are basically the same method of cooking: food is cooked quickly in a pan with sloping sides.

- If desired, replace the white wine in this recipe with additional chicken stock.

Nutritional Analysis (Per Serving)
- Calories: 200
- Protein: 23 g
- Fat: 7 g
- Carbohydrates: 12 g
- Fiber: 2 g
- Sodium: 461 mg
- Cholesterol: 83 mg

Veal Paprikash

2 tbsp	vegetable oil	25 mL
1 lb	grain-fed veal scallops or boneless beef sirloin, cut into thin strips	500 g
4 cups	quartered mushrooms (about 12 oz/375 g)	1 L
1	large onion, halved lengthwise and thinly sliced	1
2	cloves garlic, minced	2
4 tsp	sweet Hungarian paprika	20 mL
1/2 tsp	dried marjoram	2 mL
1/2 tsp	salt	2 mL
1/4 tsp	pepper	1 mL
1 tbsp	all-purpose flour	15 mL
3/4 cup	chicken stock	175 mL
1/2 cup	sour cream	125 mL
	Salt and pepper	

SERVES 4

1. In a large nonstick skillet, heat half the oil over high heat; stir-fry veal in 2 batches, each for 3 minutes or until browned but still pink inside. Transfer to a plate along with pan juices; keep warm.

2. Reduce heat to medium. Add remaining oil. Add mushrooms, onion, garlic, paprika, marjoram, salt and pepper; cook, stirring often, for 7 minutes or until lightly colored.

3. Sprinkle mushroom mixture with flour; pour in stock. Cook, stirring, for 2 minutes or until thickened. Stir in sour cream. Return veal and accumulated juices to pan; cook 1 minute more or until heated through. Adjust seasoning with salt and pepper to taste; serve immediately.

Nutritional Analysis (Per Serving)
- Calories: 266
- Protein: 30 g
- Fat: 11 g
- Carbohydrates: 12 g
- Fiber: 2 g
- Sodium: 462 mg
- Cholesterol: 107 mg

Calves Liver with Balsamic Vinegar

1 1/2 lbs	calves liver, very thinly sliced	750 g
1/4 cup	all-purpose flour	50 mL
1/4 cup	butter	50 mL
1/2 tsp	salt	2 mL
1/4 tsp	freshly ground black pepper	1 mL
1/3 cup	balsamic vinegar	75 mL
3 tbsp	finely chopped sage	45 mL

SERVES 6

1. Lightly dust liver in flour, shaking off the excess. In a skillet large enough to hold all the pieces, melt butter over heat until sizzling. Add liver and sauté for 1 1/2 minutes on each side or until cooked, but still pink inside. Season with salt and pepper. Transfer liver to warm platter.

2. Add vinegar to pan and scrape up any brown bits. Bring to a boil and cook 1 or 2 minutes until thickened. Return liver to pan. Turn it over once or twice and cook for another 1 or 2 minutes. Add sage and serve liver with sauce poured over.

Nutritional Analysis (Per Serving)
- Calories: 250
- Protein: 21.2 g
- Fat: 13.1 g
- Carbohydrates: 11.8
- Fiber: 1.4 g
- Sodium: 344 mg
- Cholesterol: 373 mg

Veal Scallops with Sage

2 lbs	veal scallops	1 kg
4 oz	prosciutto, thinly sliced	125 g
20 to 24	sage leaves, washed and dried	20 to 24
3 tbsp	unsalted butter	45 mL
½ tsp	salt	2 mL
¼ tsp	freshly ground black pepper	1 mL
¾ cup	Marsala or dry white wine	175 mL

SERVES 6

1. With a kitchen mallet or rolling pin, gently pound the veal until thin, being careful not to tear the meat. Trim each scallop to a fairly squarish shape. Lay one piece of prosciutto on top of each piece of veal, folding in the sides if necessary to make it neat.

2. Place a sage leaf at the center of each piece of prosciutto and, using a wooden cocktail stick, securely fasten the sage leaf and the prosciutto to the veal.

3. In a large skillet, melt butter over medium-high heat until sizzling. Add the veal and sauté for about 2 minutes on each side, seasoning with salt and pepper as they cook. Transfer veal to a serving platter and keep warm. Discard toothpicks.

4. Splash the Marsala into the skillet and scrape up any bits on the bottom. Bring to a gentle boil, reduce heat and simmer for a couple of minutes until sauce is glossy and slightly thickened. Pour over the veal and serve immediately.

Nutritional Analysis (Per Serving)
- Calories: 460
- Protein: 45.0 g
- Fat: 23.2 g
- Carbohydrates: 5.4
- Fiber: 1.2 g
- Sodium: 621 mg
- Cholesterol: 160 mg

Braised Roasted Veal

2 lb	veal leg (top portion)	1 kg
½ tsp	each crumbled dried rosemary and thyme	2 mL
Pinch	dried tarragon	Pinch
1	stalk celery, chopped	1
1	medium onion, chopped	1
1	medium carrot, diced	1
⅓ cup	water	75 mL
¼ cup	vinegar	50 mL
¼ cup	white wine	50 mL
1 tsp	grated lemon zest	5 mL
1 tbsp	lemon juice	15 mL

SERVES 8
Preheat oven to 475°F (240°C) • Roasting pan

1. Place veal in roasting pan; sprinkle with rosemary, thyme and tarragon. Place celery, onion and carrot around veal. Roast in preheated oven for 10 minutes.

2. Reduce temperature to 375°F (190°C). Add water, vinegar, wine, lemon zest and juice. Cover and roast for 1 hour. Remove from pan and cool. Chill. Slice to serve.

Nutritional Analysis (Per Serving)
- Calories: 144
- Protein: 25 g
- Fat: 4 g
- Carbohydrates: 0 g
- Fiber: 0 g
- Sodium: 83 mg
- Cholesterol: 100 mg

Tuscan Roast Veal with Rosemary and White Wine

2 oz	pancetta, finely diced, or bacon (see tip, at right)	60 g
¼ cup	finely chopped fresh parsley	50 mL
2	cloves garlic, minced	2
1 tsp	grated lemon zest	5 mL
	Salt and freshly ground black pepper	
3 lbs	leg of veal roast, well trimmed, tied	1.5 kg
2 tbsp	olive oil	25 mL
1 tbsp	chopped fresh rosemary or 1½ tsp (7 mL) dried rosemary, crumbled	15 mL
1 cup	dry white wine, divided	250 mL
1 cup	chicken or veal stock, divided	250 mL

You will be delighted by the tantalizing aromas of rosemary and garlic wafting through your kitchen whenever you prepare this distinctive roast — ideal for a special occasion.

SERVES 6 TO 8

Preheat oven to 350°F (180°C) • Roasting pan

1. In a bowl, combine pancetta, parsley, garlic and zest; season with salt and pepper. Stuff into cavity of roast, as evenly as possible. (Prepare earlier in the day and refrigerate to allow flavors to penetrate veal.)

2. Place veal in pan. Brush with oil; season with rosemary, salt and pepper. Place in oven and roast, uncovered, for 30 minutes. Add ½ cup (125 mL) each wine and stock to roasting pan. Tent loosely with foil and continue to roast for 1½ hours more, adding more wine and stock to the pan as necessary, until meat thermometer registers 170°F (80°C).

3. Transfer meat to serving platter and keep warm. Pour remaining wine and stock into roasting pan and place on stovetop over high heat. Bring to a boil, scraping up any brown bits from bottom of pan. Strain into a saucepan and boil until partially reduced. Slice veal into slices and drizzle with some of the pan juices. Serve remainder in a sauceboat.

Tip

• Pancetta is unsmoked Italian bacon that is available in supermarket deli counters.

Nutritional Analysis (Per Serving)
- Calories: 280
- Protein: 43.5 g
- Fat: 7.8 g
- Carbohydrates: 1.3 g
- Fiber: 0.3 g
- Sodium: 347 mg
- Cholesterol: 155 mg

Veal Meat Loaf

1 tbsp	olive oil	15 mL
1	onion, finely chopped	1
1	large clove garlic, finely chopped	1
½ tsp	dried thyme or marjoram leaves	2 mL
1 tsp	salt	5 mL
¼ tsp	freshly ground black pepper	1 mL
1	egg	1
¼ cup	chicken stock	50 mL
1 tsp	grated lemon zest	5 mL
½ cup	dry seasoned bread crumbs	125 mL
2 tbsp	finely chopped fresh parsley	25 mL
1½ lbs	lean ground veal or chicken	750 g

SERVES 6
Preheat oven to 350°F (180°C) • 9-by 5-inch (2 L) loaf pan

1. In a large nonstick skillet, heat oil over medium heat; cook onion, garlic, thyme, salt and pepper, stirring often, for 3 minutes or until softened. Let cool slightly.

2. In a bowl, beat together egg, stock and lemon zest. Stir in onion mixture, bread crumbs, parsley and veal. Using a wooden spoon, gently mix until evenly combined.

3. Press mixture lightly into loaf pan. Bake in preheated oven for 1 hour or until meat thermometer registers 170°F (80°C). Let stand for 5 minutes. Drain pan juices; turn out onto a plate a cut into thick slices.

Nutritional Analysis (Per Serving)
- Calories: 245
- Protein: 24.2 g
- Fat: 11.3 g
- Carbohydrates: 9.7 g
- Fiber: 0.7 g
- Sodium: 593 mg
- Cholesterol: 128 mg

Dijon Mustard Pork Medallions

1	pork tenderloin (about 1 lb/500 g), cut crosswise into 8 pieces	1
	Salt and freshly ground black pepper	
½ cup	plain yogurt or sour cream	125 mL
1 tbsp	Dijon mustard	15 mL
1	clove garlic, minced	1

Sublime is the only way to describe pork served with this wonderfully creamy mustard sauce.

SERVES 4
Nonstick cooking spray

1. Trim pork and discard fat. To make medallions, place pork, cut-side down, on a flat surface. Cover with waxed paper. Flatten gently with heel of hand, meat mallet or rolling pin to ¼ inch (1 cm) thick.

2. Heat nonstick skillet over medium-high heat. Lightly spray with cooking spray. Sauté medallions, in batches, for 3 minutes per side or until a hint of pink remains inside. Remove from skillet to a warm plate. Sprinkle lightly with salt and pepper.

3. In a small bowl, combine yogurt, mustard and garlic. Serve a spoonful with each medallion.

Nutritional Analysis (Per Serving)
- Calories: 157
- Protein: 25.8 g
- Fat: 4.1 g
- Carbohydrates: 2.9 g
- Fiber: 0.2 g
- Sodium: 253 mg
- Cholesterol: 73 mg

Company Pork Roast with Fruit Stuffing

STUFFING

1 tbsp	margarine or butter	15 mL
1/3 cup	chopped green onions	75 mL
1 tsp	ground cumin	5 mL
1/2 tsp	curry powder	2 mL
1 cup	chopped mixed dried fruits, such as apricots, prunes, apples, cranberries	250 mL
1/2 cup	soft bread crumbs	125 mL
1 tsp	grated orange rind	5 mL
1	egg, beaten	1
	Salt and pepper	
3 lbs	boneless pork loin roast	1.5 kg
2 tsp	vegetable oil	10 mL
1	large clove garlic, minced	1
1 tsp	rubbed sage	5 mL
1/2 tsp	dried thyme	2 mL
1 tbsp	all-purpose flour	15 mL
1/2 cup	white wine or chicken stock	125 mL
3/4 cup	chicken stock	175 mL

SERVES 10

Preheat oven to 350°F (180°C) • Roasting pan with rack

1. *Stuffing:* In a small skillet, melt butter over medium heat. Add green onions, cumin and curry powder; cook, stirring, for 2 minutes or until softened.

2. In a bowl combine onion mixture, dried fruits, bread crumbs, orange rind and egg; season with salt and pepper.

3. Remove strings from pork roast; unfold roast and trim excess fat. Place pork roast, boned side up, on work surface. Cover with plastic wrap and pound using a meat mallet to flatten slightly. Season with salt and pepper; spread stuffing down center of meat. Roll the pork around the stuffing and tie securely at 6 intervals with butcher's string.

4. Place roast on rack in roasting pan. In a small bowl, combine oil, garlic, sage and thyme; spread over pork roast and season with salt and pepper.

5. Roast in preheated oven for 1 1/2 to 1 3/4 hours or until meat thermometer registers 160°F (70°C).

6. Remove roast to cutting board; tent with foil and let stand for 10 minutes before carving.

7. Pour off fat in pan. Place over medium heat; sprinkle with flour. Cook, stirring, for 1 minute or until lightly colored. Add wine or stock; cook until partially reduced. Add stock and bring to a boil, scraping any brown bits from bottom of pan. Season with salt and pepper to taste. Strain sauce through a fine sieve into a warm sauceboat. Cut pork into thick slices and serve accompanied with gravy.

Tip

• It may appear that you have too much stuffing when you first tie the pork. But once all the strings are in place, it's easy to enclose the meat completely around the fruit mixture.

Nutritional Analysis (Per Serving)
- Calories: 258
- Protein: 32 g
- Fat: 8 g
- Carbohydrates: 12 g
- Fiber: 1 g
- Sodium: 173 mg
- Cholesterol: 119 mg

Coorg-Style Pork Curry

1 tbsp	vegetable oil	15 mL
1½ tbsp	coriander powder	22 mL
1¼ tsp	cayenne powder	6 mL
¼ tsp	turmeric	1 mL
1½ tsp	salt	7 mL
1½ lbs	pork tenderloin, cut into 1-inch (2.5 cm) pieces	750 g
1 tsp	cumin seeds	5 mL
1 tsp	whole cloves	5 mL
1 tsp	black peppercorns or to taste	5 mL
½ tsp	mustard seeds	2 mL
1	large onion, chopped into chunks	1
18	cloves garlic	18
1	piece peeled gingerroot, ½ inch by 1 inch (1 cm by 2.5 cm), chopped into chunks	1
1 tbsp	cider vinegar	15 mL
2 tbsp	lime or lemon juice	25 mL

Coorg is one of two areas in India where pork dishes abound. This dish is typical of the cooking there.

SERVES 6

1. In a large saucepan, combine oil, coriander, cayenne, turmeric and salt. Add pork and marinate for 15 minutes.

2. In a spice grinder, grind cumin seeds, cloves, black peppercorns and mustard seeds into a powder.

3. In a blender, combine onion, garlic, ginger and spice powder. Purée until smooth.

4. Add onion mixture to pork. Mix well. Bring to a boil over medium-high heat. Cover pan. Reduce heat to maintain a gentle boil and cook, stirring occasionally, until pork is thoroughly cooked, 20 to 30 minutes.

5. Add vinegar. Remove from heat. Add lime juice and mix well.

Nutritional Analysis (Per Serving)
- Calories: 185
- Protein: 25.1 g
- Fat: 5.0 g
- Carbohydrates: 10.0 g
- Fiber: 1.5 g
- Sodium: 253 mg
- Cholesterol: 72 mg

Pork Vindaloo

1 tbsp	cumin seeds	15 mL
2 tsp	coriander seeds	10 mL
1 tbsp	clarified butter or ghee (see tip, at right)	15 mL
1	onion, finely chopped	1
8	cloves garlic, minced	8
1 tbsp	minced gingerroot	15 mL
1	piece cinnamon stick, about 2 inches (5 cm)	1
6	whole cloves	6
½ tsp	salt	2 mL
2 tsp	mustard seeds	10 mL
¼ tsp	cayenne pepper	1 mL
2 lbs	stewing pork, cut into 1-inch (2.5 cm) cubes	1 kg
4	bay leaves	4
½ cup	red wine vinegar	125 mL

Make Ahead

This dish must be assembled the night before it is cooked as it needs to be marinated overnight. Follow preparation directions and refrigerate overnight. The next day, transfer to stoneware and cook as directed.

SERVES 8
Slow cooker

1. In a skillet, over medium heat, cook cumin and coriander seeds, stirring constantly, until they release their aroma and just begin to turn golden. Remove pan from heat and transfer seeds to a mortar or a cutting board. Using a pestle or a rolling pin, crush seeds coarsely. Set aside.

2. In a skillet, heat butter or ghee over medium heat. Add onion, garlic and gingerroot and cook for 1 minute. Add cumin and coriander seeds, cinnamon, cloves, salt, mustard seeds and cayenne and cook for 1 more minute. Remove from heat. Let cool.

3. Place pork in a mixing bowl. Add bay leaves and contents of pan. Add vinegar and stir to combine. Cover and marinate overnight in refrigerator. The next day, transfer to slow cooker stoneware, cover and cook on Low for 8 to 10 hours or on High for 4 to 5 hours, until pork is tender. Discard bay leaves, cinnamon stick and whole cloves.

Tip

• Ghee is a type of clarified butter that is highly valued in Indian cooking as it can be heated to a very high temperature. It is available in grocery stores specializing in Indian ingredients and will keep, refrigerated, for as long as a year.

Nutritional Analysis (Per Serving)
• Calories: 181
• Protein: 26 g
• Fat: 6 g
• Carbohydrates: 4 g
• Fiber: 1 g
• Sodium: 225 mg
• Cholesterol: 82 mg

Pork Stew

3 tbsp	olive oil	45 mL
3 lbs	lean stewing pork, cut into 2-inch (5 cm) chunks	1.5 kg
3	cloves garlic, minced	3
1	onion, finely chopped	1
1	celery stalk, finely chopped	1
2	carrots, scraped and finely chopped	2
1/4 cup	chopped flat-leaf parsley	50 mL
3 tbsp	chopped pancetta	45 mL
2	branches fresh rosemary, leaves only, finely chopped	2
1 cup	robust dry red wine	250 mL
1/2 cup	beef stock	125 mL
1 1/2 cups	canned Italian plum tomatoes, chopped, with juice	375 mL
1/2 tsp	red pepper flakes (optional)	2 mL
1/2 tsp	salt	2 mL
1/4 tsp	freshly ground black pepper	1 mL

SERVES 4 TO 6

1. In a Dutch oven or large skillet, heat olive oil over medium heat. Add pork and, in batches if necessary, brown on all sides, transferring to a plate or bowl when done.

2. Add garlic, onion, celery, carrots, parsley, pancetta, rosemary and, if necessary, another 1 tbsp (15 mL) of olive oil; sauté for about 5 minutes.

3. Return pork to the pan and mix to combine well with the vegetables and herbs. Add red wine; cook for about 5 minutes. Add stock and cook for another 5 minutes.

4. Add tomatoes and their juice, red pepper flakes, salt and pepper; stir and bring to a gentle boil. Immediately reduce heat and simmer stew until sauce is thickened and meat is tender, about 1 1/2 hours.

Nutritional Analysis (Per Serving)
- Calories: 565
- Protein: 58.6 g
- Fat: 26.1 g
- Carbohydrates: 14.3
- Fiber: 3.6 g
- Sodium: 709 mg
- Cholesterol: 179 mg

Braised Cabbage with Ham and Cheese

1 tbsp	vegetable oil	15 mL
1	small onion, thinly sliced	1
2	cloves garlic, minced	2
1 tsp	dried oregano leaves	5 mL
1 tsp	ground cumin	5 mL
6 cups	shredded cabbage, lightly packed, or 1 lb (500 g) packaged coleslaw mix	1.5 L
1	can (19 oz/540 mL) chili-style stewed tomatoes, including juice	1
1 1/2 cups	cubed smoked ham or firm tofu (1/2-inch/ 1 cm cubes)	375 mL
1 cup	shredded Cheddar cheese	250 mL

SERVES 4 TO 6

12-cup (3 L) casserole dish with lid

1. In casserole dish, combine oil, onion, garlic, oregano and cumin. Microwave, covered, on High for 2 to 3 minutes or until onion is softened. Add cabbage and tomatoes with juice. Microwave, covered, on High for 10 to 14 minutes, stirring once, until cabbage is tender.

2. Stir in ham. Microwave, covered, on High for 2 to 3 minutes longer or until heated through.

3. Sprinkle with cheese and microwave, covered, on High for 1 to 2 minutes or until cheese melts. Let stand, covered, for 3 minutes before serving.

Nutritional Analysis (Per Serving)
- Calories: 238
- Protein: 17.7 g
- Fat: 13.2 g
- Carbohydrates: 13.7 g
- Fiber: 3.5 g
- Sodium: 713 mg
- Cholesterol: 48 mg

Savory Lamb Chops

2 tbsp	oil and vinegar dressing	25 mL
1 tbsp	Dijon mustard	15 mL
1½ lbs	lamb chops, thawed if frozen	750 g
2 tbsp	prepared sun-dried tomato pesto	25 mL

Tasty, elegant, simple and quick to make, this recipe is a keeper. Serve with steamed green beans.

SERVES 4
Preheat broiler or grill

1. In a bowl, combine oil and vinegar dressing and mustard.
2. Pat lamb chops dry. Brush both sides with mixture.
3. Place on broiling pan about 6 inches (15 cm) from heat. Cook, turning once, until desired degree of doneness, 8 to 10 minutes. Serve topped with a dollop of pesto.

Tip
- For an easy extra, add 1 tsp (5 mL) dried Italian seasoning to oil and vinegar dressing before brushing lamb chops.

Nutritional Analysis (Per Serving)
- Calories: 317
- Protein: 37.5 g
- Fat: 17.6 g
- Carbohydrates: 1.6 g
- Fiber: 0.4 g
- Sodium: 198 mg
- Cholesterol: 97 mg

Grilled Lamb Chops with Mustard

1 tbsp	whole-grain mustard	15 mL
1 tsp	Dijon mustard	5 mL
1 tbsp	olive oil	15 mL
½ tsp	dried thyme	2 mL
½ tsp	crumbled dried rosemary	2 mL
¼ tsp	black pepper	1 mL
4	lamb chops, 1 inch (2.5 cm) thick (about 1¼ lbs/625 g)	4
	Salt to taste	
1 tbsp	lemon juice	15 mL
	Few sprigs fresh parsley, chopped	
2	green onions, finely chopped	2

SERVES 2
Preheat grill or broiler

1. In a small bowl, stir together the mustards, olive oil, thyme, rosemary and black pepper until smooth. Generously brush both sides of the chops with this mixture and let rest at room temperature for about 30 minutes.
2. Grill or broil lamb chops to your preference (3 to 4 minutes each side for medium rare). Sprinkle salt and lemon juice on the chops. Serve immediately, garnished with chopped parsley and green onions.

Nutritional Analysis (Per Serving)
- Calories: 458
- Protein: 57.7 g
- Fat: 8.7 g
- Carbohydrates: 3.8 g
- Fiber: 1.4 g
- Sodium: 257 mg
- Cholesterol: 147 mg

Grilled Lamb Chops with Sautéed Peppers and Zucchini

¼ cup	balsamic or red wine vinegar	50 mL
2 tbsp	olive oil, divided	25 mL
1 tbsp	Dijon mustard	15 mL
1 tsp	dried thyme leaves	5 mL
1 tsp	minced garlic	5 mL
⅛ tsp	black pepper	0.5 mL
8 to 12	bone-in, center-cut loin lamb chops, trimmed of fat (about 1½ lb/750 g in total)	8 to 12
1½ cups	sliced zucchini	375 mL
1½ cups	julienned red bell peppers	375 mL
1 cup	sliced sweet onion	250 mL

> *Try this impressive dish for your next dinner party. Your guests need never know how easy it is to make!*

SERVES 4

Preheat broiler or barbecue

1. In a large bowl, blend together vinegar, 1 tbsp (15 mL) of the oil, mustard, thyme, garlic and pepper. Transfer 2 to 3 tbsp (25 to 45 mL) of the mixture to a small bowl; set aside.

2. Place chops on broiling pan or grill; spoon reserved vinaigrette on top. Cook, turning once, for 8 to 10 minutes or until cooked to desired doneness.

3. Meanwhile, in a large nonstick skillet, heat remaining 1 tbsp (15 mL) oil over medium-high heat. Add zucchini, peppers and onion; stir-fry for 6 to 8 minutes or until tender-crisp. Add remaining vinaigrette to pan; cook, stirring, for 1 to 2 minutes or until heated through.

Tips

- For extra-easy cleanup, line the broiler pan with foil.

- If weather permits, grill chops on the barbecue; you'll improve their flavor — and enjoy some time outdoors!

- To cook the vegetables on the grill, place vegetables and sauce in a heavy-duty foil packet and barbecue for about 10 minutes, turning once.

Nutritional Analysis (Per Serving)
- Calories: 233
- Protein: 19 g
- Fat: 12 g
- Carbohydrates: 12 g
- Fiber: 2 g
- Sodium: 158 mg
- Cholesterol: 148 mg

Grilled Lamb Chops with Minted Yogurt

6	lamb chops, $1/4$ to $1/2$ inch (5 mm to 1 cm) thick, about 1 lb (500 g) in all	6
1 tbsp	olive oil	15 mL
$1/2$ tsp	dried oregano	2 mL
$1/4$ tsp	freshly ground black pepper	1 mL
$1/2$ cup	thinly sliced onions	125 mL
$1/2$ cup	yogurt	125 mL
1	clove garlic, pressed	1
2 tbsp	chopped fresh mint (or $1/2$ tsp/2 mL dried)	25 mL
1 tbsp	lemon juice	15 mL
1 tsp	extra virgin olive oil	5 mL
	Salt and pepper to taste	
$1/2$ tsp	dried oregano	2 mL

SERVES 2

Preheat grill or broiler

1. Brush lamb chops with olive oil and lay out on a flat plate. Sprinkle with $1/2$ tsp (2 mL) oregano and pepper; top with the onions, pressing down into the meat. Cover and let marinate at room temperature for 20 minutes.

2. In a small bowl, combine yogurt, garlic, mint, lemon juice, olive oil, salt and pepper. Mix to integrate well, cover and let rest up to 30 minutes, unrefrigerated. (This sauce can be prepared in advance and refrigerated. It must be allowed a 30-minute "warm-up" to room temperature and a stir before being served.)

3. Grill or broil lamb chops (with any onions that happen to stick on) for 2 to 3 minutes each side or until done to your liking. Sprinkle with dried oregano just before taking off the grill.

4. Spread a thick quantity of the yogurt sauce on each of 2 warmed plates. Transfer 3 chops onto the middle of sauce on each plate and serve immediately.

Nutritional Analysis (Per Serving)
- Calories: 408
- Protein: 44.6 g
- Fat: 20.9 g
- Carbohydrates: 10.4 g
- Fiber: 1.0 g
- Sodium: 149 mg
- Cholesterol: 106 mg

Curried Lamb Chops

6	loin lamb chops, 1½ inches (4 cm) thick	6
2 tbsp	white wine vinegar	25 mL
1 tsp	salt	5 mL
¼ tsp	black pepper	1 mL
2 tsp	vegetable oil	10 mL
1 tsp	curry powder	5 mL
1 tsp	finely chopped gingerroot	5 mL
1	clove garlic, minced	1
¼ tsp	ground cloves	1 mL
¼ tsp	ground cinnamon	1 mL
¾ cup	water, divided	175 mL
1	medium onion, chopped	1
2 tbsp	all-purpose flour	25 mL
2 tbsp	currants	25 mL
1	kiwi fruit, peeled and sliced	1
1	orange, peeled and sliced	1

Here's a dish that may seem exotic, but it's easy to make from ingredients that are readily available. It demonstrates how the use of fruit, herbs and spices can add zest to the simplest recipes. Here, oranges, kiwi fruit, currants, curry powder and gingerroot are used to give lamb chops an Eastern aura.

SERVES 6

1. Place lamb chops in shallow pan. Combine vinegar, salt and pepper; spoon over chops. Set aside for 5 minutes.

2. In a heavy skillet, cook oil, curry, ginger root, garlic and seasonings until mixture bubbles. Add ½ cup (125 mL) water and onion. Cook over medium heat for about 5 minutes.

3. Sprinkle flour over lamb chops; add chops to onion in skillet. Cook for about 4 minutes per side or until chops lose pink color. Stir in remaining water and currants. Cook, covered, over low heat for about 30 minutes or until chops are tender. Add kiwi fruit and oranges and cook for about 3 minutes.

Tips

- For a richer-tasting sauce, use white wine or beef broth instead of the water in this recipe.

- Lamb provides high-quality protein and is a good source of iron.

- Serve with Cool Cucumber Salad (see recipe, page 86).

Nutritional Analysis (Per Serving)
- Calories: 217
- Protein: 25 g
- Fat: 8 g
- Carbohydrates: 11 g
- Fiber: 1 g
- Sodium: 502 mg
- Cholesterol: 148 mg

Herbed Butterflied Leg of Lamb

½ cup	packed basil leaves	125 mL
½ cup	packed parsley leaves	125 mL
3	green onions, coarsely chopped	3
2	cloves garlic, chopped	2
2 tbsp	Russian-style mustard	25 mL
2 tbsp	balsamic vinegar	25 mL
2 tbsp	olive oil	25 mL
1	3-lb (1.5 kg) butterflied leg of lamb, trimmed	1

This is a terrific dish, especially in early summer, when fresh herbs first appear in the markets. Serve it with steamed asparagus or fiddleheads followed by fresh strawberries or a lemon dessert.

SERVES 4 TO 5

1. In a food processor, combine basil, parsley, green onions and garlic. Process until finely chopped.
2. Add mustard, vinegar and oil to food processor and blend in.
3. Place lamb in a shallow dish. Spoon marinade over lamb and turn to coat all sides. Cover and marinate, refrigerated, for 3 hours or overnight.
4. Arrange lamb fat side up on lightly greased broiler rack set over oven pan.
5. Roast in preheated 375°F (190°C) toaster oven for 25 to 30 minutes, or until meat thermometer registers 140°F (60°C) for medium-rare. Cover loosely with foil and let stand for 5 to 10 minutes before carving across the grain.

Nutritional Analysis (Per Serving)
- Calories: 305
- Protein: 35.2 g
- Fat: 16.1 g
- Carbohydrates: 3.4 g
- Fiber: 0.9 g
- Sodium: 198 mg
- Cholesterol: 108 mg

Barbecued Butterflied Leg of Lamb

1	2-lb (1 kg) butterflied leg of lamb, trimmed	1
1 tsp	minced garlic	5 mL
2 tbsp	lemon juice	25 mL
2 tbsp	chopped fresh oregano (or 2 tsp/10 mL dried)	25 mL
2 tbsp	chopped fresh mint (or 2 tsp/10 mL dried)	25 mL
1 tbsp	olive oil	15 mL
	Black pepper	

This simple Greek-style marinade is the perfect companion to grilled lamb, which is best served medium-rare.

SERVES 6

1. Place lamb in a large shallow dish, fat side down. Spread with garlic. Sprinkle with lemon juice, oregano, mint and olive oil. Season with pepper to taste.
2. Cover and marinate in refrigerator, turning once or twice, for 2 hours or overnight. Remove from refrigerator 30 minutes before grilling.
3. Preheat barbecue or broiler. For medium-rare, barbecue on greased grill for 10 to 12 minutes per side, depending on thickness of lamb or, if using a meat thermometer, until the internal temperature of lamb registers 140° to 150°F (60° to 65°C).

Nutritional Analysis (Per Serving)
- Calories: 177
- Protein: 26 g
- Fat: 7 g
- Carbohydrates: 1 g
- Fiber: 0 g
- Sodium: 96 mg
- Cholesterol: 96 mg

Roasted Leg of Lamb with Crunchy Garlic Topping

1 tbsp	margarine	15 mL
2 tsp	crushed garlic	10 mL
1/3 cup	finely chopped onion	75 mL
1/2 cup	dry bread crumbs	125 mL
1/4 cup	crushed bran cereal*	50 mL
1/4 cup	chopped fresh parsley	50 mL
1/3 cup	chicken stock	75 mL
1	leg of lamb (2 1/2 to 3 lb/1.25 to 1.5 kg), deboned	1
1/3 cup	red wine	75 mL
1/3 cup	beef stock	75 mL

* Use a wheat bran breakfast cereal

SERVES 6 TO 8
Preheat oven to 375°F (190°C)

1. In large nonstick skillet, melt margarine; sauté garlic and onion until softened. Add bread crumbs, cereal, parsley and chicken stock; mix until well combined. If too dry, add more chicken stock.

2. Place lamb in roasting pan and pat bread crumb mixture over top. Pour wine and beef stock into pan. Cover and bake for 20 minutes. Uncover and bake for 15 to 20 minutes or until meat thermometer registers 140°F (60°C) for rare or until desired doneness. Serve with pan juices.

Tips

- If you suspect the lamb will be tough, marinate it in milk, turning occasionally, for at least 3 hours before baking.

- When using margarine, choose a soft (non-hydrogenated) version to limit consumption of trans fats.

Nutritional Analysis (Per Serving)
- Calories: 227
- Protein: 25 g
- Fat: 9 g
- Carbohydrates: 6 g
- Fiber: 1 g
- Sodium: 197 mg
- Cholesterol: 77 mg

Tapenade-Crusted Lamb Racks

1	lemon	1
½ cup	pitted black olives	125 mL
2 tbsp	drained capers	25 mL
1 tbsp	olive oil	15 mL
1	clove garlic, sliced	1
1 tsp	fresh thyme leaves (or ½ tsp/2 mL dried)	5 mL
2	frenched lamb racks, about 1 lb 6 oz (620 g) in total	2
	Fresh thyme sprigs	

Make Ahead

Tapenade can be refrigerated, covered, for up to 2 days.

> *In this recipe, lamb racks are treated to a coating of tapenade, a traditional French olive paste that's usually served atop slices of toasted baguette.*

SERVES 4

Preheat oven to 450°F (230°C) • Rimmed baking sheet or shallow roasting pan

1. Cut 4 thin slices from lemon; set aside. Squeeze 2 tsp (10 mL) juice from rest of lemon. In a mini chopper, food processor or blender, combine lemon juice, olives, capers, olive oil, garlic and thyme; process until finely minced and well combined.

2. Place lamb racks, meaty-side up, on baking sheet; spread olive mixture over top of each lamb rack. Roast in preheated oven, uncovered, for 20 minutes (rare), 25 minutes (medium-rare), or until a meat thermometer inserted into meaty part of lamb (not touching any bones) registers 140 or 150°F (60 or 65°C).

3. Remove lamb from oven; transfer to a warm serving platter. Let stand, loosely covered with foil, for 10 minutes. To serve, slice lamb between bones into individual chops. Serve garnished with reserved lemon slices and fresh thyme.

Tips

- Don't use canned olives for this recipe; the flavor won't be nearly as good. Look for kalamata or other black olives in the deli section of your supermarket. To remove pits, use an olive or cherry pitter or simply smash each olive with the flat side of a large knife, then carefully peel the flesh from the pit.

- Roast lamb in less than 30 minutes? It's possible if you serve lamb racks, those neat strips of chops that are available in the frozen meat section of your supermarket. They're perfect for entertaining — easily prepared and quick to cook. For a larger crowd, simply double the recipe.

- For best results, cook lamb so that it's still pink in the middle. If possible, buy frozen lamb racks that have been "frenched," or had the bones cleaned of excess fat.

Nutritional Analysis (Per Serving)
- Calories: 260
- Protein: 32.7g
- Fat: 13.7 g
- Carbohydrates: 1.4 g
- Fiber: 0.5 g
- Sodium: 284 mg
- Cholesterol: 84 mg

Easy Skillet Lamb Shanks

1 tbsp	canola or vegetable oil	15 mL
6	lamb shanks (about 3½ lbs/1.75 kg in total), thawed if frozen, patted dry	6
2	large onions, sliced	2
1½ cups	beef stock	375 mL
2 tbsp	tomato paste	25 mL
2 tbsp	mint jelly	25 mL
1 tbsp	Worcestershire sauce	15 mL
1 tbsp	balsamic vinegar	15 mL
1 tsp	dried rosemary	5 mL
¼ tsp	salt	1 mL
¼ tsp	black pepper	1 mL
	Chopped fresh parsley	

Make Ahead

Lamb shanks can be cooked, cooled then refrigerated for up to 2 days. Reheat, covered, in a 350°F (180°C) oven for 45 to 60 minutes or until piping hot and bubbly.

Here's the ultimate in comfort food: meaty, succulent lamb shanks in a flavorful sauce.

SERVES 6

Deep skillet with lid or Dutch oven large enough to hold lamb shanks in one layer

1. In the skillet, heat oil over medium-high heat. Cook lamb shanks in batches, turning often, for 3 to 5 minutes or until browned on all sides. Remove shanks to a plate as each batch browns.

2. Add onions to oil remaining in skillet; cook over medium heat, stirring, for 4 to 6 minutes or until onions are golden brown. Stir in stock, tomato paste, mint jelly, Worcestershire sauce, vinegar, rosemary, salt and pepper. Increase heat to high; bring to a boil, scraping up any brown bits from bottom of skillet.

3. Return lamb shanks to skillet, along with any juices that have accumulated on plate, arranging shanks in a single layer and spooning some of the sauce over each. Reduce heat to low; simmer, tightly covered, basting and turning lamb shanks occasionally, for 1½ hours or until lamb shanks are very tender.

4. With a slotted spoon, remove lamb shanks to a warm serving dish; keep warm. Bring contents of skillet to a boil over high heat; boil, stirring occasionally, for 5 minutes or until sauce is reduced in volume and slightly thickened. Spoon over lamb shanks; serve sprinkled with parsley.

Tip

- Lamb shanks from New Zealand are available in most large supermarkets; look for them in the frozen meat department. If your supermarket doesn't have them, they should — so kick up a fuss!

Nutritional Analysis (Per Serving)
- Calories: 417
- Protein: 33.8 g
- Fat: 24.1 g
- Carbohydrates: 15.3 g
- Fiber: 2.0 g
- Sodium: 455 mg
- Cholesterol: 114 mg

Lamb with Peppers

2 cups	dry white wine	500 mL
2 tbsp	crumbled thyme	25 mL
3 tbsp	olive oil	45 mL
3	cloves garlic, finely chopped	3
1 tbsp	grated lemon zest	15 mL
3 lbs	boneless shoulder of lamb, trimmed of excess fat, cut into 1-inch (2.5 cm) chunks	1.5 kg
1/4 cup	olive oil	50 mL
1	large onion, chopped	1
3 tbsp	chopped flat-leaf parsley	45 mL
2	dried hot chilies, crumbled (use rubber gloves when handling)	2
3	cloves garlic, finely chopped	3
1 cup	*passata* (puréed, sieved tomatoes) or canned ground or crushed tomatoes	250 mL
1 1/2 cups	chicken stock	375 mL
3/4 tsp	salt	4 mL
1/4 tsp	freshly ground black pepper	1 mL
2	red bell peppers, seeded and cut into strips	2
1	yellow bell pepper, seeded and cut into strips	1
1	green pepper, seeded and cut into strips	1

SERVES 4 TO 6

1. In a large bowl, whisk together the white wine, thyme, 3 tbsp (45 mL) of oil, garlic and lemon zest. Add chunks of lamb and toss to coat. Cover with plastic wrap and refrigerate 8 hours or overnight.

2. In a large heavy casserole or Dutch oven, heat olive oil over medium heat. With tongs, transfer lamb to a plate lined with a few thicknesses of paper towel. (Reserve marinade.) Pat lamb dry and brown in batches in casserole, transferring to a bowl when done. Add more oil as needed to finish browning lamb.

3. Add chopped onion, parsley, chilies and garlic; sauté for a few minutes or until onion is softened. (Do not allow garlic to brown.) Add reserved marinade and bring to a boil, scraping up any brown bits. Add cooked lamb, tomatoes, stock, salt and pepper; return to a boil. Reduce heat and simmer mixture for 1 1/2 to 2 hours or until meat is tender.

4. Just before the lamb is completely cooked, warm a little more olive oil in a nonstick skillet. Add strips of peppers and sauté for about 3 minutes or until slightly cooked but not softened. Add to casserole and allow lamb to simmer for another few minutes.

Tips

- You can prepare the dish a day ahead with good results. Be sure to allow enough time (overnight if possible) to marinate the lamb.

- If shoulder of lamb is not available, use boneless leg of lamb and reduce final cooking time by about 30 minutes.

Nutritional Analysis (Per Serving)
- Calories: 679
- Protein: 32.1 g
- Fat: 48.4 g
- Carbohydrates: 17.1
- Fiber: 4.1 g
- Sodium: 550 mg
- Cholesterol: 120 mg

Lamb Braised in Yogurt, Tomatoes and Onions

1 cup	plain nonfat yogurt, at room temperature	250 mL
1 tsp	cornstarch	5 mL
2 lbs	boneless lamb, cut into bite-size pieces	1 kg
1½ cups	minced onions	375 mL
1 cup	chopped tomatoes	250 mL
⅓ cup	cilantro, chopped	75 mL
1½ tbsp	minced peeled gingerroot	22 mL
1 tbsp	minced garlic	15 mL
1 tbsp	minced green chilies, preferably serranos	15 mL
1 tbsp	coriander powder	15 mL
1½ tsp	cumin powder	7 mL
¾ tsp	cayenne pepper	4 mL
¾ tsp	turmeric	4 mL
2 tsp	salt or to taste	10 mL
2 tbsp	vegetable oil	25 mL
1 tsp	garam masala	5 mL
3 tbsp	cilantro, chopped, for garnish	45 mL

SERVES 8

1. Stir yogurt to a creamy consistency. Add cornstarch and stir together.

2. In a saucepan, combine lamb, onions, tomatoes, ⅓ cup (75 mL) cilantro, ginger, garlic, chilies, coriander powder, cumin, cayenne pepper, turmeric, salt, yogurt mixture and oil. Mix well, preferably with your hands. Marinate for 30 minutes at room temperature.

3. Cover and bring to a boil over medium-high heat. Reduce heat to maintain a gentle boil. Cook, stirring occasionally, until meat is fork-tender, about 1 hour. If too much liquid remains after meat is cooked, uncover, increase heat and reduce until gravy is thickened.

4. Remove from heat and sprinkle with garam masala. Cover and let stand for 5 minutes for flavors to permeate. Stir mixture. Garnish with 3 tbsp (45 mL) cilantro.

Nutritional Analysis (Per Serving)
- Calories: 226
- Protein: 25.4 g
- Fat: 9.8 g
- Carbohydrates: 8.6 g
- Fiber: 1.3 g
- Sodium: 681 mg
- Cholesterol: 73 mg

Cardamom-Scented Lamb

2 tbsp	vegetable oil	25 mL
¼ cup	cardamom seeds, removed from pods and crushed	50 mL
2 lbs	boneless lamb, cut into bite-size pieces	1 kg
1 lb	fresh spinach, washed and chopped (about 4 cups/1 L)	500 g
1 cup	chopped tomatoes	250 mL
2 tsp	coriander powder	10 mL
1½ tsp	salt or to taste	7 mL
½ tsp	freshly ground black pepper	2 mL
1½ tbsp	all-purpose flour	22 mL

This is a classic Sindhi dish. Its soupy, lightly spiced consistency is considered very nourishing.

SERVES 8

1. In a large saucepan, heat oil over medium-high heat. Stir in cardamom seeds and sauté until fragrant, about 1 minute.

2. Add lamb and spinach. Reduce heat to medium. Cover and cook until spinach loses all moisture, 4 to 5 minutes. Uncover and brown lamb for 8 to 10 minutes.

3. Add tomatoes and cook until moisture is evaporated, 10 minutes longer.

4. Sprinkle with coriander, salt and pepper. Mix well and brown for 2 minutes longer.

5. Pour in 2 cups (500 mL) water. Bring to a boil over medium-high heat. Reduce heat to low. Cover and simmer until lamb is tender, 45 minutes to 1 hour.

6. Stir flour with 4 tbsp (60 mL) water to make a smooth paste. Gradually pour over lamb, stirring continuously. When thickened, remove from heat.

Tip

- The spinach is used for flavor and as a thickener. It will be barely visible.

Nutritional Analysis (Per Serving)
- Calories: 205
- Protein: 24.1 g
- Fat: 9.8 g
- Carbohydrates: 4.9 g
- Fiber: 1.9 g
- Sodium: 521 mg
- Cholesterol: 72 mg

Lamb Souvlaki

1 lb	lean boneless lamb	500 g
¼ cup	freshly squeezed lemon juice	50 mL
¼ cup	olive oil	50 mL
2 to 4	cloves garlic, minced	2 to 4
	Salt and freshly ground black pepper	

The usual meat for this Greek favorite is lamb, although I also like it with pork. Either way, chunks of meat are marinated in a lemon juice, oil and herb mixture before being skewered and grilled. Vegetable chunks, such as green pepper or onion, can be added.

SERVES 4
Wooden skewers

1. Trim lamb and discard fat. Cut into 1-inch (2.5 cm) chunks. Set aside.
2. In a bowl, whisk together lemon juice, oil, garlic, salt and pepper. Add meat and stir to coat. Marinate for up to 24 hours in the refrigerator or at room temperature for 30 minutes.
3. If using wooden skewers, soak them in cold water for at least 10 minutes to prevent charring during cooking.
4. Remove meat from marinade. Reserve marinade for basting (see tip, below).
5. Thread meat on four skewers. Broil under preheated broiler 6 inches (15 cm) from heat. Turn and baste halfway through with cooked marinade. Or grill on preheated broiler over medium-high heat for 5 minutes per side for rare and 7 minutes per side for medium.

Tips

- If you are basting with the lemon marinade in which the raw meat has been marinating, bring it to a boil for 5 minutes to kill any harmful bacteria left from marinating raw meat.
- Boneless pork loin or tenderloin may replace the lamb.

Nutritional Analysis (Per Serving)
- Calories: 155
- Protein: 23.0 g
- Fat: 6.1 g
- Carbohydrates: 0.5 g
- Fiber: 0 g
- Sodium: 72 mg
- Cholesterol: 72 mg

Grilled Keftas with Yogurt Mint Sauce

1 lb	ground lamb or beef (or a combination)	500 g
¼ cup	finely chopped parsley	50 mL
1 tsp	dried oregano	5 mL
¼ tsp	freshly ground black pepper	1 mL
1	onion	1
1 cup	yogurt	250 mL
2	cloves garlic, pressed	2
¼ cup	chopped fresh mint (or 1 tsp/5 mL dried)	50 mL
2 tbsp	lemon juice	25 mL
1 tsp	extra virgin olive oil	5 mL
	Salt and pepper to taste	
	Extra salt	

The people of the eastern Mediterranean have invented many savory recipes for minced meat, most of them venerable descendants of original recipes from Afghanistan and Persia.

SERVES 4

1. Put minced meat into a bowl and spread it out. Sprinkle with parsley, oregano and pepper. Grate the onion through the grater's largest holes directly onto the meat, so as to catch all the onion juices. Knead the meat and its condiments actively for at least 3 minutes, until everything is well distributed and the meat has paled in color. Cover and refrigerate for at least 30 minutes (or up to 2 hours).

2. In a small bowl, combine yogurt, garlic, mint, lemon juice, oil, salt and pepper. Mix to integrate well, cover and let rest up to 30 minutes, unrefrigerated. (This sauce can wait in the fridge for several hours; it must be allowed a 30-minute "warm up" to room temperature and a stir before being served.)

3. Form the chilled meat into patties just ½ inch (1 cm) thick and 2½ to 3 inches (6 to 8 cm) in diameter. You should get 8 of them. Grill, broil or fry them as you would hamburgers (3 minutes each side for medium-rare, 4 minutes for medium, etc.). Serve immediately with salt on the side and the yogurt sauce for spooning at table.

Tip

- It is important to mix the meat properly (at least 3 minutes of active kneading), and to let it stay in the fridge for 30 minutes, making it firmer and therefore easier to form into patties.

Nutritional Analysis (Per Serving)
- Calories: 388
- Protein: 22.9 g
- Fat: 27.9 g
- Carbohydrates: 10.3 g
- Fiber: 1.0 g
- Sodium: 700 mg
- Cholesterol: 85 mg

Greek Feta Burgers

½ cup	chopped onions	125 mL
1 cup	chopped mushrooms	250 mL
2 oz	feta cheese, crumbled	50 g
1 lb	lean ground lamb or beef	500 g
¼ cup	chopped chives	50 mL
3 tbsp	chopped oregano (or 1 tsp/5 mL dried)	45 mL
2 tbsp	barbecue sauce	25 mL
2 tbsp	bread crumbs	25 mL
2 tsp	crushed garlic	10 mL
1	egg	1

Make Ahead

Prepare burgers a day ahead or freeze for up to 3 weeks. Cook just before serving.

SERVES 4 TO 5

Start barbecue or preheat oven to 450°F (230°C)

1. In nonstick skillet sprayed with vegetable spray, sauté onions and mushrooms until softened and browned, approximately 4 minutes. Add cheese and set aside.

2. In a bowl, mix lamb, chives, oregano, barbecue sauce, bread crumbs, garlic and egg until well combined. Add onion mixture and form into 4 or 5 burgers.

3. Place burgers on greased grill and barbecue, or place on rack or baking sheet and bake for 10 to 15 minutes, or until no longer pink inside, turning once.

Tips

- Ground veal, chicken or pork can be substituted.
- These burgers can also be sautéed in a nonstick skillet sprayed with vegetable spray.

Nutritional Analysis (Per Serving)
- Calories: 260
- Protein: 23 g
- Fat: 15 g
- Carbohydrates: 6 g
- Fiber: 1 g
- Sodium: 200 mg
- Cholesterol: 150 mg

Vegetarian Meals

Stir-Fried Vegetables with Tofu

2 tbsp	vegetable oil	25 mL
1	large onion, cut into wedges	1
3	medium carrots, sliced diagonally	3
3	celery stalks, sliced diagonally	3
1/4	small cabbage, sliced thinly	1/4
1 cup	snow peas, trimmed	250 mL
1 cup	sliced mushrooms	250 mL
1 cup	firm tofu, cubed	250 mL
1/2 cup	vegetable broth or tomato juice	125 mL
1 tbsp	cornstarch	15 mL
1 tsp	finely chopped ginger root (or 1/2 tsp/2 mL ground ginger)	5 mL
1/4 tsp	black pepper	1 mL

Ginger root adds zest to this tasty dish.

SERVES 6

1. In a wok or large heavy skillet, heat oil over high heat. When oil is very hot, add onion, carrot and celery; cover and steam for 5 minutes. Add cabbage, snow peas, mushrooms and tofu; steam, covered, for 5 minutes longer.

2. Mix together chicken broth, cornstarch, ginger and pepper; pour over vegetable mixture. Stir-fry for 1 minute or until sauce thickens.

Tip

- Tofu, a source of protein and some calcium, is made from soy milk, in much the same way that cheese is made from animal milk. Tofu is best stored in water in a covered container in the refrigerator. Change the water daily to keep tofu fresh for 1 week.

Nutritional Analysis (Per Serving)
- Calories: 151
- Protein: 9 g
- Fat: 8 g
- Carbohydrates: 12 g
- Fiber: 4 g
- Sodium: 96 mg
- Cholesterol: 0 mg

Puffed Tofu and Vegetables

	Vegetable oil for frying	
1	medium soft tofu cake (about 10 oz/300 g)	1
1 tbsp	vegetable oil	15 mL
1	clove garlic, crushed	1
1/2 tsp	crushed red pepper flakes	2 mL
1	small carrot, sliced	1
1	medium onion, cut into wedges	1
1/2	small cucumber, peeled and sliced	1/2
1 1/2 cups	sliced bok choy	375 mL
8	snow peas	8
1/4 cup	water	50 mL
1 tbsp	dry sherry	15 mL

SAUCE

1/4 cup	water	50 mL
1 tsp	tamari or soy sauce	5 mL
1 tsp	cornstarch	5 mL
Pinch	granulated sugar	Pinch

Tofu is frequently used in Asian cuisine. In this recipe, it's fried first to give it a golden brown color, then stir-fried with garlic and vegetables.

SERVES 4

1. Heat 1/4 inch (5 mm) oil in a wok or skillet. Cut tofu into 4 slices; fry until light golden brown. Transfer to paper towel-lined plate to drain excess oil. Place in hot water for 5 minutes; drain again on paper towel-lined plate.

2. In same wok or skillet, heat 1 tbsp (15 mL) oil; stir-fry garlic and tofu pieces. Remove garlic. Sprinkle tofu with red pepper flakes; remove from wok and keep warm.

3. Stir-fry carrot and onion for 2 minutes. Add cucumber, bok choy and snow peas; stir-fry for 2 minutes. Add water and sherry; cover and cook for 1 to 2 minutes.

4. *Sauce:* Combine water, tamari sauce, cornstarch and sugar; add to wok and cook until thickened. Transfer to serving dish and top with tofu.

Tip

- Don't judge tofu by how it tastes on its own. Tofu is bland almost to the point of being tasteless. However, it has a remarkable affinity for other foods and spices and takes on their flavors when combined in cooking.

Nutritional Analysis (Per Serving)
- Calories: 159
- Protein: 8 g
- Fat: 11 g
- Carbohydrates: 9 g
- Fiber: 3 g
- Sodium: 76 mg
- Cholesterol: 0 mg

Tofu Vegetable Quiche

2 cups	coarsely chopped vegetables, such as bell pepper or zucchini	500 mL
½ cup	finely chopped onion	125 mL
2	eggs	2
1	package (19 oz/550 g) silken tofu, drained	1
	Salt and freshly ground black pepper	

SERVES 4

Preheat oven to 350°F (180°C) • 10-inch (25 cm) quiche pan or deep plate, lightly greased

1. In a large nonstick skillet, over medium-high heat, cook vegetables and onion for 10 minutes or until tender (add water if sticking occurs). Place in prepared pan.
2. In a food processor or blender, purée eggs and tofu until smooth and creamy. Add salt and pepper to taste. Pour tofu mixture over reserved vegetables.
3. Bake in preheated oven for 50 minutes or until knife inserted in the center comes out clean. Cut into 4 wedges and serve.

Nutritional Analysis (Per Serving)
- Calories: 170
- Protein: 14.9 g
- Fat: 9.1 g
- Carbohydrates: 9.6 g
- Fiber: 2.1 g
- Sodium: 43 mg
- Cholesterol: 107 mg

Spinach Crustless Quiche

1	package (10 oz/300 g) frozen chopped spinach, thawed	1
1	red bell pepper, finely chopped	1
4	eggs	4
1 cup	cottage cheese	250 mL
	Salt and freshly ground black pepper	

SERVES 4

Preheat oven to 325°F (160°C) • 10-inch (25 cm) pie plate, greased

1. Drain spinach by pressing out moisture with a slotted spoon. Spread half in prepared pie plate. Sprinkle with red pepper.
2. In a large bowl, beat eggs and cottage cheese. Add salt and pepper to taste. Stir in remaining spinach. Pour into pie plate.
3. Bake in preheated oven for 40 minutes or until knife inserted in center comes out clean. Remove from oven. Let stand for 5 minutes before cutting into 4 wedges.

A wonderful lunch or vegetarian dinner, this crustless quiche is an excellent source of calcium and a good source of iron.

Nutritional Analysis (Per Serving)
- Calories: 157
- Protein: 15.3 g
- Fat: 7.8 g
- Carbohydrates: 6.6 g
- Fiber: 2.4 g
- Sodium: 340 mg
- Cholesterol: 222 mg

Spinach Frittata

6	eggs, beaten	6
1 tbsp	vegetable oil	15 mL
½ cup	diced onion	125 mL
1 tsp	dried Italian seasoning	5 mL
½ tsp	salt	2 mL
	Freshly ground black pepper	
1	package (10 oz/300 g) frozen chopped spinach, thawed and squeezed dry, or 1 package (10 oz/300 g) spinach, washed, stems removed and chopped	1
¼ cup	grated Parmesan cheese	50 mL
2 tbsp	prepared sun-dried tomato pesto	25 mL

A frittata is an Italian omelet in which the ingredients are cooked with the eggs rather than being folded into them, French-style.

SERVES 2

Preheat oven to 425°F (220°C) • Ovenproof skillet with heatproof handle and lid (see tip, below)

1. In a bowl, lightly beat eggs. Set aside.
2. In an ovenproof skillet, heat oil over medium heat. Add onion and cook, stirring, until softened, about 3 minutes. Stir in Italian seasoning, salt, and black pepper to taste. Add spinach and stir well.
3. Reduce heat to low. Cover and cook until spinach is wilted, about 5 minutes. Slowly pour eggs over spinach. Increase heat to medium. Cover and cook until mixture begins to form a crust on the bottom, 2 to 3 minutes.
4. Sprinkle with Parmesan cheese and transfer pan to preheated oven. Bake, uncovered, until eggs are set but frittata is still soft in the center, about 3 minutes. Cut into wedges and serve topped with a dollop of pesto.

Tip

• If the handle of your skillet is not ovenproof, wrap it in aluminum foil.

Nutritional Analysis (Per Serving)
• Calories: 448   • Protein: 28.5 g   • Fat: 31.3 g
• Carbohydrates: 13.2 g   • Fiber: 4.6 g   • Sodium: 1186 mg
• Cholesterol: 652 mg

Zucchini Frittata

2 cups	sliced zucchini	500 mL
1	small onion, minced	1
1 tbsp	butter or margarine	15 mL
1½ tsp	olive oil	7 mL
6	eggs, beaten	6
1 tbsp	chopped fresh parsley	15 mL
1 tsp	ground fennel (see tip, at right)	5 mL
½ tsp	ground dried rosemary	2 mL
½ tsp	salt	2 mL
¼ tsp	freshly ground black pepper	1 mL
2 tbsp	shredded Cheddar cheese	25 mL

Make this Italian-style omelette when zucchini is in season or vary the recipe using other vegetables — mushrooms, red or green bell peppers and broccoli would also work well.

SERVES 6
Preheat broiler • Ovenproof skillet

1. In a large ovenproof skillet over medium-high heat, cook zucchini and onion in butter and olive oil for about 5 minutes or until tender.

2. In another bowl, combine eggs, parsley, fennel, rosemary, salt and pepper; pour over vegetables. Cook over medium heat, without stirring, until bottom of mixture has set but top is still soft. Sprinkle cheese on top. Place under preheated broiler for about 3 minutes or until cheese is melted and top is brown.

Tips

- If the handle of your skillet is not ovenproof, wrap it in aluminum foil.

- If you don't have ground fennel in your cupboard, use a generous teaspoon (5 mL) of fennel seeds in this recipe. Toast them over medium heat in a dry pan until they release their aroma, then crush finely before adding to the eggs. The flavor will be even better than if you had used the ground spice.

- This meatless light meal is best served with lower-fat accompaniments. A side salad or Italian Broiled Tomatoes (see recipe, page 340) and a fruit dessert will complete the meal.

Nutritional Analysis (Per Serving)
- Calories: 126
- Protein: 7 g
- Fat: 9 g
- Carbohydrates: 3 g
- Fiber: 1 g
- Sodium: 294 mg
- Cholesterol: 221 mg

Black Bean, Corn and Leek Frittata

1½ tsp	vegetable oil	7 mL
2 tsp	minced garlic	10 mL
¾ cup	chopped leeks	175 mL
½ cup	chopped red bell peppers	125 mL
½ cup	canned or frozen corn kernels, drained	125 mL
½ cup	canned black beans, rinsed and drained	125 mL
⅓ cup	chopped fresh coriander	75 mL
2	eggs	2
3	egg whites	3
⅓ cup	2% milk	75 mL
¼ tsp	salt	1 mL
¼ tsp	freshly ground black pepper	1 mL
2 tbsp	grated Parmesan cheese	25 mL

Make Ahead

Combine entire mixture early in the day. Cook just before serving.

SERVES 4 TO 6

1. In a nonstick saucepan sprayed with vegetable spray, heat oil over medium-high heat. Add garlic, leeks and red peppers; cook 4 minutes or until softened. Remove from heat; stir in corn, black beans and coriander.

2. In a bowl whisk together whole eggs, egg whites, milk, salt and pepper. Stir in cooled vegetable mixture.

3. Spray a 12-inch (30 cm) nonstick frying pan with vegetable spray. Heat over medium-low heat. Pour in frittata mixture. Cook 5 minutes, gently lifting sides of frittata to let uncooked egg mixture flow under frittata. Sprinkle with Parmesan. Cover and cook another 3 minutes or until frittata is set. Slip frittata onto serving platter.

4. Cut into wedges and serve immediately.

Tips

- Here's a great variation on the traditional omelet — but with less fat and cholesterol.
- Replace beans and vegetables with other varieties of your choice.
- Coriander can be replaced with dill, parsley or basil.

Nutritional Analysis (Per Serving)
- Calories: 101
- Protein: 7 g
- Fat: 4 g
- Carbohydrates: 10 g
- Fiber: 2 g
- Sodium: 253 mg
- Cholesterol: 74 mg

Cheese and Mushroom Oven Omelette

4	eggs, separated	4
2 tbsp	milk	25 mL
	Salt and freshly ground black pepper	
1 tbsp	butter	15 mL
3 cups	sliced assorted mushrooms	750 mL
3	green onions, chopped	3
¼ cup	light or herb cream cheese	50 mL
⅓ cup	shredded Cheddar cheese	75 mL
2 oz	smoked ham, cut into thin strips, or 3 slices bacon, cooked crisp and crumbled	60 g

Versatile mushrooms star in this terrific dish that's perfect to serve for brunch or a light supper.

SERVES 2 TO 3

Preheat oven to 350°F (180°C) • Well-buttered 9- or 10-inch (23 or 25 cm) pie plate, sprinkled with 1 tbsp (15 mL) fine dry bread crumbs

1. In a small bowl, beat egg yolks with milk; season with salt and pepper. In a bowl, using an electric mixer, beat egg whites until stiff peaks form. Slowly beat in yolk mixture on low speed until blended into egg whites. Pour into prepared pie plate. Bake for 15 minutes or until just set in the center.

2. Meanwhile, in a large nonstick skillet, melt butter over medium-high heat. Cook mushrooms and green onions, stirring, for 5 minutes or until tender and liquid is evaporated. Remove from heat; stir in cream cheese until smooth.

3. Spoon evenly over omelette; sprinkle with cheese and ham. Bake for 8 minutes more or until cheese is melted.

Tips

• Use a variety of white and exotic mushrooms such as shiitake, portobello and oyster.

• Herbed soft goat cheese can replace the cream cheese.

Nutritional Analysis (Per Serving)
• Calories: 446 • Protein: 31.5 g • Fat: 30.8 g
• Carbohydrates: 10.9 g • Fiber: 2.5 g • Sodium: 809 mg
• Cholesterol: 511 mg

Individual Salsa Fresca Omelettes

SALSA FRESCA

1 cup	diced seeded tomatoes	250 mL
1 cup	diced cucumber	250 mL
1/3 cup	chopped red onions	75 mL
1/4 cup	chopped fresh cilantro or parsley	50 mL
2 tbsp	lime juice	25 mL
	Salt and black pepper to taste	

OMELETTES

4	eggs	4
1 tbsp	water	15 mL
	Salt and black pepper to taste	
1 tsp	butter or vegetable oil	5 mL

This is an easy meal for older children or teens to prepare for themselves and the family. The ingredients can easily be doubled to serve 4.

SERVES 2

1. *Salsa Fresca:* In a bowl, combine tomatoes, cucumber, red onions, cilantro, lime juice, salt and pepper. Let stand for 10 minutes. Drain well.

2. *Omelettes:* In a bowl, beat together eggs, water, salt and pepper. In a small (8-inch/20 cm) nonstick skillet over medium-high heat, melt 1/2 tsp (2 mL) of the butter. Making 1 omelette at a time, pour half of the egg mixture into pan. As eggs begin to set at edges, use a spatula to gently push cooked portions to the center, tilting pan to allow uncooked egg to flow into empty spaces.

3. When eggs are almost set on the surface but still look moist, fill half the omelette with some of the Salsa Fresca. Slip spatula under unfilled side, fold over filling and slide omelette onto plate. Top with additional Salsa Fresca. Repeat with remaining butter, egg mixture and Salsa Fresca.

Variation

- Dress up your omelette with chopped ham, green onions and shredded cheese.

Tips

- If you don't have time to make the salsa, use a commercially prepared salsa instead. Use about 1/2 cup (125 mL) salsa per omelette.

- The Salsa Fresca is rich in vitamins and antioxidants, which work to help the body get rid of cell-damaging free radicals.

Nutritional Analysis (Per Serving)
- Calories: 185
- Protein: 13 g
- Fat: 12 g
- Carbohydrates: 6 g
- Fiber: 1 g
- Sodium: 161 mg
- Cholesterol: 431 mg

Best-Ever Scrambled Eggs

4	eggs	4
¼ cup	cream or milk	50 mL
¼ tsp	salt	1 mL
	Freshly ground black pepper	
1 tbsp	butter	15 mL

SERVES 2

1. In a bowl, whisk together eggs, cream, salt, and black pepper to taste. Set aside.
2. In a saucepan, melt butter over low heat. Add egg mixture and cook just until eggs begin to set, about 2 minutes. Begin to stir, scraping up set bits from the bottom, and stir constantly until the mixture is setting but still moist, about 3 minutes. Remove from heat and serve immediately.

Tips

- For a little bit of spice, add a pinch of cayenne pepper with the salt and pepper.
- Double or triple this recipe as required.

Variations

- *Scrambled Eggs with Smoked Salmon:* Accompany eggs with 2 slices smoked salmon per serving and garnish with 1 tbsp (15 mL) finely chopped green onion or chives.
- *Mexican-Style Scrambled Eggs:* Add 1 tsp (5 mL) finely chopped jalapeño pepper (alternatively, add hot pepper sauce to beaten eggs, to taste), ¼ cup (50 mL) cooked or thawed corn kernels and ¼ cup (50 mL) diced cured chorizo sausage to saucepan along with the butter. Stir in 2 tbsp (25 mL) salsa after the eggs are cooked. Be sure to use cured cooked chorizo sausage (which is hard) as the uncooked variety will not cook in this recipe. Serve with sliced tomatoes in season.
- *Scrambled Eggs with Pesto:* Just before serving, stir 1 to 2 tbsp (15 to 25 mL) basil pesto into the eggs.
- *Scrambled Eggs with Fine Herbs:* Sprinkle cooked eggs with any combination of the following mixture of fresh herbs, to taste: finely chopped parsley, chives, basil, tarragon, marjoram and thyme.

Nutritional Analysis (Per Serving)

- Calories: 304
- Protein: 13.2 g
- Fat: 26.8 g
- Carbohydrates: 2.1 g
- Fiber: 0 g
- Sodium: 486 mg
- Cholesterol: 482 mg

Cheese-Baked Eggs

¾ cup	shredded Swiss cheese	175 mL
6	eggs	6
⅔ cup	milk or light (5%) cream	150 mL
	Salt and freshly ground black pepper	
	Finely chopped fresh parsley or basil, optional	

This is the easiest and the very best way to cook eggs without watching them!

SERVES 4 TO 6

Preheat oven to 350°F (180°C)
8-inch (2 L) baking pan, greased

1. Sprinkle cheese over bottom of prepared pan. Break eggs over cheese.

2. Whisk together milk and salt and pepper to taste. Pour over eggs.

3. Bake in a preheated oven for 15 minutes or until eggs are just set. Sprinkle with chopped parsley, if using.

Tip

- Any of the hard cheeses that shred well may replace Swiss. Use Cheddar or Monterey Jack for Mexican-style, Asiago or Provolone when you want to go Italian or small dollops of chèvre for a French influence.

Nutritional Analysis (Per Serving)
- Calories: 172
- Protein: 13.2 g
- Fat: 11.7 g
- Carbohydrates: 2.8 g
- Fiber: 0 g
- Sodium: 134 mg
- Cholesterol: 275 mg

Indian Scrambled Eggs

8	eggs	8
1 tsp	salt or to taste	5 mL
¼ tsp	freshly ground black pepper	1 mL
3 tbsp	vegetable oil	45 mL
1 tsp	cumin seeds	5 mL
1 cup	chopped onion	250 mL
2 tsp	finely chopped green chilies, preferably serranos	10 mL
1 cup	chopped tomato	250 mL
½ tsp	cayenne pepper	2 mL
¼ tsp	turmeric	1 mL
¼ cup	cilantro, chopped	50 mL
	Tomato wedges and cilantro sprigs, for garnish	

SERVES 4 TO 6

1. In a bowl, gently whisk eggs, salt and pepper. Do not beat.
2. In a large skillet, heat oil over medium-high heat and add cumin seeds. Stir in onion and green chilies and sauté until golden, 3 to 4 minutes.
3. Add tomato and sauté, stirring continuously, for 1 minute. Stir in cayenne, turmeric and cilantro. Cook for 1 minute longer. Reduce heat to medium-low and slowly add egg mixture. Cook, stirring gently, until eggs are soft and creamy, 3 to 4 minutes. Do not overcook.
4. Serve garnished with tomato wedges and cilantro sprigs.

Nutritional Analysis (Per Serving)
- Calories: 215
- Protein: 10.8 g
- Fat: 16.3 g
- Carbohydrates: 6.2g
- Fiber: 1.1 g
- Sodium: 570 mg
- Cholesterol: 341 mg

Indian Omelet

6	eggs	6
1 tsp	salt	5 mL
¼ tsp	freshly ground black pepper	1 mL
2 to 3 tbsp	vegetable oil, divided	25 to 45 mL
¾ cup	chopped onion, divided	175 mL
¾ cup	chopped tomato, divided	175 mL
2 tsp	chopped green chilies, preferably serranos, divided	10 mL
¼ cup	cilantro, chopped, divided	50 mL

SERVES 4

1. In a bowl, beat together eggs, salt, pepper and 2 tbsp (25 mL) water until blended.
2. In a large nonstick skillet, heat 1 tbsp (15 mL) of the oil over medium heat. Pour one-quarter of the eggs into skillet. Scatter one-quarter each of the onion, tomato, chilies and cilantro evenly on top. Cook, without stirring, until edges can be lifted with spatula, about 2 minutes. Fold over to form semicircle. Cook for 30 seconds longer.
3. Transfer to platter and keep warm. Repeat to make remaining 3 omelets, adding enough oil between batches to prevent sticking.

Nutritional Analysis (Per Serving)
- Calories: 222
- Protein: 10.0 g
- Fat: 17.7 g
- Carbohydrates: 5.5 g
- Fiber: 0.9 g
- Sodium: 679 mg
- Cholesterol: 320 mg

Egg Curry

2 tbsp	vegetable oil	25 mL
2 cups	finely chopped onions (2 to 3)	500 mL
1 tbsp	minced peeled gingerroot	15 mL
1 tbsp	minced garlic	15 mL
1 tbsp	minced green chilies	15 mL
1½ tbsp	coriander powder	22 mL
¾ tsp	turmeric	4 mL
½ tsp	cayenne pepper	2 mL
½ tsp	cumin powder	2 mL
1	can (28 oz/796 mL) tomatoes, puréed with liquid	1
1½ tsp	salt or to taste	7 mL
12	hard-cooked eggs, peeled and halved	12
½ tsp	garam masala	2 mL
	Juice of 1 lime or lemon	
¼ cup	cilantro, chopped	50 mL

SERVES 8

1. In a large saucepan, heat oil over medium-high heat. Sauté onions until beginning to color, 4 to 6 minutes. Reduce heat to medium and sauté until browned, 8 to 10 minutes. Stir in ginger, garlic and chilies and cook for 2 minutes.

2. Stir in coriander, turmeric, cayenne pepper and cumin. Cook for 2 to 3 minutes, stirring continuously.

3. Pour in tomatoes and salt. Mix well. Reduce heat to low, cover and simmer, stirring occasionally, until gravy is thickened, 8 to 10 minutes.

4. Place halved eggs in single layer in pan. Spoon gravy on top of eggs and simmer, uncovered, for 5 minutes longer.

5. Remove from heat. Sprinkle with garam masala and lime juice. Cover and let stand for 5 minutes.

6. Garnish with cilantro to serve.

Nutritional Analysis (Per Serving)
- Calories: 183
- Protein: 10.8 g
- Fat: 11.3 g
- Carbohydrates: 10.5 g
- Fiber: 2.1 g
- Sodium: 542 mg
- Cholesterol: 320 mg

Whole Baked Masala Cauliflower

1	medium cauliflower (about 1½ lbs/750 g)	1
3 tbsp	vegetable oil, divided	45 mL
2 cups	finely chopped onions (2 to 3)	500 mL
2 tsp	minced green chilies, preferably serranos	10 mL
1 tsp	minced peeled gingerroot	5 mL
1 tsp	minced garlic	5 mL
1 cup	finely chopped tomato or 1 can (14 oz/398 mL) diced tomatoes, liquid reserved	250 mL
1½ tsp	coriander powder	7 mL
¾ tsp	cumin powder	4 mL
½ tsp	turmeric	2 mL
1½ tsp	salt or to taste	7 mL
2 tbsp	coarsely chopped garlic	25 mL

Make Ahead

Cauliflower and gravy can be prepared a day ahead and refrigerated. Let cauliflower come to room temperature and warm gravy before assembling for baking.

This elegant dish from north India is particularly wonderful in the cooler months, when cauliflower is at its best.

SERVES 8

Preheat oven to 350°F (180°C) • 13-by 9-inch (3 L) baking dish

1. Remove leaves from cauliflower. In a large saucepan filled with about 3 inches (7.5 cm) water, place cauliflower, stem side down. Cover and bring to a boil over medium-high heat. Reduce heat to medium and cook for 2 minutes. Remove from heat and let stand, covered, for 3 minutes longer to steam. Remove cauliflower carefully from water and place in a colander under cool running water to stop further cooking. Set aside to drain. Cauliflower should be tender-crisp.

2. Meanwhile, in a small saucepan, heat 2 tbsp (25 mL) of the oil over medium-high heat. Sauté onions until golden, about 10 minutes.

3. Stir in chilies, ginger and garlic. Reduce heat to medium and continue to cook until onions are browned, 5 to 8 minutes longer.

4. Mix in tomatoes or drained canned tomatoes, reserving liquid. Cook until tomatoes can be mashed with back of spoon, about 5 minutes.

5. Stir in coriander, cumin, turmeric and salt. Cook for 2 to 3 minutes. If using fresh tomatoes, add ¾ cup (175 mL) water; if canned, add reserved tomato liquid. Reduce heat to low. Cover and simmer for 10 minutes. Gravy should be thick.

6. Place cauliflower in baking dish. Spoon gravy in between florets, taking care cauliflower does not break apart. Cover completely with remaining gravy. Bake in preheated oven until cauliflower is tender, about 20 minutes.

7. In a small saucepan, heat remaining oil over medium heat. Sauté garlic until golden, about 2 minutes. Pour on top of cauliflower just before serving.

8. Serve either in baking dish or transfer carefully, without breaking, to a serving platter.

Nutritional Analysis (Per Serving)
- Calories: 88
- Protein: 2.2 g
- Fat: 5.4 g
- Carbohydrates: 9.5 g
- Fiber: 2.8 g
- Sodium: 461 mg
- Cholesterol: 0 mg

Side Dishes

Roasted Asparagus

1 lb	asparagus	500 g
1	clove garlic, minced	1
1 tbsp	olive oil	15 mL
1 tbsp	balsamic vinegar	15 mL
	Salt and freshly ground black pepper	

SERVES 6

heat oven to 450°F (230°C) • Baking dish, greased

1. Break asparagus stalks at natural breaking point. Toss with garlic, oil, vinegar, salt and pepper. Place in prepared baking dish.
2. Roast in preheated oven, uncovered, turning once, for 20 minutes or until asparagus is tender.

Tip

- Choose asparagus carefully, selecting firm, vivid green stalks with tightly closed tips and cook them as soon as possible.

Nutritional Analysis (Per Serving)
- Calories: 31
- Protein: 1.1 g
- Fat: 2.3g
- Carbohydrates: 2.3 g
- Fiber: 1.0 g
- Sodium: 1 mg
- Cholesterol: 0 mg

Roasted Asparagus with Coriander Butter

1½ lbs	slender asparagus	750 g
2 tbsp	butter	25 mL
1 tsp	ground coriander	5 mL
	Fresh chervil sprigs or chopped fresh parsley	

Make Ahead

Asparagus can be refrigerated (washed, trimmed, wrapped in a damp tea towel and sealed in a plastic bag) for up to 24 hours.

Roasting the asparagus here concentrates its flavor, while the aromatic butter provides a spicy yet subtle accent.

SERVES 6

Preheat oven to 400°F (200°C)
Baking sheet

1. Trim woody ends of asparagus by breaking them off where they snap naturally. Spread asparagus out more or less in a single layer on baking sheet.
2. In a small saucepan, heat butter and coriander over medium-high heat until butter melts and starts to bubble. Drizzle evenly over asparagus. Bake in preheated oven, turning with a spatula halfway through cooking time, for 15 to 18 minutes or until asparagus is tender. Transfer to a warm serving platter; sprinkle with chervil. Serve at once.

Nutritional Analysis (Per Serving)
- Calories: 50
- Protein: 1.6 g
- Fat: 4.0 g
- Carbohydrates: 3.2 g
- Fiber: 1.5 g
- Sodium: 41 mg
- Cholesterol: 10 mg

Stir-Fried Asparagus with Garlic, Shallots and Toasted Chili Oil

2 tbsp	Toasted Chili Oil (see recipe, below right)	25 mL
4	medium shallots, thinly sliced	4
1 tbsp	minced garlic	15 mL
1 lb	asparagus, trimmed and cut into 2-inch (5 cm) lengths	500 g
3 tbsp	water or chicken stock	45 mL
	Salt and pepper to taste	

In season, this combination of asparagus, garlic and chili makes a wonderful spring treat. The water or stock steams the asparagus to a tender crispness. If you like spicy food, add dried chili flakes along with the shallots.

SERVES 4

1. Heat a nonstick wok or skillet over high heat for 30 seconds. Add chili oil, shallots and garlic; sauté 2 minutes or until the shallots are soft and beginning to color. Add asparagus and continue to cook until it begins to soften and color, about 2 to 3 minutes.

2. Add water or stock; continue to cook until all the moisture has evaporated. Season with salt and pepper and toss to mix well. Transfer to a warm platter and serve immediately.

Nutritional Analysis (Per Serving)
- Calories: 98
- Protein: 2.6 g
- Fat: 6.9 g
- Carbohydrates: 8.4 g
- Fiber: 1.4 g
- Sodium: 31 mg
- Cholesterol: 0 mg

Toasted Chili Oil

In a heavy skillet or small saucepan, heat 2 tbsp (25 mL) chili flakes until toasted and almost smoking. Carefully pour in 2 cups (500 mL) vegetable oil and heat for 1 minute. Remove from heat and allow the flavors to infuse for at least 20 minutes. Transfer to a sterilized glass jar or bottle and refrigerate for up to 2 months. Makes about 2 cups (500 mL).

Asparagus with Lemon and Garlic

½ lb	asparagus, trimmed	250 g
2 tsp	vegetable oil	10 mL
1 tsp	crushed garlic	5 mL
¼ cup	diced sweet red pepper	50 mL
1	green onion, sliced	1
2 tbsp	white wine	25 mL
4 tsp	lemon juice	20 mL
2 tbsp	chicken stock	25 mL
	Pepper	

Make Ahead

Make this early in day if it is to be served cold, to allow the asparagus a chance to marinate.

SERVES 4

1. Steam or boil asparagus just until tender-crisp. Do not overcook. Drain and set aside.
2. In large nonstick skillet, heat oil; sauté garlic and red pepper until softened.
3. Reduce heat and add green onion, wine, lemon juice, chicken stock, pepper to taste and asparagus. Cook for 1 minute. Place asparagus mixture in serving dish.

Nutritional Analysis (Per Serving)
- Calories: 46
- Carbohydrates: 4 g
- Cholesterol: 0 mg
- Protein: 2 g
- Fiber: 1 g
- Fat: 2 g
- Sodium: 29 mg

Asparagus with Parmesan and Toasted Almonds

1½ lbs	asparagus	750 g
¼ cup	sliced blanched almonds	50 mL
2 tbsp	margarine or butter	25 mL
2	cloves garlic, finely chopped	2
¼ cup	freshly grated Parmesan cheese	50 mL
	Salt and freshly ground black pepper	

SERVES 6

1. Snap off asparagus ends; cut spears on the diagonal into 2-inch (5 cm) lengths. In a large nonstick skillet, bring ½ cup (125 mL) water to a boil; cook asparagus for 2 minutes (start timing when water returns to a boil) or until just tender-crisp. Run under cold water to chill; drain and reserve.
2. Dry the skillet and place over medium heat. Add almonds and toast, stirring often, for 2 to 3 minutes or until golden. Remove and reserve.
3. Increase heat to medium-high. Add butter to skillet; cook asparagus and garlic, stirring, for 4 minutes or until asparagus is just tender.
4. Sprinkle with Parmesan; season with salt and pepper. Transfer to serving bowl; top with almonds.

Nutritional Analysis (Per Serving)
- Calories: 107
- Carbohydrates: 7 g
- Cholesterol: 14 mg
- Protein: 5 g
- Fiber: 2 g
- Fat: 8 g
- Sodium: 113 mg

Asparagus with Caesar Dressing

1 lb	asparagus, trimmed	500 g
2 tsp	crushed garlic	10 mL
1 tbsp	Dijon mustard	15 mL
1 tbsp	lemon juice	15 mL
2 tbsp	olive oil	25 mL
1 tbsp	grated Parmesan cheese	15 mL

Make Ahead

Make dressing at any time. Just before serving, cook asparagus.

SERVES 4

1. Steam or microwave asparagus until just tender. Drain and place on serving dish.
2. In small bowl, mix garlic, mustard, lemon juice and oil until combined; pour over asparagus. Sprinkle with cheese.

Nutritional Analysis (Per Serving)
- Calories: 101
- Protein: 4 g
- Fat: 7 g
- Carbohydrates: 6 g
- Fiber: 2 g
- Sodium: 76 mg
- Cholesterol: 1 mg

Individual Asparagus and Goat Cheese Flan

1 lb	asparagus (about 24 stems), bottom 1½ inches (4 cm) trimmed	500 g
4 oz	softened goat cheese	125 g
2	eggs, beaten	2
2	green onions, chopped into ¼-inch (5 mm) pieces	2
1 tbsp	lemon juice	15 ml
¼ tsp	salt	1 mL
¼ tsp	freshly ground black pepper	1 mL
1 tsp	olive oil	5 mL
2 tbsp	pine nuts	25 mL

Asparagus is the most elegant of vegetables and, happily for us, it is available year-round. In the south of France, where they only eat it in season (spring), they make a delicious omelette with the thinnest stalks. Here's a take on their omelettes that works with any size asparagus. It ends up saucy and tart — a perfect appetizer for a dinner party.

SERVES 4

Four ½-cup (125 mL) ramekins • Baking sheet • Preheat oven to 400°F (200°C)

1. Bring a large pot of water to a boil. Add trimmed asparagus, return to a boil and cook for 3 minutes. Drain. Rinse under cold water; drain. Cut into 1½-inch (4 cm) pieces; set aside.
2. In a bowl mix goat cheese with eggs until combined but still lumpy. Stir in asparagus, green onions, lemon juice, salt and pepper. Brush bottom of ramekins with oil. Divide asparagus mixture between ramekins; sprinkle evenly with pine nuts.
3. Transfer ramekins to baking sheet. Bake 15 to 18 minutes or until set around edges but still slightly runny just at the center. Do not unmold. Serve immediately in ramekins.

Nutritional Analysis (Per Serving)
- Calories: 194
- Protein: 12.0 g
- Fat: 14.4 g
- Carbohydrates: 5.6 g
- Fiber: 1.9 g
- Sodium: 326 mg
- Cholesterol: 129 mg

Braised Shanghai Bok Choy with Oyster Mushrooms and Garlic Sauce

1 tbsp	cornstarch	15 mL
1 tsp	sesame oil	5 mL
1 tbsp	oyster sauce	15 mL
1 tbsp	chicken stock	15 mL
1 tbsp	vegetable oil	15 mL
2 cups	oyster mushrooms, torn into bite-sized pieces	500 mL
1 tsp	minced garlic	5 mL
1 tsp	minced ginger root	5 mL
4	medium Shanghai bok choy or regular bok choy, cut lengthwise into quarters	4
1/3 cup	chicken stock	75 mL
	Salt and pepper to taste	

Prized for its tender texture, Shanghai bok choy is a close cousin of regular bok choy, with spoon-shaped leaves and thinner stalks on the same bulbous base. The main difference is its color — a paler green than regular bok choy. It's sold in bundles of 4 to 5 heads and is at its best when no more than 5 or 6 inches (12.5 or 15 cm) tall.

SERVES 4

1. In a small bowl, combine ingredients for sauce; mix well and set aside.

2. In a wok or deep skillet, heat oil over medium-high heat for about 30 seconds. Add mushrooms, garlic and ginger root; sauté until mushrooms are golden, about 1 to 2 minutes. Add bok choy; toss and cook briefly. Add chicken stock; bring to boil. Turn heat to low; cover and allow to braise for 2 to 3 minutes or until vegetables are tender.

3. Stir in sauce ingredients and cook until slightly thickened. Season to taste with salt and pepper. Transfer to a platter and serve immediately.

Nutritional Analysis (Per Serving)
- Calories: 92
- Protein: 4.8 g
- Fat: 5.1 g
- Carbohydrates: 9.4 g
- Fiber: 2.7 g
- Sodium: 261 mg
- Cholesterol: 0 mg

Pan-Fried Baby Bok Choy with Sesame Oil and Ginger

1 lb	baby bok choy	500 g
1 tbsp	vegetable oil	15 mL
1 tbsp	minced ginger root	15 mL
3 tbsp	water or chicken stock	45 mL
1 tsp	sesame oil	5 mL
	Salt and pepper to taste	

Bok choy, a juicy and refreshing Chinese white cabbage, is also packed with vitamins and nutrients. For additional flavor, cook this dish in the same pan in which your meat or fish has been cooked.

SERVES 4

1. With a heavy knife, cut bok choy across the bottom to separate stems. Cut each stem in half lengthwise and wash thoroughly.

2. In a nonstick pan, heat oil for 30 seconds. Add ginger root and sauté until fragrant, about 1 minute. Add bok choy and cook until it begins to color and the leaves turn bright green, about 2 to 3 minutes. Add water or stock and sesame oil; cook until all the liquid has evaporated.

3. Transfer to a platter, season with salt and pepper and serve immediately.

Nutritional Analysis (Per Serving)
- Calories: 56
- Protein: 1.8 g
- Fat: 4.7 g
- Carbohydrates: 2.8 g
- Fiber: 1.1 g
- Sodium: 101 mg
- Cholesterol: 0 mg

Orange Broccoli

2 tbsp	orange juice	25 mL
2 tsp	lemon juice	10 mL
1 tbsp	vegetable oil	15 mL
1½ tsp	granulated sugar	7 mL
½ tsp	crushed dried basil	2 mL
¼ tsp	coarsely ground black pepper	1 mL
¼ tsp	Dijon mustard	1 mL
1	bunch broccoli florets, blanched	1
2 tbsp	unsalted shelled sunflower seeds, toasted	25 mL

Citrus juice, mustard, herbs and spices give broccoli a new taste.

SERVES 6

1. Whisk first 7 ingredients until blended.

2. Drizzle mixture over broccoli. Cover and heat until warm. Sprinkle with sunflower seeds.

Tips

- If you don't have sunflower seeds on hand, substitute toasted nuts such as pine nuts, walnuts or almonds.

- The snappy combination of broccoli and fruit juices is rich in folic acid as well as vitamin C.

Nutritional Analysis (Per Serving)
- Calories: 57
- Protein: 2 g
- Fat: 4 g
- Carbohydrates: 4 g
- Fiber: 2 g
- Sodium: 25 mg
- Cholesterol: 0 mg

Orange Broccoli with Red Pepper

1/3 cup	orange juice	75 mL
1/2 tsp	cornstarch	2 mL
1 tbsp	olive oil	15 mL
4 cups	small broccoli florets and stalks, cut into 1 1/2- by 1/2-inch (4 by 1 cm) lengths	1 L
1	sweet red pepper, cut into 2- by 1/2-inch (5 by 1 cm) strips	1
1	clove garlic, minced	1
1 tsp	grated orange rind	5 mL
1/4 tsp	salt	1 mL
1/4 tsp	pepper	1 mL

SERVES 4

1. In a glass measuring cup, stir together orange juice and cornstarch until smooth; reserve.
2. Heat oil in a large nonstick skillet over high heat. Add broccoli, red pepper and garlic; cook, stirring, for 2 minutes.
3. Add orange juice mixture; cover and cook 1 to 2 minutes or until vegetables are tender-crisp. Sprinkle with orange rind; season with salt and pepper. Serve immediately.

Nutritional Analysis (Per Serving)
- Calories: 78
- Protein: 3 g
- Fat: 4 g
- Carbohydrates: 10 g
- Fiber: 3 g
- Sodium: 161 mg
- Cholesterol: 0 mg

Broccoli and peppers are a winning combination, providing excellent sources of vitamins A and C and folic acid.

Broccoli with Feta Cheese and Red Pepper

4 cups	chopped broccoli florets and 2-inch (5 cm) stalk pieces	1 L
2 tsp	vegetable oil	10 mL
2 tsp	crushed garlic	10 mL
3/4 cup	diced onion	175 mL
1/3 cup	sliced black olives	75 mL
1 cup	diced tomatoes	250 mL
2 tbsp	chicken stock	25 mL
1 tsp	dried oregano (or 2 tbsp/25 mL chopped fresh)	5 mL
1 1/2 oz	feta cheese, crumbled	40 g

SERVES 4

1. Steam or microwave broccoli just until barely tender. Drain and set aside.
2. In nonstick skillet, heat oil; sauté garlic and onion just until softened, approximately 3 minutes. Add broccoli, olives, tomatoes, chicken stock and oregano; cook for 3 minutes. Place in serving dish. Sprinkle with feta cheese.

Tip
- For a change, substitute asparagus for the broccoli, and goat cheese for the feta.

Nutritional Analysis (Per Serving)
- Calories: 111
- Protein: 5 g
- Fat: 6 g
- Carbohydrates: 11 g
- Fiber: 4 g
- Sodium: 270 mg
- Cholesterol: 9 mg

"Little" Broccoli Gratin

1	bunch broccoli	1
2 tbsp	olive oil	25 mL
1/2 tsp	salt	2 mL
1/4 tsp	freshly ground black pepper	1 mL
1 tbsp	minced fresh chili pepper or 1/4 tsp (1 mL) hot pepper flakes	15 mL
1 cup	thickly sliced red onion	250 mL
8 oz	button mushrooms, trimmed and halved	250 g
1 tbsp	raisins	15 mL
1 tsp	white wine vinegar	5 mL
8 oz	bocconcini cheese, cut into 1/4-inch (0.5 cm) rounds	250 g
1/2 cup	walnut pieces	125 mL

> *The "little" part of this recipe refers to a fine-chopping technique that enhances the taste and texture of broccoli.*

SERVES 4 TO 6
Preheat broiler • 10-inch (25 cm) pie plate or baking dish

1. Separate florets of broccoli from the large stalks. (Reserve stalks for another use.) Chop florets into tiny match-head-sized bits. (You should get just over 2 cups/500 mL.) Bring a pot of salted water to a boil. Add broccoli; bring back to boil and cook for about 2 minutes. Drain through a fine wire strainer. Rinse under cold water; drain well and set aside.

2. In a large frying pan, heat oil, salt and pepper over high heat for 1 minute. Add chilies, onions and mushrooms; stir-fry for 3 minutes or until vegetables start to brown. Add raisins and vinegar; cook, stirring, for 30 seconds. Stir in broccoli; remove from heat.

3. Transfer contents of frying pan to a pie plate, spreading evenly to make a flat layer about 1/2 inch (1 cm) deep. Place rounds of bocconcini on top so that most of the surface is covered. Sprinkle the walnut pieces over the uncovered spots.

4. Broil 3 to 4 minutes until cheese is melted and walnuts have turned dark brown. Serve immediately in its baking dish to be portioned at table.

Tip

- This salad can be served immediately or it can wait up to 2 hours, covered and unrefrigerated.

Variation

- If you wish, replace the bocconcini with the same weight of mozzarella nuggets — cut 1/4 inch (0.5 cm) thick — for a slightly saltier result.

Nutritional Analysis (Per Serving)
- Calories: 301
- Protein: 17.5 g
- Fat: 21.0 g
- Carbohydrates: 14.7 g
- Fiber: 4.8 g
- Sodium: 472 mg
- Cholesterol: 26 mg

Jalapeño Broccoli

1 tsp	salt	5 mL
1	head broccoli, trimmed and separated into spears	1
1 tbsp	balsamic vinegar	15 mL
2 to 3 tbsp	olive oil	25 to 45 mL
2	fresh jalapeño peppers, thinly sliced (with or without seeds, depending on desired hotness)	2
¼ cup	toasted pine nuts	50 mL
	Few sprigs fresh coriander or parsley, chopped	

The stubby, lush green chilies that take their name from the Mexican city of Jalapa have become as common in our markets as they are in their home country.

SERVES 4 TO 5

1. Bring a pot of water to the boil and add salt. Add broccoli spears and boil over high heat for 3 to 5 minutes (depending on desired tenderness). Drain and transfer broccoli to bowl of ice cold water for 30 seconds. Drain and lay out the cooked spears decoratively on a presentation plate. Drizzle evenly with balsamic vinegar.

2. In a small frying pan, heat olive oil over medium heat for 30 seconds. Add sliced jalapeño peppers (with seeds, if using) and stir-fry for 2 to 3 minutes until softened. Take peppers with all the oil from the pan, and distribute evenly over broccoli. Garnish with pine nuts and herbs.

Nutritional Analysis (Per Serving)
- Calories: 190
- Protein: 7.3 g
- Fat: 15.1 g
- Carbohydrates: 10.8 g
- Fiber: 5.7 g
- Sodium: 629 mg
- Cholesterol: 0 mg

Herb-Glazed Brussels Sprouts

¼ cup	coarsely chopped fresh mint	50 mL
¼ cup	coarsely chopped fresh basil	50 mL
¼ cup	olive oil	50 mL
2 tbsp	fresh lemon juice	25 mL
1 tbsp	Dijon mustard	15 mL
¼ tsp	salt	1 mL
¼ tsp	black pepper	1 mL
2 lbs	small Brussels sprouts, stems and outer leaves trimmed (if necessary) and a slit cut in stem end of each	1 kg
	Fresh mint or basil leaves and/or grated lemon zest	

SERVES 6

1. In a mini chopper or in a bowl and using a whisk, combine mint, basil, olive oil, lemon juice, mustard, salt and pepper; process or whisk until well combined.

2. In a saucepan of boiling salted water, cook Brussels sprouts for 3 to 5 minutes or until just tender but still a little crisp. (Check by cutting one in half.) Drain well; return to saucepan.

3. Spoon dressing over Brussels sprouts; stir gently to combine. Spoon into a warm serving dish; sprinkle with mint or basil leaves and/or lemon zest. Serve at once.

Nutritional Analysis (Per Serving)
- Calories: 147
- Protein: 5.1 g
- Fat: 9.5 g
- Carbohydrates: 13.9 g
- Fiber: 5.6 g
- Sodium: 162 mg
- Cholesterol: 0 mg

Brussels Sprouts with Parmesan Cheese Sauce

1½ lbs	Brussels sprouts, ends trimmed and cut in half lengthwise	750 g
2 tbsp	butter	25 mL
2 tbsp	all-purpose flour	25 mL
1⅓ cups	milk	325 mL
¼ cup	freshly grated Parmesan cheese	50 mL
1 tsp	grated lemon zest	5 mL
	Salt	
	Freshly grated nutmeg	

Make Ahead

Prepare recipe as directed, cover and refrigerate. To reheat, microwave, covered, on High for 4 to 7 minutes, stirring once, until piping hot.

Brussels sprouts cook up perfectly in the microwave. This do-ahead recipe helps cut down on last-minute dinner preparation and is ideal for holiday meals.

SERVES 6

8-cup (2 L) casserole dish with lid • 8-cup (2 L) glass measure

1. Place Brussels sprouts in casserole dish and add ⅓ cup (75 mL) water. Microwave, covered, on High for 5 to 8 minutes, stirring once, until just tender and bright green. Let stand, covered, while making sauce.

2. In glass measure, melt butter, uncovered, on High for 30 to 45 seconds or until bubbling. Blend in flour. Whisk in milk. Microwave, uncovered, on High for 3 to 4 minutes, whisking once, until sauce comes to a full rolling boil and thickens.

3. Add Parmesan cheese and lemon zest. Season with salt and nutmeg to taste. Drain Brussels sprouts well and pour sauce over top.

Variation

- Substitute cauliflower for the Brussels sprouts. Separate 1 cauliflower into florets (about 6 cups/1.5 L). Place in casserole dish with ⅓ cup (75 mL) water. Microwave, covered, on High for 6 to 9 minutes, stirring once, until just tender. Prepare sauce as directed. Drain cauliflower and toss with sauce.

Tips

- Milk-based sauces tend to boil over in the microwave, so prepare them in a large glass measure.

- To cook whole Brussels sprouts in the microwave, trim ends and cut a small X on the bottom of each sprout. Add ⅓ cup (75 mL) water. Microwave, covered, on High for 6 to 9 minutes, stirring once, until just tender and bright green.

- Serve this lemon-accented cream sauce with other cooked vegetables, such as cauliflower or broccoli.

Nutritional Analysis (Per Serving)
- Calories: 132
- Protein: 6.4 g
- Fat: 7.1 g
- Carbohydrates: 12.5 g
- Fiber: 3.4 g
- Sodium: 198 mg
- Cholesterol: 51 mg

Braised Cabbage

3	slices back bacon, diced	3
1	small onion, sliced	1
1/4 cup	finely diced carrot	50 mL
4 cups	grated cabbage	1 L
1	bay leaf	1
Pinch	dried thyme	Pinch
1/4 cup	chicken broth	50 mL
	Freshly ground black pepper	

Most people imagine coleslaw and cabbage rolls when thinking of cabbage, but cabbage is also a particularly delicious side dish, as long as it is not overcooked. Its taste is complemented by many seasonings, including the back bacon in this recipe.

SERVES 4

1. In a large skillet over low heat, cook bacon and onion for about 5 minutes, stirring frequently.

2. Add carrot; cover and cook for 1 minute. Stir in cabbage, bay leaf, thyme and chicken broth. Cook, covered, over low heat for about 10 minutes or until tender-crisp, stirring occasionally. Season with pepper to taste. Remove bay leaf before serving.

Tips

- When cooking cabbage, discard the tough outer leaves and remove the hard core at the base. And don't overcook; cabbage should be tender but firm.

- This recipe uses back bacon as a lower-fat alternative to side bacon. It adds a delicious flavor to cabbage, which is low in calories and high in vitamin C.

Nutritional Analysis (Per Serving)
- Calories: 71
- Protein: 3 g
- Fat: 3 g
- Carbohydrates: 9 g
- Fiber: 3 g
- Sodium: 177 mg
- Cholesterol: 11 mg

Braised Red Cabbage

1	small red cabbage (about 1½ lb/750 g)	1
⅓ cup	red wine vinegar	75 mL
1 tbsp	granulated sugar	15 mL
1 tsp	salt	5 mL
1	slice bacon, chopped	1
1 tbsp	olive oil	15 mL
⅓ cup	chopped onion	75 mL
2	Granny Smith apples, peeled, cored and cut into eighths	2
1	whole clove	1
1	small onion	1
1	bay leaf	1
½ cup	boiling water	125 mL
2 tbsp	dry red wine (optional)	25 mL

SERVES 10

Preheat oven to 325°F (160°C) • 8-cup (2 L) baking dish

1. Remove outer leaves of cabbage and discard. Cut cabbage into quarters; trim off excess white heart. Shred about ⅛ inch (3 mm) thick to make 6 cups (1.5 L). Place in bowl; toss with vinegar, sugar and salt.

2. In a large skillet, brown bacon; remove bacon, reserving drippings in pan. Set bacon aside. Add chopped onion; cook, stirring, for 2 minutes. Add apples; cook for 5 minutes.

3. Push clove into onion; add to skillet along with cabbage mixture, bay leaf, boiling water and bacon. Mix well. Pour into 8-cup (2 L) baking dish. Cover and bake in preheated oven for 2 hours, stirring occasionally. (If it becomes dry, add more water.) Remove onion and bay leaf. Stir in wine, if desired.

Tips

- The apple and the red wine vinegar in this recipe add acid, which helps the cabbage keep its rich red color.

- Vegetables, fruit and herbs create mouthwatering aromas and tastes while they gently bake together. Serve this delicious casserole with Turkey Hazelnut Roll (see recipe, page 240) for a great fall meal.

- Long, slow cooking develops the flavors in this fabulous fall or winter dish. It will reheat well and may be stored for 1 week in the refrigerator.

Nutritional Analysis (Per Serving)
- Calories: 44
- Protein: 1 g
- Fat: 1 g
- Carbohydrates: 8 g
- Fiber: 2 g
- Sodium: 40 mg
- Cholesterol: 0 mg

Stir-Fried Red Cabbage

5¹/₂ cups	thinly shredded red cabbage	1.4 L
1 tbsp	cider vinegar	15 mL
1 tsp	salt	5 mL
2 tbsp	vegetable oil	25 mL
¹/₄ tsp	salt	1 mL
¹/₄ tsp	freshly ground black pepper	1 mL
1 tsp	whole fennel seeds	5 mL
1	small green bell pepper, cut into thin strips	1
1 tbsp	cider vinegar	15 mL
	Few sprigs fresh dill, chopped	

Slightly tart, startlingly red-purple cabbage adds welcome sparkle and flavor (not to mention nutrition) to any vegetarian table. The fennel seeds and fresh dill add character without drawing away any of the assertiveness of the humble cabbage.

SERVES 4 TO 6

1. In a saucepan, cover cabbage with cold water; add vinegar and salt. Place on high heat for 7 to 8 minutes until just coming to a boil. Drain cabbage, refresh under cold water and drain again.

2. In a large frying pan, heat oil over high heat for 30 seconds. Add salt, pepper and fennel seeds and stir-fry for 1 minute, or until the seeds start to pop. Add green pepper strips and stir-fry for 1 minute until pepper wilts.

3. Add drained cabbage and stir-fry for 3 to 4 minutes until all the cabbage is shiny and warm through.

4. Remove from heat. Add cider vinegar and half of the chopped dill. Toss well to mix. Transfer to a serving dish and garnish with the remaining dill.

Tip

- This dish can be served warm, or it can wait for up to 2 hours, covered and unrefrigerated, to be served at room temperature.

Nutritional Analysis (Per Serving)
- Calories: 79
- Protein: 1.4 g
- Fat: 5.7 g
- Carbohydrates: 7.2 g
- Fiber: 2.3 g;
- Sodium: 591 mg
- Cholesterol: 0 mg

Preeti's Cabbage with Peanuts

2 tbsp	vegetable oil	25 mL
1½ tsp	mustard seeds	7 mL
25 to 30	fresh curry leaves (optional)	25 to 30
3 to 4	green chilies, preferably serranos, cut into ¾-inch (2 cm) pieces	3 to 4
8 cups	finely sliced cabbage	2 L
¾ cup	finely sliced red or green bell pepper	175 mL
¾ tsp	salt or to taste	4 mL
⅓ cup	skinned raw peanuts, dry roasted in skillet	75 mL

With its jewel-like colors, this dish is as much a treat for the eyes as it is for the palate.

SERVES 8

Large wok or skillet with tight-fitting lid

1. In a large wok or skillet, heat oil over high heat until a couple of mustard seeds thrown in start to sputter. Add remaining mustard seeds and cover quickly.

2. When the seeds stop popping in a few seconds, uncover, reduce heat to medium and add curry leaves, if using, and chilies. Sauté for 30 seconds.

3. Add cabbage, bell pepper and salt. Stir-fry until cabbage is softened, 3 to 4 minutes.

4. Fold in peanuts and cook for 1 minute.

Nutritional Analysis (Per Serving)
- Calories: 77
- Protein: 2.3 g
- Fat: 5.4 g
- Carbohydrates: 6.4 g
- Fiber: 2.6 g
- Sodium: 274 mg
- Cholesterol: 0 mg

Savoy Cabbage Sauté

1 tsp	canola oil or vegetable oil	5 mL
1	3 oz (75 g) piece salt pork or back bacon, cut into ⅛-inch (3 mm) cubes	1
1	onion, halved and thinly sliced	1
2 tsp	maple syrup	10 mL
1 tsp	Chinese five-spice powder	5 mL
1	head Savoy cabbage, cored and coarsely shredded (about 12 cups/3 L)	1
⅓ cup	chicken stock	75 mL
1 tsp	fresh lemon juice	5 mL
½ tsp	salt	2 mL
½ tsp	black pepper	2 mL

SERVES 6 TO 8

Large deep skillet with lid or Dutch oven

1. In skillet or Dutch oven, heat oil over medium-high heat. Add salt pork; cook, stirring often, for 5 minutes or until well browned. Reduce heat to medium; add onion, maple syrup and Chinese five-spice powder. Cook, stirring often, for 5 minutes or until onion is soft and starts to brown.

2. Stir in cabbage and chicken stock. Cook, tightly covered and stirring occasionally, for 5 to 7 minutes or until cabbage is tender. Add lemon juice, salt and pepper; stir well. Spoon into a warm serving dish. Serve at once.

Nutritional Analysis (Per Serving)
- Calories: 83
- Protein: 5.1 g
- Fat: 3.0 g
- Carbohydrates: 10.5 g
- Fiber: 3.3 g
- Sodium: 390 mg
- Cholesterol: 7 mg

Cauliflower and Red Pepper

1	head cauliflower, florets only	1	
2	red bell peppers, roasted, skinned and cut into thick strips	2	
¼ tsp	salt	1 mL	
¼ tsp	black pepper	1 mL	
2 tbsp	lemon juice	25 mL	
1 tbsp	Dijon mustard	15 mL	
1 tsp	vegetable oil	5 mL	
1 tsp	black mustard seeds	5 mL	
½ tsp	turmeric	2 mL	
½ tsp	whole coriander seeds	2 mL	
2	cloves garlic	2	
2 tbsp	olive oil	25 mL	

SERVES 6

1. Blanch cauliflower florets in a large saucepan of boiling water for 5 to 6 minutes, until just cooked. Drain, refresh in iced water, drain again and transfer to a bowl. Add red peppers to cauliflower. Sprinkle with salt and pepper and toss.

2. In a small bowl whisk together the lemon juice and Dijon mustard until blended. Set aside.

3. In a small frying pan heat vegetable oil over medium heat for 1 minute. Add mustard seeds, turmeric and coriander seeds, and stir-fry for 2 to 3 minutes, or until the seeds begin to pop. With a rubber spatula, scrape cooked spices from the pan into the lemon-mustard mixture. Squeeze garlic through a garlic press and add to the mixture. Add olive oil and whisk until the dressing has emulsified.

4. Add dressing to the cauliflower-red pepper mixture. Toss gently but thoroughly to dress all the pieces evenly. Transfer to a serving bowl, propping up the red pepper ribbons to properly accent the yellow-tinted cauliflower. This salad benefits greatly from a 1- or 2-hour wait, after which it should be served at room temperature.

Tips

- A colorful, emphatically dressed combination of lush red pepper and the oft-neglected cauliflower, this salad travels well on picnics in the summer, just as it helps to liven up a cozy dinner in winter.

- This is an excellent source of vitamins A and C.

Nutritional Analysis (Per Serving)
- Calories: 83
- Protein: 2 g
- Fat: 6 g
- Carbohydrates: 7 g
- Fiber: 2 g
- Sodium: 142 mg
- Cholesterol: 0 mg

Grilled Eggplant with Goat Cheese

1	eggplant (about 1 lb/500 g)	1	
1 tsp	salt	5 mL	
2 tbsp	olive oil	25 mL	
4 oz	soft goat cheese	125 g	
1 tbsp	olive oil	15 mL	
1 tbsp	balsamic vinegar	15 mL	
1 tsp	drained capers	5 mL	
	Freshly ground black pepper to taste		
	Few sprigs fresh basil and/or parsley, chopped		

This beautiful (if slightly calorific) dish takes a little while to prepare; but it can be done in two stages and is guaranteed to fetch compliments.

SERVES 4

Preheat broiler and, if using, start barbecue (see tip, below)
• Baking sheet

1. Cut off top ½ inch (1 cm) of the eggplant and discard. Slice 12 perfect round slices, about ¼ inch (0.5 cm) thick. Sprinkle salt on both sides of the eggplant slices, and let rest 10 minutes.

2. Rinse salt off the slices and pat dry. Brush each side of slices with the olive oil. Lay them out on a baking sheet and broil them 6 to 7 minutes on the first side, until soft. Flip them, and broil the second side for 2 to 3 minutes.

3. Remove from broiler. Arrange eggplant slices on the baking sheet in 4 clusters of 3 slices each. Divide the cheese into 4 equal portions and form each into a patty; place one patty in the center of each cluster. Sprinkle each cluster evenly with the olive oil.

4. Return to the broiler and broil for 2 to 3 minutes until the cheese is melted and has started to brown a little.

5. With a spatula, carefully lift each cluster onto a plate. Sprinkle with the vinegar, capers, black pepper and chopped herb(s). Serve immediately.

Tip

• In barbecue season, it is best to grill the eggplant slices instead of broiling them (Step 2). Grill 4 to 5 minutes on one side, turn over and grill another 3 minutes. You'll still need the broiler for the final gratin.

Nutritional Analysis (Per Serving)
• Calories: 222   • Protein: 7.2 g   • Fat: 18.8 g
• Carbohydrates: 7.6 g   • Fiber: 2.8 g   • Sodium: 752 mg
• Cholesterol: 0 mg

Braised Endive and Tomato Gratinée

2	medium endives	2
2 tbsp	water	25 mL
1 tbsp	olive oil	15 mL
4	black olives, pitted and cut into thirds	4
2	cloves garlic, thinly sliced	2
2	sun-dried tomatoes, cut into thirds	2
1	ripe tomato, cut into $\frac{1}{2}$-inch (1 cm) wedges	1
Pinch	dried oregano leaves	Pinch
Pinch	dried basil leaves	Pinch
$\frac{1}{4}$ tsp	salt	1 mL
$\frac{1}{8}$ tsp	freshly ground black pepper	0.5 mL
2 oz	sharp cheese, shredded (such as Pecorino, Parmesan or old Cheddar)	60 g
	Few sprigs fresh basil or parsley, chopped	

Endive is plentiful and available throughout the year. Here's a recipe that combines endive with sunbelt flavors and uses the ancient French culinary method of braising or slow cooking.

SERVES 2

1. Place endives into a small shallow pot with a lid. Add water, olive oil, olives, garlic, sun-dried tomatoes, tomato, oregano, basil, salt and pepper; cook over high heat for 1 to 2 minutes or until bubbling. Push the tomato wedges to the bottom of the pot around the endives, pushing the other ingredients into the ensuing liquid. Reduce heat to minimum, cover and cook undisturbed for 35 minutes or until soft and pierceable. (The recipe can prepared to this point up to 2 hours in advance.)

2. Carefully transfer endives to a small ovenproof dish. (They should fit snugly.) Cover endives with sauce. With a sharp knife, slice the endives halfway down and open up the cuts so that they are somewhat butterflied. Sprinkle shredded cheese evenly on the butterflied surfaces. Place under a hot broiler for 3 to 4 minutes, until the cheese is bubbling and beginning to char. Lift the endives carefully with a spatula onto 2 plates and pour sauce around them. Garnish with chopped basil or parsley. Serve immediately.

Nutritional Analysis (Per Serving)
- Calories: 257
- Protein: 13.9 g
- Fat: 18.2 g
- Carbohydrates: 11.4 g
- Fiber: 3.9 g
- Sodium: 930 mg
- Cholesterol: 22 mg

Endive with Walnuts and Pancetta

3 tbsp	olive oil	45 mL
¼ lb	pancetta, finely chopped	125 g
2	cloves garlic, finely chopped	2
6	Belgian endives, washed, trimmed and cut in half lengthwise	6
½ cup	dry white wine	125 mL
¼ tsp	salt	1 mL
¼ tsp	freshly ground black pepper	1 mL
1 cup	grated Parmigiano-Reggiano	250 mL
1 cup	walnut halves, chopped (reserve a few, unchopped, for garnish)	250 mL

SERVES 4 TO 6

6-cup (1.5 L) gratin dish or other ovenproof dish

1. In a large skillet, heat the olive oil over medium heat. Add pancetta and garlic; cook for 3 minutes. Do not let garlic brown. Add endives; cook for 3 minutes, turning once or twice with tongs. Arrange endives cut-side down. Pour in wine; sprinkle with salt and pepper. Cover skillet, reduce heat to medium-low and cook 10 minutes or until endives are tender. Preheat broiler.

2. Transfer cooked endives and skillet contents to gratin dish. Sprinkle with grated Parmigiano-Reggiano. Broil for 2 minutes or until cheese is lightly browned. Sprinkle with chopped walnuts. Serve immediately, garnished with halved walnuts.

Tips

- This simple side dish requires the freshest walnuts — so buy them unshelled if available.
- To boost the flavor, briefly toast unchopped walnuts in the oven on a baking sheet; keep a careful eye on them, since they can burn quickly.

Nutritional Analysis (Per Serving)
- Calories: 390
- Protein: 16.9 g
- Fat: 32.6 g
- Carbohydrates: 6.5
- Fiber: 3.6 g
- Sodium: 753 mg
- Cholesterol: 26 mg

Green Beans and Diced Tomatoes

8 oz	green beans, trimmed	250 g
1½ tsp	vegetable oil	7 mL
1 tsp	crushed garlic	5 mL
¾ cup	chopped onion	175 mL
⅓ cup	chopped sweet red or yellow pepper	75 mL
1½ cups	diced tomatoes	375 mL
½ tsp	dried basil (or 1 tbsp/ 15 mL fresh)	2 mL
½ tsp	dried oregano	2 mL
2 tbsp	chicken stock	25 mL
2 tsp	lemon juice	10 mL
2 tsp	grated Parmesan cheese (optional)	10 mL

Make Ahead

If serving cold, prepare early in day and allow flavors to blend.

SERVES 4

1. Steam or microwave green beans just until tender. Set aside.
2. In nonstick skillet, heat oil; sauté garlic, onion and red pepper just until tender.
3. Add green beans, tomatoes, basil, oregano, stock and lemon juice; cook for 2 minutes, stirring constantly. Serve sprinkled with Parmesan (if using).

Tip
- Snow peas or asparagus can replace the green beans.

Nutritional Analysis (Per Serving)
- Calories: 65
- Protein: 2 g
- Fat: 2 g
- Carbohydrates: 10 g
- Fiber: 3 g
- Sodium: 55 mg
- Cholesterol: 1 mg

Green Beans with Cashews

1 lb	green beans, trimmed	500 g
2 tbsp	olive oil	25 mL
½ cup	slivered red onion	125 mL
⅓ cup	raw cashews	75 mL
¼ tsp	salt	1 mL
¼ tsp	freshly ground black pepper	1 mL
	Few sprigs fresh parsley, chopped	

The simple addition of cashews and red onions to this dish transforms ordinary green beans into a formidable companion to any gourmet main course.

SERVES 4

1. Blanch green beans in a pot of boiling water for 5 minutes. Drain and immediately refresh in a bowl of ice-cold water. Drain and set aside.
2. In a large frying pan, heat olive oil over medium-high heat for 30 seconds. Add onions, cashews, salt and pepper and stir-fry for 2 to 3 minutes, until the onions are softened. Add cooked green beans, increase heat to high, and stir-fry actively for 2 to 3 minutes, until the beans feel hot to the touch. (Take care that you don't burn any cashews in the process.) Transfer to a serving plate and garnish with chopped parsley. Serve immediately.

Nutritional Analysis (Per Serving)
- Calories: 168
- Protein: 3.9 g
- Fat: 12.2 g
- Carbohydrates: 13.7 g
- Fiber: 4.4 g
- Sodium: 155 mg
- Cholesterol: 0 mg

Braised Green Beans and Fennel

¼ cup	olive oil	50 mL
½ tsp	salt	2 mL
¼ tsp	freshly ground black pepper	1 mL
1 tsp	whole fennel seeds	5 mL
12 oz	green beans, trimmed	375 g
1	large or 2 small fennel bulbs, trimmed, cored, and cut into ½-inch (1 cm) slices (see tip, at right)	1
1	small carrot, scraped and sliced into ¼ -inch (0.5 cm) rounds	1
6	cloves garlic, thinly sliced	6
1 cup	water	250 mL
1 tbsp	balsamic vinegar	15 mL
	Few sprigs fennel greens, chopped	

This recipe works beautifully as a warm-up starter salad, or as a side vegetable to grilled meat or fish. Green beans provide the bulk, but it is the fresh fennel that gives it character.

SERVES 6

1. In a large, deep frying pan, heat olive oil, salt and pepper over high heat for 1 minute. Add fennel seeds; stir-fry 1 minute or until just browning. Add green beans, fennel and carrots; stir-fry 3 minutes or until all the vegetables are shiny and beginning to sizzle. Add garlic; stir-fry for 1 more minute.

2. Immediately add water and vinegar; cook 2 minutes or until bubbling. Reduce heat to medium-low, cover pan tightly and cook 20 minutes.

3. Place a strainer over a bowl and strain contents of the pan. Transfer the strained vegetables onto a platter and keep warm. Transfer the liquid that has collected in the bowl back into the pan; bring to a boil and cook 6 to 7 minutes or until thick and syrupy.

4. Spoon the reduced sauce over the vegetables, garnish with the chopped fennel greens and serve immediately.

Tip

- The fennel bulb always comes attached to woody branches and thin leaves that look like dill. You'll need the leaves for the final garnish, so cut them off and set them aside. Cut off and discard the woody branches. Quarter the bulb vertically, then cut out and discard the hard triangular sections of core. What remains is the usable part of the fennel.

Nutritional Analysis (Per Serving)
- Calories: 144
- Protein: 2.2 g
- Fat: 11.1 g
- Carbohydrates: 11.4 g
- Fiber: 4.3 g
- Sodium: 264 mg
- Cholesterol: 0 mg

Spanish Green Beans

1½ lbs	green beans, washed and trimmed	750 g
2 tbsp	olive oil	25 mL
3 cups	sliced button mushrooms (about 8 oz/250 g)	750 mL
1	clove garlic, minced	1
8 oz	cooked salad shrimp (optional), thawed if frozen	250 g
4 oz	prosciutto, trimmed of excess fat and coarsely chopped	125 g
¼ tsp	black pepper	1 mL
Pinch	salt (optional)	Pinch

Make Ahead

Green beans can be washed, trimmed then refrigerated, wrapped in a damp tea towel and sealed in a plastic bag, for up to 24 hours.

SERVES 6

1. In a large saucepan of boiling salted water, cook beans for 6 to 8 minutes or until just tender; drain well. Keep warm.

2. In a large skillet, heat oil over medium-high heat. Add mushrooms and garlic; cook, stirring, for 3 minutes or until mushrooms are golden and tender. Stir in beans, shrimp, prosciutto and pepper. Reduce heat to medium-low; cook, stirring gently, for 2 minutes or until heated through. If desired, season to taste with salt and additional pepper. Serve at once or let cool to room temperature.

Nutritional Analysis (Per Serving)
- Calories: 156
- Protein: 15.8 g
- Fat: 6.5 g
- Carbohydrates: 10.4 g
- Fiber: 4.3 g
- Sodium: 383 mg
- Cholesterol: 68 mg

Bitter Greens with Paprika

1	bunch rapini or dandelion greens, washed, bottom 2 inches (5 cm) of stalks trimmed	1
2 tbsp	olive oil	25 mL
1 tsp	sweet paprika	5 mL
¼ tsp	turmeric	1 mL
¼ tsp	salt	1 mL
¼ tsp	freshly ground black pepper	1 mL
3	cloves garlic, thinly sliced	3
2 tbsp	freshly squeezed lemon juice	25 mL
1 tsp	drained capers	5 mL

Suitable as a starter or as a side dish with grilled or roasted meat, this hyper-nutritious dish has taste to spare.

SERVES 3 OR 4

1. Cut stalks of greens in half. Bring a pot of salted water to a boil and add the lower half of stalks. Let water return to boil and cook for 3 minutes. Add upper half of stalks (with the leaves); return to boil and cook for 3 minutes. Rinse under cold water; drain and set aside.

2. In a large frying pan, combine oil, paprika, turmeric, salt and pepper. Cook, stirring, over high heat for 1 minute. Add garlic; stir-fry for 30 seconds. Add drained greens; stir-fry for 2 minutes, folding from the bottom up to distribute garlic and spices evenly. Reduce heat to medium. Stir in lemon juice; cook, stirring, for 2 minutes. Stir in capers. Serve immediately.

Nutritional Analysis (Per Serving)
- Calories: 92
- Protein: 2.9 g
- Fat: 7.1 g
- Carbohydrates: 6.4 g
- Fiber: 3.0 g
- Sodium: 191 mg
- Cholesterol: 0 mg

Golden Mushroom Sauté

1 tsp	olive oil	5 mL
1	medium onion, chopped	1
2	cloves garlic, minced	2
1¼ lb	chanterelle or portobello mushrooms, sliced	625 g
½ lb	small button mushrooms	250 g
3	sun-dried tomatoes, softened and chopped	3
¾ cup	chicken broth	175 mL
½ cup	dry white wine	125 mL
2 tbsp	lemon juice	25 mL
1 tbsp	sweet Hungarian paprika	15 mL
½ tsp	caraway seeds	2 mL
	Salt and black pepper	
2 tbsp	chopped fresh parsley	25 mL

This sauté has a great mix of herbs and spices, and the result is spectacular flavor with little fat.

SERVES 8

1. In a large skillet, heat oil over medium heat; cook onion, stirring, for 2 minutes. Add garlic, chanterelle and button mushrooms and tomatoes; cook for 2 to 3 minutes.

2. Add chicken broth, wine, lemon juice, paprika and caraway seeds; bring to a boil. Simmer over low heat for about 15 minutes or until slightly thickened, stirring occasionally. Season with salt and pepper to taste. Sprinkle with parsley.

Tip

- To soften sun-dried tomatoes, cover with boiling water and let stand for 10 minutes. Drain well.

Nutritional Analysis (Per Serving)
- Calories: 44
- Protein: 2 g
- Fat: 1 g
- Carbohydrates: 6 g
- Fiber: 2 g
- Sodium: 62 mg
- Cholesterol: 0 mg

Marinated Mushrooms

2 cups	sliced mushrooms (see tip, at right)	500 mL
2 tbsp	white vinegar	25 mL
1 tbsp	extra virgin olive oil	15 mL
2 tbsp	chopped fresh parsley	25 mL
	Salt and freshly ground black pepper	

Mix and match any mushroom — portobello, button, shiitake, oyster — all can be marinated using this recipe.

SERVES 4

1. Place mushrooms in a shallow container.

2. In a small bowl, whisk together vinegar, oil, parsley, salt and pepper. Pour over mushrooms. Let stand at room temperature for several hours before serving. Drain before serving.

Tip

- Choose the freshest mushrooms — firm and evenly colored, unbroken and with tightly closed caps. If the gills are showing, they are past their prime. To prepare, wipe with a damp paper towel or a mushroom brush.

Nutritional Analysis (Per Serving)
- Calories: 44
- Protein: 1.4 g
- Fat: 3.5 g
- Carbohydrates: 2.5 g
- Fiber: 0.7 g
- Sodium: 3 mg
- Cholesterol: 0 mg

Fennel Mushroom Stir-Fry

1	fennel bulb (about 1 lb/500 g)	1
3 tbsp	olive oil	45 mL
¼ tsp	salt	1 mL
¼ tsp	freshly ground black pepper	1 mL
½ cup	roughly chopped red onion	125 mL
½	red bell pepper, roughly chopped	½
2½ cups	trimmed and halved mushrooms	625 mL
1 tbsp	freshly squeezed lemon juice	15 mL

Bold, crunchy and colorful, this simple stir-fry gains its appeal from its large-chunk vegetables and its simple flavoring, which allows the subtle licorice of the fennel to shine through. It can be enjoyed hot from the pan, or at room temperature on a party buffet.

SERVES 4

1. Remove and discard any branches shooting up from the fennel bulb (they are fibrous and inedible). Cut the bulb in half, and trim away triangles of hard core. Chop remaining fennel in large chunks. Set aside.
2. In a large frying pan, heat olive oil over high heat for 30 seconds. Add salt, pepper, onions and red pepper. Stir-fry for 1 minute. Add fennel and stir-fry for3 to 4 minutes, until the vegetables are slightly charred. Add mushrooms and stir-fry actively (the pan will be crowded by now) for 3 minutes, until mushrooms are slightly browned and soft. Remove from heat and stir in lemon juice. Transfer to a presentation dish and serve.

Nutritional Analysis (Per Serving)
- Calories: 133
- Protein: 2.7 g
- Fat: 10.5 g
- Carbohydrates: 9.2 g
- Fiber: 2.8 g
- Sodium: 171 mg
- Cholesterol: 0 mg

Basil and Roasted Red Pepper Stuffed Mushrooms

14 oz	large stuffing mushrooms (approximately 16)	400 g
¾ cup	packed basil leaves	175 mL
½ tsp	minced garlic	2 mL
1½ tbsp	olive oil	20 mL
2 tbsp	water	25 mL
1½ tbsp	toasted pine nuts	20 mL
1 tbsp	grated Parmesan cheese	15 mL
¼ cup	light cream cheese	50 mL
2 tbsp	finely diced roasted red peppers	25 mL

Make Ahead

Prepare filling up to a day ahead. Fill mushrooms early in the day and cover. Bake just before serving.

SERVES 6

Preheat oven to 425°F (220°C) • Baking sheet sprayed with vegetable spray

1. Wipe mushrooms clean and gently remove stems; reserve for another purpose. Put caps on baking sheet.
2. Put basil, garlic, olive oil, water, pine nuts, Parmesan and cream cheese into food processor; process until finely chopped, scraping down sides of bowl once. Process until smooth. Add red peppers and combine just until mixed.
3. Divide mixture evenly among mushroom caps. Bake for 15 minutes or until hot.

Nutritional Analysis (Per Serving)
- Calories: 95
- Protein: 4 g
- Fat: 7 g
- Carbohydrates: 4 g
- Fiber: 1 g
- Sodium: 65 mg
- Cholesterol: 9 g

Portobello Mushrooms with Goat Cheese

2 tbsp	olive oil	25 mL
6 oz	portobello mushrooms, trimmed and sliced ½ inch (1 cm) thick	175 g
1 tbsp	finely chopped garlic	15 mL
2 tsp	balsamic vinegar	10 mL
¼ tsp	salt	1 mL
⅛ tsp	freshly ground black pepper	0.5 mL
¼ tsp	drained green peppercorns (optional)	1 mL
2 oz	goat cheese	50 g
2 tsp	pine nuts	10 mL
	Several lettuce leaves	
2 tsp	olive oil	10 mL

Exotic-sounding name notwithstanding, portobello mushrooms are nothing more than overgrown regular mushrooms. But for some alchemical reason their taste is very different (more meaty) from those lowly buttons. As a result, they are usually associated with "wild" (or "fancy") mushrooms and are very much in demand. Luckily, they are available everywhere, often, quite conveniently, already trimmed and sliced into attractive ½-inch (1 cm) slices.

SERVES 2

Preheat broiler • Baking sheet

1. In a nonstick frying pan, heat 2 tbsp (25 mL) olive oil over high heat for 1 minute. Add mushroom slices in one layer; cook 2 to 3 minutes or until nicely browned (they will absorb all the oil). Turn and cook second side for under a minute. Add garlic, 1 tsp (5 mL) of the balsamic vinegar, salt and pepper; continue cooking for 1 minute to brown the garlic somewhat.

2. Remove from heat. Arrange on baking sheet in 2 flat piles about 3 inches (7.5 cm) wide. Sprinkle evenly with green peppercorns, if using. Divide the goat cheese in two; make each half into a thick disc, about 1 inch (2.5 cm) wide. Place a disc of cheese on each pile of mushrooms. Sprinkle the pine nuts evenly over the piles, some on the cheese and some on the surrounding mushrooms. (The recipe can wait at this point up to 1 hour, covered and unrefrigerated).

3. Broil the mushrooms for just under 4 minutes or until the cheese is soft and a little brown, and the pine nuts are dark brown.

4. Line 2 plates with lettuce. Carefully lift each pile off the baking sheet and transfer as intact as possible onto the lettuce. Sprinkle about 1 tsp (5 mL) olive oil and ½ tsp (2 mL) balsamic vinegar over each portion and serve immediately.

Tip

- Green peppercorns are sold packed in brine; leftovers will keep if refrigerated in their original brine. While optional, they are delicious in this recipe.

Nutritional Analysis (Per Serving)
- Calories: 314
- Protein: 10.5 g
- Fat: 28.4 g
- Carbohydrates: 7.3 g
- Fiber: 2.1 g
- Sodium: 443 mg
- Cholesterol: 22 mg

Cheesy Pesto Stuffed Mushrooms

14 oz	large stuffing mushrooms (approximately 16)	350 g
¾ cup	packed basil leaves	175 mL
1½ tbsp	olive oil	20 mL
1½ tbsp	toasted pine nuts (see tip, page 340)	20 mL
1 tbsp	grated Parmesan cheese	15 mL
½ tsp	minced garlic	2 mL
2 tbsp	chicken stock or water	25 mL
¼ cup	5% ricotta cheese	50 mL

Make Ahead

Prepare filling up to a day ahead. Fill mushrooms early in the day. Bake just before serving.

SERVES 6

Preheat oven to 425°F (220°C) • Baking sheet sprayed with vegetable spray

1. Wipe mushrooms clean and gently remove stems; reserve for another purpose. Put caps on baking sheet.
2. Put basil, olive oil, pine nuts, Parmesan and garlic in food processor; process until finely chopped, scraping down sides of bowl once. Add stock through the feed tube and process until smooth. Add ricotta and process until mixed.
3. Divide mixture evenly among mushroom caps. Bake for 10 to 15 minutes or until hot.

Nutritional Analysis (Per Serving)
- Calories: 75
- Protein: 4 g
- Fat: 6 g
- Carbohydrates: 4 g
- Fiber: 1 g
- Sodium: 49 mg
- Cholesterol: 4 mg

Mushrooms Stuffed with Spinach and Ricotta Cheese

2 cups	fresh spinach	500 mL
16	medium mushrooms	16
1 tbsp	vegetable oil	15 mL
2 tsp	crushed garlic	10 mL
¼ cup	finely chopped onions	50 mL
⅓ cup	ricotta cheese	75 mL
1 tbsp	grated Parmesan cheese	15 mL
	Salt and pepper	

Make Ahead

Prepare early in day and refrigerate. Bake just before serving.

SERVES 8

Preheat oven to 400°F (200°C)

1. Rinse spinach and shake off excess water. With just the water clinging to leaves, cook until wilted. Drain and squeeze out excess moisture; chop finely and set aside.
2. Remove stems from mushrooms. Place caps on baking sheet. Dice half of the stems and reserve. Use remaining stems for another use.
3. In small nonstick saucepan, heat oil; sauté garlic, onions and diced stems until softened. Add spinach and cook for 1 minute. Remove from heat.
4. Add ricotta, half the Parmesan, and salt and pepper to taste; mix well and carefully fill mushroom caps. Sprinkle with remaining Parmesan. Bake for 8 to 10 minutes or just until mushrooms release their liquid.

Nutritional Analysis (Per Serving)
- Calories: 51
- Protein: 2 g
- Fat: 3 g
- Carbohydrates: 3 g
- Fiber: 1 g
- Sodium: 33 mg
- Cholesterol: 5 mg

Mushrooms Stuffed with Goat Cheese and Leeks

16	medium mushrooms	16
1 tsp	vegetable oil	5 mL
1$\frac{1}{2}$ tsp	minced garlic	7 mL
$\frac{1}{3}$ cup	finely chopped leeks	75 mL
$\frac{1}{3}$ cup	finely chopped red peppers	75 mL
$\frac{1}{3}$ cup	crumbled goat cheese	75 mL
3 tbsp	light cream cheese	45 mL
2 tbsp	chopped fresh oregano (or $\frac{1}{2}$ tsp/2 mL dried)	25 mL
2 tbsp	finely chopped green onions (about 1 medium)	25 mL

Make Ahead

Stuff mushrooms up to a day ahead. Keep refrigerated. Bake just before serving.

SERVES 4 TO 6
Preheat oven to 425°F (220°C)

1. Remove stems from mushrooms; set caps aside and dice stems.
2. In small nonstick saucepan sprayed with vegetable spray, heat oil over medium heat; add diced mushroom stems, garlic, leeks and peppers. Cook for 5 minutes, or until softened. Remove from heat.
3. Add goat and cream cheeses, oregano and green onions; mix well. Carefully stuff mixture into mushroom caps. Place in a baking dish and bake for 15 to 20 minutes or just until mushrooms release their liquid.

Nutritional Analysis (Per Serving)
- Calories: 72
- Protein: 4 g
- Fat: 5 g
- Carbohydrates: 4 g
- Fiber: 1 g
- Sodium: 175 mg
- Cholesterol: 18 mg

Mushrooms with Creamy Feta Cheese and Dill Stuffing

16	medium mushrooms	16
1 tsp	vegetable oil	5 mL
1$\frac{1}{2}$ tsp	minced garlic	7 mL
$\frac{1}{3}$ cup	finely chopped onions	75 mL
$\frac{1}{3}$ cup	finely chopped red or green peppers	75 mL
$\frac{1}{3}$ cup	crumbled feta cheese	75 mL
3 tbsp	5% ricotta cheese	45 mL
2 tbsp	chopped fresh dill (or 1 tsp/5 mL dried)	25 mL
2 tbsp	finely chopped green onions (about 1 medium)	25 mL

Make Ahead

Stuff mushrooms up to a day ahead. Keep refrigerated. Bake just before serving.

SERVES 4 TO 6
Preheat oven to 425°F (220°C)

1. Remove stems from mushrooms; set caps aside and dice stems.
2. In small nonstick saucepan sprayed with vegetable spray, heat oil over medium heat; add diced mushroom stems, garlic, onions and peppers. Cook for 5 minutes, or until softened. Remove from heat.
3. Add feta and ricotta cheeses, dill and green onions; mix well. Carefully stuff mixture into mushroom caps. Place in a baking dish and bake for 15 to 20 minutes or just until mushrooms release their liquid.

Nutritional Analysis (Per Serving)
- Calories: 67
- Protein: 4 g
- Fat: 4 g
- Carbohydrates: 4 g
- Fiber: 1 g
- Sodium: 162 mg
- Cholesterol: 14 mg

New Orleans Braised Onions

2 to 3	large Spanish onions	2 to 3
6 to 9	whole cloves	6 to 9
½ tsp	salt	2 mL
½ tsp	cracked black peppercorns	2 mL
Pinch	ground thyme	Pinch
	Grated zest and juice of 1 orange	
½ cup	condensed beef broth, undiluted	125 mL
	Finely chopped fresh parsley, optional	
	Hot pepper sauce, optional	

SERVES 10
Slow cooker

1. Stud onions with cloves. Place in slow cooker stoneware and sprinkle with salt, peppercorns, thyme and orange zest. Pour orange juice and beef broth over onions, cover and cook on Low for 8 hours or on High for 4 hours, until onions are tender.

2. Keep onions warm. In a saucepan over medium heat, reduce cooking liquid by half.

3. When ready to serve, cut onions into quarters. Place on a deep platter and cover with sauce. Sprinkle with parsley, if desired, and pass the hot pepper sauce, if desired.

Tip

- This is a great dish to serve with roasted poultry or meat. If your guests like spice, pass hot pepper sauce at the table.

Nutritional Analysis (Per Serving)
- Calories: 20
- Protein: 1 g
- Fat: 0 g
- Carbohydrates: 4 g
- Fiber: 1 g
- Sodium: 188 mg
- Cholesterol: 0 mg

Peppery Red Onions

4	large red onions, quartered	4
1 tbsp	extra-virgin olive oil	15 mL
1 tsp	dried oregano leaves	5 mL
¼ cup	water or chicken or vegetable stock	50 mL
	Salt and pepper, to taste	
	Hot pepper sauce, to taste (see tip, at right)	

SERVES 4 TO 6
Slow cooker

1. In slow cooker stoneware, combine all ingredients except hot sauce. Stir thoroughly, cover and cook on Low for 8 hours or on High for 4 hours, until onions are tender.

2. Toss well with hot sauce and serve.

Tip

- Use your favorite hot sauce, such as Tabasco, Louisiana Hot Sauce or Piri Piri, or try other more exotic brands to vary the flavors in this recipe.

Nutritional Analysis (Per Serving)
- Calories: 49
- Protein: 1 g
- Fat: 2 g
- Carbohydrates: 7 g
- Fiber: 1 g
- Sodium: 7 mg
- Cholesterol: 0 mg

Sautéed Skillet Peppers

1	each green, red and yellow bell pepper	1
2 tsp	olive oil	10 mL
1	clove garlic, sliced	1
	Salt and freshly ground black pepper	
2 tbsp	freshly grated Parmesan cheese	25 mL

SERVES 4

1. Remove and discard seeds from peppers. Cut peppers into long strips.
2. In a nonstick skillet, heat oil over medium heat. Add garlic and cook for 30 seconds. Add pepper slices. Reduce heat to medium-low. Cover and cook for 15 minutes or until peppers are tender and no longer moist, stirring occasionally. Season lightly with salt and pepper.
3. Sprinkle with cheese. Cover and cook on low for 5 minutes or until cheese is melted.

Nutritional Analysis (Per Serving)
- Calories: 63
- Protein: 2.1 g
- Fat: 3.2 g
- Carbohydrates: 7.5 g
- Fiber: 2.2 g
- Sodium: 49 mg
- Cholesterol: 2 mg

Piedmont Peppers

6	red bell peppers, halved and seeded, stems left intact	6
6	plum tomatoes, peeled and quartered	6
12	anchovy fillets, rinsed and roughly chopped	6
4	cloves garlic, thinly sliced	4
1/2 cup	extra virgin olive oil	125 mL
	Salt and freshly ground black pepper	
12	whole leaves flat-leaf parsley	12

Within this simple preparation resides the essence of rustic Italian cooking: startlingly fresh ingredients, simply paired and quickly put together.

SERVES 4 TO 6

13- by 9-inch (3 L) baking dish, oiled • Preheat oven to 350°F (180°C)

1. Lay peppers in prepared baking dish, cut-side up, in one layer. Into each pepper cavity, place two pieces of tomato. Sprinkle with chopped anchovies, making sure each pepper gets the equivalent of a whole anchovy fillet. Evenly distribute the sliced garlic among the peppers. Carefully pour the olive oil over the peppers. Sprinkle with just a little bit of salt (because of anchovies) and lots of freshly ground black pepper.
2. Roast in the top half of preheated oven for 1 hour or until the peppers are tender. Cool slightly. Serve warm, garnished with parsley leaves.

Nutritional Analysis (Per Serving)
- Calories: 288
- Protein: 6.1 g
- Fat: 23.3 g
- Carbohydrates: 16.8
- Fiber: 5.1 g
- Sodium: 427 mg
- Cholesterol: 10 mg

Rapini with Balsamic Vinegar

1	bunch rapini, washed, bottom 1½ inches (4 cm) of stalks trimmed	1
1 tsp	salt	5 mL
3 tbsp	balsamic vinegar	45 mL
2 tbsp	extra virgin olive oil	25 mL
	Freshly ground black pepper to taste	
	Few sprigs fresh basil or parsley, chopped	
¼ cup	thinly sliced red onion	50 mL
1 tsp	drained capers	5 mL
3 tbsp	shaved Parmesan or Pecorino cheese	45 mL

SERVES 4

1. Prepare rapini. Cut off the top 2½ inches (6 cm) — the part that has the leaves and the flowers — and set aside. Cut the remaining stalks into 1-inch (2.5 cm) pieces.

2. In a large pot, bring 1½ inches (4 cm) of water to a boil. Add salt and chopped stalks and cook, uncovered, for 8 minutes, until tender. Add the reserved tops and cook, uncovered, for another 8 minutes. Drain, refresh with cold water, and drain again.

3. Transfer drained rapini to a serving plate and spread out. In a small bowl, combine vinegar, olive oil, pepper to taste and chopped basil or parsley. Evenly dress the rapini with this sauce. Scatter slices of red onion and capers over the rapini, and top with shaved cheese.

Nutritional Analysis (Per Serving)
- Calories: 108
- Protein: 4.3 g
- Fat: 8.2 g
- Carbohydrates: 6.5 g
- Fiber: 2.8 g
- Sodium: 697 mg
- Cholesterol: 3 mg

Sautéed Spinach with Lemon

3 lbs	fresh spinach	1.5 kg
3 tbsp	olive oil	45 mL
3	cloves garlic, finely chopped	3
	Salt and freshly ground black pepper to taste	
1	lemon, cut into wedges	1

This method also works well with Swiss chard, rapini, green beans and zucchini.

SERVES 4 TO 6

1. Trim and wash spinach. Put the spinach in a large saucepan with just the water that clings to the leaves after washing. Cook, covered, over high heat until steam begins to escape from beneath lid. Remove lid, toss spinach and cook 1 minute longer or until tender. Remove from heat. Drain; return to pot. Cook over medium-high heat, shaking the pot, until moisture evaporates.

2. Add olive oil, garlic and salt and pepper to taste. Cook, stirring, for 2 minutes. Do not let garlic brown. Serve immediately, sprinkled with lemon juice and freshly ground black pepper.

Nutritional Analysis (Per Serving)
- Calories: 153
- Protein: 6.7 g
- Fat: 11.7 g
- Carbohydrates: 8.8 g
- Fiber: 6.2 g
- Sodium: 184 mg
- Cholesterol: 0 mg

Sautéed Spinach with Pine Nuts

2 tsp	olive oil	10 mL
¼ cup	pine nuts	50 mL
1	package (10 oz/300 g) fresh spinach, trimmed	1
1 tsp	minced garlic	5 mL
1 tsp	lemon juice	5 mL
⅛ tsp	ground nutmeg	0.5 mL
	Black pepper	

This is an easy way to add flavor to spinach. You can substitute Swiss chard, kale, rapini or mustard greens for the spinach. If you don't have pine nuts, try pecans or walnuts.

SERVES 4

1. In a large nonstick skillet, heat 1 tsp (5 mL) of the oil over medium heat. Add pine nuts and cook, stirring constantly, for 2 to 3 minutes or until golden. Remove pine nuts from pan and set aside.

2. Add remaining oil to pan. Add spinach in several bunches (it will cook down quickly), stirring constantly. Add garlic and cook for 1 to 2 minutes. Stir in lemon juice and nutmeg. Season with pepper to taste. Add reserved pine nuts. Cook until heated through.

Tip

- Stir-frying vegetables is a great way to preserve nutrients. When boiled, vegetables can lose up to 45% of vitamin C; they lose only 5% when stir-fried.

Nutritional Analysis (Per Serving)
- Calories: 90
- Protein: 4 g
- Fat: 8 g
- Carbohydrates: 4 g
- Fiber: 3 g
- Sodium: 48 mg
- Cholesterol: 0 mg

Spinach Fancy

1	package (10 oz/300 g) fresh spinach	1
3 tbsp	raisins	45 mL
Pinch	dried mint	Pinch
Pinch	ground fennel	Pinch
Pinch	dried oregano	Pinch
1 tbsp	butter or margarine	15 mL
2 tbsp	water	25 mL
1 tsp	lemon juice	5 mL
½ tsp	salt	2 mL
Pinch	black pepper	Pinch
	Lemon slices	

No one will have to tell you to eat your spinach anymore! You will be more than willing to enjoy this tasty dish, which is particularly good with fish.

SERVES 5

1. Wash spinach and dry thoroughly; remove stems and chop.

2. In a large skillet over medium heat, cook raisins, mint, fennel and oregano in butter. Add spinach and water; cover and steam for 2 to 3 minutes or until wilted. Drain liquid. Sprinkle with lemon juice, salt and pepper; toss well. Serve with lemon slices.

Nutritional Analysis (Per Serving)
- Calories: 50
- Protein: 2 g
- Fat: 2 g
- Carbohydrates: 7 g
- Fiber: 1 g
- Sodium: 180 mg
- Cholesterol: 6 mg

Spinach Florentine

1 cup	water	250 mL
½ tsp	salt	2 mL
4 cups	finely chopped fresh spinach, packed down	1 L
2 tbsp	olive oil	25 mL
¼ tsp	salt	1 mL
¼ tsp	freshly ground black pepper	1 mL
3	cloves garlic, finely chopped	3
3	sun-dried tomatoes, finely sliced	3
2 tbsp	chopped fresh tarragon or 1 tsp (5 mL) dried	25 mL
1 cup	shredded mozzarella cheese	250 mL
1 tbsp	grated Parmesan cheese	15 mL

A spinach recipe for those who prefer their vitamins and Popeye-like strength from palate teasers. Perked up with garlic and sun-dried tomato and mantled with two kinds of cheese, this bundle of tasty greens is as irresistible as it is nutritious.

SERVES 4

1. In a large saucepan, bring water to a rolling boil over high heat. Add salt. Add spinach, cover, and cook for 2 minutes until spinach has greatly reduced in volume and is bright green. Drain and refresh with cold water. (Let drain on its own, without pressing down.)

2. In a large frying pan, heat olive oil over high heat for 30 seconds. Add salt, pepper and garlic; stir-fry for 30 seconds. Add sun-dried tomatoes and stir-fry for another 30 seconds. Add spinach and tarragon, and stir-fry for 1 minute, folding the ingredients together. Reduce heat to medium.

3. Spread spinach out over bottom of pan. Sprinkle evenly with mozzarella and Parmesan. Cover pan and let cook until cheese melts, about 1 to 2 minutes. Remove from heat and keep covered. Serve as soon as possible.

Variation

- This dish can be turned into Eggs Florentine — the café-brunch fave — if served under poached or fried eggs. This quantity of spinach can cater to 2 large appetites if split in half and served with 2 eggs each, or 4 modest ones if divided into quarters with an egg atop each serving.

Nutritional Analysis (Per Serving)
- Calories: 195
- Protein: 11.4 g
- Fat: 14.6 g
- Carbohydrates: 5.6 g
- Fiber: 1.4 g
- Sodium: 684 mg
- Cholesterol: 22 mg

Spinach Roll with Cheese Dill Filling

ROLL

1	package (10 oz/300 g) frozen chopped spinach, thawed and squeezed dry	1
2	egg yolks	2
1/2 cup	light sour cream	125 mL
1/3 cup	chopped fresh dill	75 mL
1/3 cup	all-purpose flour	75 mL
4	egg whites	4
Pinch	salt	Pinch
1 tbsp	grated Parmesan cheese	15 mL

FILLING

3/4 cup	5% ricotta cheese	175 mL
2 oz	softened light cream cheese	50 g
2 tbsp	grated Parmesan cheese	25 mL
3 tbsp	chopped green onions	45 mL
3 tbsp	chopped roasted red peppers	45 mL
2 tbsp	chopped fresh dill	25 mL
2 tbsp	2% milk	25 mL

Make Ahead

Prepare filling up to 1 day in advance. Bake roll (to the end of Step 3) early in the day. Can be refrigerated for up to 2 days.

SERVES 6 TO 8

Preheat oven to 350°F (180°C) • 10- by 15-inch (25 by 37.5 cm) jelly roll pan lined with parchment paper and sprayed with vegetable spray

1. In a food processor, purée spinach, egg yolks, sour cream, dill and flour until smooth. Transfer to a large bowl.

2. In a large bowl using an electric mixer, beat egg whites with salt until stiff peaks form. Stir one-quarter of egg whites into spinach mixture. Fold in remaining egg whites. Spoon onto prepared jelly roll pan and smooth top with spatula. Bake 10 to 12 minutes or until tester comes out clean. Let cool 5 minutes. Sprinkle with 1 tbsp (15 mL) Parmesan.

3. Invert jelly roll pan onto a clean tea towel. Remove pan and gently remove parchment paper. Roll up spinach roll and tea towel along short end, keeping tea towel inside the roll. Allow to cool completely.

4. *Make the filling:* In a bowl using an electric mixer or whisk, beat together ricotta, cream cheese and 1 tbsp (15 mL) of the Parmesan until smooth. Stir in green onions, roasted red peppers, dill and milk. Unroll spinach roll. Sprinkle with remaining 1 tbsp (15 mL) Parmesan. Spread with ricotta filling. Tightly re-roll and place on serving dish.

5. Serve at room temperature. Cut into 1-inch (2.5 cm) slices with a serrated knife.

Tips

- If ricotta mixture seems dry, add an extra 1 or 2 tbsp (15 or 25 mL) 2% milk.

- Roll carefully, using a tea towel to assist you. Keep the towel inside the roll until it cools. Be sure to remove the towel before filling!

- Roll may crack. Don't worry; just keep rolling.

Nutritional Analysis (Per Serving)
- Calories: 126
- Protein: 11 g
- Fat: 4 g
- Carbohydrates: 9 g
- Fiber: 2 g
- Sodium: 250 mg
- Cholesterol: 69 mg

Crustless Dill Spinach Quiche with Mushrooms and Cheese

10 oz	fresh spinach	300 g
2 tsp	vegetable oil	10 mL
1 tsp	minced garlic	5 mL
¾ cup	chopped onions	175 mL
¾ cup	chopped mushrooms	175 mL
⅔ cup	5% ricotta cheese	150 mL
⅔ cup	2% cottage cheese	150 mL
⅓ cup	grated Cheddar cheese	75 mL
2 tbsp	grated Parmesan cheese	25 mL
1	whole egg	1
1	egg white	1
3 tbsp	chopped fresh dill (or 2 tsp/10 mL dried)	45 mL
¼ tsp	ground black pepper	1 mL

SERVES 6

Preheat oven to 350°F (180°C) • 8-inch (2 L) springform pan sprayed with vegetable spray

1. Wash spinach and shake off excess water. In the water clinging to the leaves, cook the spinach over high heat just until it wilts. Squeeze out excess moisture, chop and set aside.

2. In large nonstick skillet, heat oil over medium heat; add garlic, onions and mushrooms and cook for 5 minutes or until softened. Remove from heat and add chopped spinach, ricotta, cottage, Cheddar and Parmesan cheeses, whole egg, egg white, dill and pepper; mix well. Pour into prepared pan and bake for 35 to 40 minutes or until knife inserted in center comes out clean.

Make Ahead

Prepare mixture early in the day. Bake just before serving. Great reheated gently the next day.

Nutritional Analysis (Per Serving)
- Calories: 134
- Protein: 13 g
- Fat: 7 g
- Carbohydrates: 6 g
- Fiber: 2 g
- Sodium: 259 mg
- Cholesterol: 54 mg

Snow Peas with Sesame Seeds

1 tbsp	vegetable oil	15 mL
1½ tsp	crushed garlic	7 mL
1 lb	snow peas, trimmed	500 g
½ cup	diced sweet red peppers	125 mL
2 tsp	sesame oil	10 mL
1½ tsp	sesame seeds, toasted	7 mL
4	medium green onions, sliced	4

SERVES 4

1. In nonstick skillet, heat vegetable oil; sauté garlic, snow peas and red peppers until tender-crisp.

2. Add sesame oil and seeds and green onions; cook for 1 minute. Serve immediately.

Tips

- This dish is also great with asparagus instead of snow peas.

- Other nuts, such as toasted pine nuts, can be substituted.

Make Ahead

If serving cold as a salad, prepare early in the day and stir just before serving.

Nutritional Analysis (Per Serving)
- Calories: 112
- Protein: 4 g
- Fat: 6 g
- Carbohydrates: 10 g
- Fiber: 3 g
- Sodium: 8 mg
- Cholesterol: 0 mg

Lemon-Herb Snow Peas

1 tbsp	butter or margarine, melted	15 mL
1 tsp	freshly grated lemon zest	5 mL
½ tsp	dried tarragon or 1 tbsp (15 mL) fresh	2 mL
1 lb	snow peas, trimmed	500 g
	Salt and freshly ground black pepper	

A simply delicious way to dress up snow peas.

SERVES 4

1. In a small dish, combine butter, lemon zest and tarragon. Set aside.
2. In a large saucepan, cook snow peas in boiling water for 2 minutes or until tender-crisp. Drain well. Transfer to a warm serving bowl. Add butter mixture and toss to coat. Season lightly with salt and pepper.

Nutritional Analysis (Per Serving)
- Calories: 78
- Protein: 3.6 g
- Fat: 3.1 g
- Carbohydrates: 9.6 g
- Fiber: 3.2 g
- Sodium: 35 mg
- Cholesterol: 8 mg

Pea Tops with Pancetta and Tofu

1	3-inch (7.5 cm) square medium tofu	1
2 tbsp	vegetable oil, divided	25 mL
	Salt and pepper to taste	
1 tsp	sesame oil	5 mL
2	slices pancetta or prosciutto, finely chopped	2
2 tsp	minced garlic	10 mL
8 oz	pea tops or arugula	250 g
2 tbsp	chicken stock or vegetable stock	25 mL

SERVES 4

1. Slice tofu into pieces ½ inch (1 cm) thick by 1½ inches (3.5 cm) square.
2. In a nonstick skillet, heat 1 tbsp (15 mL) oil over medium-high heat for 30 seconds. Add tofu and season lightly with salt, pepper and sesame oil; fry until golden, about 1 minute per side. Remove from skillet; arrange on a platter and keep warm.
3. Add remaining oil to skillet and heat for 30 seconds. Add pancetta and garlic; fry briefly until fragrant, about 20 to 30 seconds. Add pea tops and stock; stir-fry until pea tops are just wilted. Arrange evenly over tofu and serve.

Tip
- Pea tops are the shoots of snow pea plants. They're now available almost year round in Asian markets. They are tasty in salads and have a subtle, nutty flavor when cooked. However, they are quite perishable and won't last much longer than a couple of days in your refrigerator.

Nutritional Analysis (Per Serving)
- Calories: 129
- Protein: 7.4 g
- Fat: 10.4 g
- Carbohydrates: 2.8 g
- Fiber: 1.0 g
- Sodium: 236 mg
- Cholesterol: 8 mg

Italian Broiled Tomatoes

2	large tomatoes	2
Pinch	garlic powder	Pinch
1 tbsp	chopped fresh parsley	15 mL
1 tsp	dried basil	5 mL
1/2 tsp	dried oregano	2 mL
	Freshly ground black pepper to taste	
2 tbsp	bread crumbs	25 mL

Serve this often during tomato season to accompany broiled or barbecued meat.

SERVES 4

Preheat broiler • Shallow baking pan

1. Cut tomatoes in half crosswise. Place cut side up on rack in shallow baking pan. Sprinkle lightly with garlic powder. Combine parsley, seasonings and bread crumbs. Divide mixture over surface of tomato halves.

2. Place pan about 6 inches (15 cm) below broiler. Broil for 3 to 4 minutes until tomatoes are heated through, or cook on barbecue along with meat being grilled.

Nutritional Analysis (Per Serving)
- Calories: 30
- Protein: 2 g
- Fat: 1 g
- Carbohydrates: 4 g
- Fiber: 1 g
- Sodium: 34 mg
- Cholesterol: 0 mg

Cherry Tomato and Zucchini Sauté with Basil

1 tbsp	olive oil	15 mL
3	small zucchini, halved lengthwise and thinly sliced	3
2 cups	cherry tomatoes, halved	500 mL
1/2 tsp	ground cumin (optional)	2 mL
2	green onions, sliced	2
2 tsp	balsamic vinegar	10 mL
	Salt and freshly ground black pepper	
2 tbsp	chopped fresh basil or mint	25 mL
2 tbsp	lightly toasted pine nuts (optional)	25 mL

This colorful vegetable medley is a great summer side dish.

SERVES 4

1. In a large nonstick skillet, heat oil over high heat. Add zucchini and cook, stirring, for 1 minute. Add cherry tomatoes, cumin, if using, green onions and balsamic vinegar. Cook, stirring, for 1 to 2 minutes or until zucchini is tender-crisp and tomatoes are heated through. Season with salt and pepper to taste.

2. Sprinkle with basil and pine nuts, if using, and serve immediately.

Tip

- To toast the pine nuts, place in dry skillet over medium heat, stirring, for 3 to 4 minutes.

Nutritional Analysis (Per Serving)
- Calories: 71
- Protein: 2.3 g
- Fat: 4.5 g
- Carbohydrates: 7.2 g
- Fiber: 2.4 g
- Sodium: 9 mg
- Cholesterol: 0 mg

Tomatoes Stuffed with Spinach and Ricotta Cheese

4 cups	fresh spinach	1 L
4	medium tomatoes	4
2$\frac{1}{2}$ tsp	vegetable oil	12 mL
2 tsp	crushed garlic	10 mL
$\frac{2}{3}$ cup	chopped onion	150 mL
$\frac{2}{3}$ cup	ricotta cheese	150 mL
	Salt and pepper	

TOPPING

1 tbsp	dry bread crumbs	15 mL
1 tbsp	chopped fresh parsley	15 mL
1 tsp	margarine	5 mL
1 tsp	grated Parmesan cheese	5 mL

Make Ahead

Make early in day and refrigerate. Bake just prior to serving.

SERVES 4

Preheat oven to 350°F (180°C) • Baking dish sprayed with nonstick vegetable spray

1. Rinse spinach and shake off excess water. With just the water clinging to leaves, cook until wilted. Squeeze out excess moisture; chop and set aside.

2. Slice off tops of tomatoes. Scoop out pulp, leaving shell of tomato intact. (Reserve pulp for another use.)

3. In nonstick skillet, heat oil; sauté garlic and onion until softened. Remove from heat. Add spinach, cheese, and salt and pepper to taste; mix well. Fill tomatoes with cheese mixture and place in baking dish.

4. *Topping:* Combine bread crumbs, parsley, margarine and cheese; sprinkle over tomatoes. Bake for 15 minutes or until heated through and topping is golden brown.

Tips

- For a different texture, try crushed bran cereal for the topping instead of bread crumbs.

- Use cottage cheese instead of ricotta to reduce the calories.

- If frozen spinach is used, use $\frac{2}{3}$ cup (150 mL) cooked and well drained.

- When using margarine, choose a soft (non-hydrogenated) version to limit consumption of trans fats.

Nutritional Analysis (Per Serving)
- Calories: 132
- Protein: 7 g
- Fat: 6 g
- Carbohydrates: 13 g
- Fiber: 3 g
- Sodium: 108 mg
- Cholesterol: 12 mg

Stuffed Tomatoes or Zucchini

6	small tomatoes or 2 large zucchini	6

PROVENÇAL STUFFING

2	medium onions, finely chopped	2
2	cloves garlic, finely chopped	2
2 cups	packed fresh parsley, finely chopped	500 mL
1 tbsp	olive oil	15 mL
3	slices white bread, crusts removed	3
1/3 cup	grated Parmesan cheese	75 mL

MUSHROOM STUFFING

1	medium onion, finely chopped	1
1 tbsp	butter	15 mL
1/2 lb	mushrooms, chopped (about 15)	250 g
1/2 cup	beef broth	125 mL
1 tbsp	chopped fresh dill (or 1 tsp/5 mL dried dillweed)	15 mL
3	slices white bread, crusts removed	3
	Salt and black pepper	

SERVES 6

Preheat oven to 350°F (180°C) • Baking pan

1. Halve tomatoes and hollow out using small spoon or melon baller. Slice each zucchini into six 1-inch (2.5 cm) pieces; hollow out, leaving bottom 1/4 inch (5 mm) thick. (If desired, before slicing zucchini, use vegetable peeler to cut lengthwise strips down zucchini to give striped effect.) Stuff with 1 of the stuffing mixtures.

2. *Provençal Stuffing:* In a skillet, sauté onions, garlic and parsley in olive oil for about 3 minutes; remove from heat. Finely chop bread; add to onion mixture. Stir in cheese. Fill vegetables; place in baking pan. Bake in preheated oven for 10 to 15 minutes or until heated through and lightly browned.

3. *Mushroom Stuffing:* In a skillet, sauté onion in butter for 2 minutes. Add mushrooms; cook for about 2 minutes longer. Stir in beef broth and dill; bring to a boil, stirring until slightly thickened. Remove from heat. Finely chop bread; stir into mushroom mixture. Season with salt and pepper to taste. Fill vegetables; place in baking pan. Bake in preheated oven for 10 to 15 minutes or until heated through.

Tips

- When making the Mushroom Stuffing in this recipe, experiment with the many varieties of mushrooms that are now readily available.

- Use this recipe to take advantage of fresh tomatoes or zucchini when these vegetables are in season.

STUFFED TOMATOES
Nutritional Analysis (Per Serving)
- Calories: 112
- Protein: 5 g
- Fat: 4 g
- Carbohydrates: 14 g
- Fiber: 3 g
- Sodium: 191 mg
- Cholesterol: 5 mg

STUFFED ZUCCHINIS
Nutritional Analysis (Per Serving)
- Calories: 62
- Protein: 2 g
- Fat: 2 g
- Carbohydrates: 9 g
- Fiber: 1 g
- Sodium: 191 mg
- Cholesterol: 5 mg

Summer Zucchini

4	young zucchini, preferably 2 each of green and yellow, less than 6 inches (15 cm) in length	4
3 tbsp	olive oil	45 mL
¼ tsp	salt	1 mL
¼ tsp	freshly ground black pepper	1 mL
1	red bell pepper, cut into thick strips	1
3	green onions, chopped	3
1 tbsp	freshly squeezed lemon juice	15 mL
	Few sprigs fresh basil and/or parsley, chopped	

SERVES 4

1. Trim ends of zucchini and cut into ¾-inch (2 cm) chunks. Set aside.
2. In a large frying pan, heat olive oil over high heat for 30 seconds. Add salt and pepper and stir. Add zucchini chunks and red pepper strips. Stir-fry for 4 to 6 minutes until the zucchini have browned on both sides and the red pepper has softened. Add green onions and stir-fry for 30 seconds. Transfer to a serving dish and drizzle evenly with lemon juice. Garnish with basil and/or parsley and serve immediately.

Nutritional Analysis (Per Serving)
- Calories: 121
- Protein: 1.9 g
- Fat: 10.4 g
- Carbohydrates: 6.9 g
- Fiber: 2.5 g
- Sodium: 151 mg
- Cholesterol: 0 mg

Zucchini with Bacon

12	small zucchini (about 3 lbs/1.5 kg)	12
1 tsp	salt	5 mL
½ lb	pancetta or back bacon, cut into thin strips	250 g
1	onion, sliced	1
3	cloves garlic, minced	3
2 tbsp	chopped flat-leaf parsley	25 mL
2 tbsp	chopped marjoram or oregano	25 mL
1 lb	plum tomatoes, peeled, seeded and chopped or 4 cups (1 L) canned plum tomatoes, seeded, drained and chopped	500 g
	Salt and freshly ground black pepper to taste	

SERVES 4 TO 6

1. Peel zucchini and slice into ¼-inch (5 mm) rounds. Put in a colander set in the sink; sprinkle with salt. Let stand 1 hour. Rinse under cold running water. Pat dry with paper towels.
2. In a large skillet set over medium heat, cook pancetta and onion for 5 minutes or until onion is softened. Stir in garlic, parsley and marjoram; cook, stirring occasionally, for 10 minutes or until well browned.
3. Stir in tomatoes, zucchini, a pinch of salt and plenty of freshly ground black pepper. Cook, stirring occasionally, for 15 minutes or until zucchini is tender. Serve immediately.

Tip
- This dish is very good with chicken.

Here is a preparation that will put to good use all those baskets full of small zucchini your garden produces each summer.

Nutritional Analysis (Per Serving)
- Calories: 133
- Protein: 14.7 g
- Fat: 3.0 g
- Carbohydrates: 13.7
- Fiber: 4.1 g
- Sodium: 1126 mg
- Cholesterol: 26 mg

Zucchini Boats Stuffed with Cheese and Vegetables

2 cups	fresh spinach	500 mL
16	medium mushrooms	16
1 tbsp	vegetable oil	15 mL
2 tsp	crushed garlic	10 mL
¼ cup	finely chopped onions	50 mL
⅓ cup	ricotta cheese	75 mL
1 tbsp	grated Parmesan cheese	15 mL
	Salt and pepper	

Make Ahead

Prepare early in day and refrigerate. Bake just before serving.

SERVES 8
Preheat oven to 400°F (200°C)

1. Rinse spinach and shake off excess water. With just the water clinging to leaves, cook until wilted. Drain and squeeze out excess moisture; chop finely and set aside.

2. Remove stems from mushrooms. Place caps on baking sheet. Dice half of the stems and reserve. Use remaining stems for another use.

3. In small nonstick saucepan, heat oil; sauté garlic, onions and diced stems until softened. Add spinach and cook for 1 minute. Remove from heat.

4. Add ricotta, half the Parmesan, and salt and pepper to taste; mix well and carefully fill mushroom caps. Sprinkle with remaining Parmesan. Bake for 8 to 10 minutes or just until mushrooms release their liquid.

Tip

- Cherry tomatoes can replace the mushrooms.

Nutritional Analysis (Per Serving)
- Calories: 51
- Protein: 2 g
- Fat: 3 g
- Carbohydrates: 3 g
- Fiber: 1 g
- Sodium: 33 mg
- Cholesterol: 5 mg

Grilled Vegetables

2	large bell peppers, any color, halved and seeded	2
1	eggplant, cut lengthwise into thin slices	1
	Olive oil	
	Salt and freshly ground black pepper	

Vegetables such as onion, garlic and bell pepper contain natural sugars that caramelize when grilled, giving a depth of flavor that pan sautéing could never match.

SERVES 4
Preheat barbecue

1. Brush pepper halves and eggplant slices lightly with olive oil.
2. On a rack or in a basket, grill pepper halves over medium-high heat for 20 minutes or until skin is blackened. Remove peppers to a paper or plastic bag until cool. Peel away blackened skin and cut into smaller pieces.
3. Grill sliced eggplant over medium-high heat, turning once, for 4 minutes per side or until flesh is tender. Season lightly with salt and pepper.

Nutritional Analysis (Per Serving)
- Calories: 86
- Protein: 2.1 g
- Fat: 3.8 g
- Carbohydrates: 13.1 g
- Fiber: 4.8 g
- Sodium: 6 mg
- Cholesterol: 0 mg

Sautéed Vegetables

1/4 cup	sliced onion	50 mL
1 tbsp	olive oil	15 mL
1 cup	broccoli florets	250 mL
1 cup	cauliflower florets	250 mL
1 cup	cubed zucchini	250 mL
1/2 cup	chopped raw beets	125 mL
1 cup	chicken broth	250 mL
1 cup	chopped Swiss chard or spinach (optional)	250 mL
1 cup	chopped tomatoes	250 mL
2 tbsp	water	25 mL
2 tsp	cornstarch	10 mL
	Salt and black pepper to taste	

Chopped beets add an attractive rosy red color to this dish.

SERVES 6

1. In a large skillet over medium-high heat, cook onion in hot oil for about 5 minutes. Add broccoli, cauliflower, zucchini, beets and chicken broth. Cook, covered, for about 3 minutes or until tender-crisp.
2. Stir in chard, if using, and tomatoes. Mix together water, cornstarch and seasonings; stir into vegetable mixture. Cook for about 2 minutes or until thickened.

Tip
- This colorful array of vegetables will add eye appeal to many dishes while providing lots of fiber, vitamins and minerals. The vitamin C in this recipe will enhance the absorption of iron from non-meat sources.

Nutritional Analysis (Per Serving)
- Calories: 53
- Protein: 2 g
- Fat: 3 g
- Carbohydrates: 6 g
- Fiber: 2 g
- Sodium: 124 mg
- Cholesterol: 0 mg

Company Vegetables with Toasted Almonds

4 cups	cauliflower florets (½ head)	1 L
4 cups	broccoli florets	1 L
1	red bell pepper, cut into cubes	1
1	yellow or orange bell pepper, cut into cubes	1

TOPPING

3 tbsp	butter, divided	45 mL
⅓ cup	sliced almonds	75 mL
1	clove garlic, minced	1
1 tbsp	freshly squeezed lemon juice	15 mL
2 tbsp	chopped fresh parsley	25 mL
	Salt and freshly ground black pepper	

> *Put your microwave oven to good use when preparing vegetables to serve a crowd. Arrange vegetables in dish, ready to pop in the microwave shortly before serving.*

SERVES 6 TO 8

10-cup (2.5 L) shallow baking dish or large (12-inch/30 cm) microwave-safe platter (see tip, below)

1. In baking dish or platter, alternately arrange cauliflower and broccoli, with broccoli stalks toward the outside, around outer edge of dish. Mound pepper cubes in center. Add ⅓ cup (75 mL) water. Cover with lid or plastic wrap and turn back one corner to vent. Microwave on High for 6 to 9 minutes or until vegetables are tender-crisp. Let stand, covered, while preparing topping.

2. *Topping:* In a small microwave-safe glass bowl, combine 2 tbsp (25 mL) of the butter and almonds. Microwave, uncovered, on High for 1½ to 3 minutes or until almonds are lightly toasted, stirring twice. (Can be done up to 4 hours ahead, if desired.)

3. Just before serving, add remaining butter and garlic to toasted almonds. Microwave, uncovered, on High for 45 to 60 seconds or until fragrant. Stir in lemon juice. Carefully drain water from vegetables (a plate set on top will hold vegetables in place).

4. Pour almond butter over top. Sprinkle with parsley. Season with salt and pepper to taste. Serve immediately.

Tips

- Test first to see if the dish called for fits comfortably in your microwave oven. If not, divide vegetable mixture among two 9-inch (23 cm) microwave-safe pie plates. Cover with inverted plate or plastic wrap with one corner turned back to vent. Microwave each plate on High for 4 to 6 minutes.

- Serve almond butter with other steamed vegetables, such as Brussels sprouts.

Nutritional Analysis (Per Serving)
- Calories: 112
- Protein: 4.1 g
- Fat: 7.6 g
- Carbohydrates: 9.6 g
- Fiber: 4.4 g
- Sodium: 83 mg
- Cholesterol: 13 mg

Teriyaki Sesame Vegetables

1½ tsp	vegetable oil	7 mL
1 tsp	crushed garlic	5 mL
Half	large sweet red or yellow pepper, sliced thinly	Half
Half	large sweet green pepper, sliced thinly	Half
1½ cups	snow peas	375 mL
1	large carrot, sliced thinly	1
½ tsp	sesame seeds	2 mL

SAUCE

1 tsp	crushed garlic	5 mL
1 tbsp	soya sauce	15 mL
1 tbsp	rice wine vinegar or white wine vinegar	15 mL
½ tsp	minced gingerroot	2 mL
½ tsp	sesame oil	2 mL
1 tbsp	water	15 mL
1 tbsp	brown sugar	15 mL
1½ tsp	vegetable oil	7 mL

SERVES 4

1. *Sauce:* In small saucepan, combine garlic, soya sauce, vinegar, ginger, sesame oil, water, sugar and vegetable oil; cook for 3 to 5 minutes or until thickened and syrupy.

2. In large nonstick skillet, heat oil; sauté garlic, red and green peppers, snow peas and carrot, stirring constantly, for 2 minutes.

3. Add sauce; sauté for 2 minutes or just until vegetables are tender-crisp. Place in serving dish and sprinkle with sesame seeds.

Tip

• Remember to cook over high heat and not to overcook.

Nutritional Analysis (Per Serving)

• Calories: 96
• Protein: 2 g
• Fat: 4 g
• Carbohydrates: 12 g
• Fiber: 2 g
• Sodium: 271 mg
• Cholesterol: 0 mg

Carmelo's Summer Vegetable Stew

2 lbs	ripe tomatoes	1 kg
1 tbsp	olive oil	15 mL
1	onion, finely chopped	1
1	large red or green bell pepper, seeded and cut into 1/2-inch (1 cm) pieces	1
2	medium zucchini, cut into 1/2-inch (1 cm) cubes	2
1/2 tsp	salt	2 mL
1/4 tsp	black pepper	1 mL
1/2 tsp	granulated sugar	2 mL
1	egg, beaten	1
	Fresh basil sprigs	

Make Ahead

The stew can be refrigerated, covered, for up to 3 days. Let stand at room temperature for 30 minutes before serving cold, or reheat over medium heat until piping hot.

> *Versions of this vegetable stew, known as pisto, are popular all across Spain, and it's as versatile as it is fresh-tasting. Topped with halved hard-cooked eggs, pisto makes a good vegetarian main course.*

SERVES 6 TO 8

1. Fill a large bowl with cold water. With a sharp knife, cut an "x" in the skin at the base of each tomato. In a large saucepan of boiling water, simmer tomatoes for 1 minute or until tomato skins split. With a slotted spoon, remove tomatoes from saucepan and immediately place in the bowl of cold water.

2. When tomatoes are cool enough to handle, carefully peel off skins. With a sharp knife, cut out stem ends from tomatoes; discard. Chop tomatoes coarsely; set aside.

3. In a large skillet, heat oil over medium-high heat. Add onion and pepper; cook, stirring occasionally, for 3 to 5 minutes or until onion is lightly browned. Add zucchini, salt and pepper; cook, stirring occasionally, for 3 to 5 minutes or until pepper is tender and starting to brown.

4. Add tomatoes. Reduce heat to medium-low; simmer, uncovered and stirring occasionally, for 20 to 30 minutes or until vegetables are tender and most of the liquid has evaporated.

5. Add sugar; stir well. Add egg; cook, stirring, for 2 to 3 minutes or until creamy and slightly thickened. If desired, season to taste with additional salt and pepper. Spoon into a warm serving dish; garnish with basil. Serve at once. (Alternatively, let cool and serve at room temperature, garnished with basil.)

Tip

- Although this is best made in late summer, when local tomatoes are in season, it's almost as good prepared at other times during the year using vine-ripened hothouse tomatoes sold on the stem. Let hothouse tomatoes stand at room temperature for 3 to 5 days until the stems are dry and the tomatoes are fully ripe. Never refrigerate tomatoes or their texture will become woolly.

Nutritional Analysis (Per Serving)
- Calories: 76
- Protein: 3.0 g
- Fat: 3.1 g
- Carbohydrates: 10.9 g
- Fiber: 3.0 g
- Sodium: 185 mg
- Cholesterol: 30 mg

Desserts

Raisin Honey Cookies

$\frac{1}{2}$ cup	water	125 mL
1 cup	raisins	250 mL
$\frac{1}{2}$ cup	vegetable oil	125 mL
$\frac{1}{3}$ cup	honey	75 mL
2	medium eggs	2
$\frac{1}{2}$ tsp	vanilla extract	2 mL
$1\frac{1}{2}$ cups	whole-wheat flour	375 mL
$\frac{1}{2}$ cup	chopped nuts	125 mL
$\frac{1}{4}$ cup	wheat germ	50 mL
1 tsp	cinnamon	5 mL
$\frac{1}{2}$ tsp	baking powder	2 mL
$\frac{1}{4}$ tsp	salt	1 mL
$\frac{1}{8}$ tsp	ground allspice	0.5 mL
$\frac{1}{8}$ tsp	ground cloves	0.5 mL
$\frac{1}{8}$ tsp	ground nutmeg	0.5 mL

MAKES ABOUT 40 COOKIES
Preheat oven to 350°F (180°C) • Baking sheet sprayed with baking spray

1. In a small saucepan, bring water to a boil. Stir in raisins, reduce heat and simmer for 5 minutes. Drain. Cool.
2. In a bowl, beat together oil, honey, eggs and vanilla. Stir in raisins. In another bowl, stir together whole wheat flour, nuts, wheat germ, cinnamon, baking powder, salt, allspice, cloves and nutmeg. Stir into raisin mixture. Drop by teaspoonfuls (5 mL) onto prepared baking sheet.
3. Bake for 8 minutes or until golden.

Nutritional Analysis (Per Cookie)
- Calories: 83
- Protein: 1 g
- Fat: 5 g
- Carbohydrates: 9 g
- Fiber: 0.5 g
- Sodium: 18 mg
- Cholesterol: 16 mg

Cinnamon Ginger Cookies

$\frac{1}{4}$ cup	brown sugar	50 mL
3 tbsp	margarine, melted	45 mL
2 tbsp	molasses	25 mL
2 tbsp	2% yogurt	25 mL
1 tsp	vanilla	5 mL
1 cup	all-purpose flour	250 mL
$\frac{1}{2}$ tsp	baking soda	2 mL
$\frac{1}{2}$ tsp	ginger	2 mL
$\frac{1}{2}$ tsp	cinnamon	2 mL
Pinch	nutmeg	Pinch
$1\frac{1}{2}$ tsp	brown sugar	7 mL

Make Ahead
Dough can be frozen for up to 2 weeks.

MAKES 30 COOKIES
Preheat oven to 350°F (180°C) • Baking sheet sprayed with nonstick vegetable spray

1. In bowl, combine $\frac{1}{4}$ cup (50 mL) brown sugar, margarine, molasses, yogurt and vanilla until well mixed.
2. Combine flour, baking soda, ginger, cinnamon and nutmeg; stir into bowl just until combined.
3. Using teaspoon, form dough into small balls and place on baking sheet. Press flat with fork; sprinkle with $1\frac{1}{2}$ tsp (7 mL) brown sugar. Bake for 10 to 12 minutes or until golden.

Tip
- This cookie dough can be chilled, then rolled out and cut into various patterns.

Nutritional Analysis (Per Cookie)
- Calories: 38
- Protein: 0.5 g
- Fat: 1 g
- Carbohydrates: 6 g
- Fiber: 0 g
- Sodium: 31 mg
- Cholesterol: 0 mg

Sunflower Cookies

½ cup	butter or margarine	125 mL
¾ cup	lightly packed brown sugar	175 mL
¾ cup	granulated sugar	175 mL
1	egg, beaten	1
½ tsp	vanilla	2 mL
½ tsp	baking soda	2 mL
2 tsp	hot water	10 mL
1 cup	unsalted shelled sunflower seeds	250 mL
½ cup	all-purpose flour	125 mL
½ cup	whole-wheat flour	125 mL
½ cup	large-flake rolled oats	125 mL
½ cup	chocolate chips	125 mL
½ cup	raisins	125 mL
⅓ cup	natural wheat bran	75 mL
⅓ cup	wheat germ	75 mL
1 tsp	salt	5 mL

The crunchiness of nuts and seeds and the sweetness of raisins and chocolate chips make this healthy cookie one that everyone will enjoy.

MAKES 60 COOKIES

Preheat oven to 350°F (180°C) • Cookie sheets, lightly greased

1. In a large bowl, cream butter, brown sugar and granulated sugar until fluffy. Stir in egg, vanilla and baking soda dissolved in hot water. Add sunflower seeds, flours, oats, chocolate chips, raisins, bran, wheat germ and salt; combine thoroughly.

2. Drop batter a spoonful at a time onto lightly greased or nonstick cookie sheets. Bake in preheated oven for about 10 minutes.

Tips

- Almost all cookies are ideal for freezing. They take up little space and thaw quickly. To freeze, bake cookies, cool, then wrap tightly in plastic wrap.

- Since sunflower seeds are high in fat, check them for freshness before using to ensure that they haven't become rancid.

- The nuts, seeds and raisins combined with chocolate chips make these cookies particularly appetizing and delicious. Serve with a cold glass of milk for a great after-school snack.

Nutritional Analysis (Per Cookie)
- Calories: 69
- Protein: 1 g
- Fat: 3 g
- Carbohydrates: 9 g
- Fiber: 1 g
- Sodium: 63 mg
- Cholesterol: 8 mg

Peanut Butter Chocolate Chip Cookies

½ cup	brown sugar	125 mL
⅓ cup	granulated sugar	75 mL
⅓ cup	peanut butter	75 mL
⅓ cup	2% milk	75 mL
¼ cup	soft margarine	50 mL
1	egg	1
1 tsp	vanilla	5 mL
½ cup	all-purpose flour	125 mL
⅓ cup	whole wheat flour	75 mL
1 tsp	baking soda	5 mL
⅓ cup	chocolate chips	75 mL
¼ cup	raisins	50 mL

Make Ahead

Dough can be frozen up to
2 weeks. Bake just before eating
for best flavor.

MAKES 40 COOKIES
Preheat oven to 350°F (180°C) • Baking sheets sprayed with
nonstick vegetable spray

1. In large bowl or food processor, beat together
   brown and granulated sugars, peanut butter,
   milk, margarine, egg and vanilla until well
   blended.
2. Combine all-purpose and whole wheat flours
   and baking soda; add to bowl and mix just
   until incorporated. Do not overmix. Stir in
   chocolate chips and raisins.
3. Drop by heaping teaspoonfuls (5 mL) 2 inches
   (5 cm) apart onto baking sheets. Bake for
   12 to 15 minutes or until browned.

Nutritional Analysis (Per Cookie)
- Calories: 70
- Protein: 1 g
- Fat: 3 g
- Carbohydrates: 10 g
- Fiber: 1 g
- Sodium: 51 mg
- Cholesterol: 6 mg

Oatmeal Raisin Cookies

6 tbsp	packed brown sugar	90 mL
¼ cup	butter, softened	50 mL
1	egg	1
1 tsp	vanilla extract	5 mL
½ cup	rolled oats	125 mL
½ cup	raisins	125 mL
¼ cup	whole-wheat flour	50 mL
¼ cup	wheat germ	50 mL
½ tsp	baking powder	2 mL

MAKES ABOUT 18 COOKIES
Preheat oven to 375°F (190°C) • Baking sheet sprayed with
baking spray

1. In a bowl cream brown sugar with butter. Beat
   in egg and vanilla. In another bowl, stir together
   oats, raisins, whole-wheat flour, wheat germ
   and baking powder. Stir into creamed mixture
   just until blended.
2. Drop batter by teaspoonfuls (5 mL) onto
   prepared baking sheet, leaving 2 inches (5 cm)
   between cookies. Bake for 10 to 12 minutes or
   until golden. Cool on wire racks.

Nutritional Analysis (Per Cookie)
- Calories: 49
- Protein: 0.9 g
- Fat: 2 g
- Carbohydrates: 6 g
- Fiber: 0.2
- Sodium: 56 mg
- Cholesterol: 10 mg

Oatmeal Raisin Pecan Cookies

½ cup	brown sugar	125 mL
¼ cup	soft margarine	50 mL
1	egg	1
1 tsp	vanilla	5 mL
½ cup	rolled oats	125 mL
¼ cup	whole wheat flour	50 mL
¼ cup	wheat germ	50 mL
¼ cup	pecan pieces	50 mL
¼ cup	raisins	50 mL
½ tsp	baking powder	2 mL

Make Ahead

Dough can be frozen for up to 2 weeks.

MAKES 30 COOKIES
Preheat oven to 350°F (180°C) • Baking sheets sprayed with nonstick vegetable spray

1. In large bowl or food processor, beat together sugar, margarine, egg and vanilla until well blended.
2. Add rolled oats, flour, wheat germ, pecans, raisins and baking powder; mix just until incorporated.
3. Drop by heaping teaspoonfuls (5 mL) 2 inches (5 cm) apart onto baking sheets. Bake for 12 to 15 minutes or until browned.

Tip
- These cookies are soft and chewy if baked for a shorter time, crisp if baked longer.

Nutritional Analysis (Per Cookie)
- Calories: 57
- Protein: 1 g
- Fat: 3 g
- Carbohydrates: 8 g
- Fiber: 0 g
- Sodium: 27 mg
- Cholesterol: 7 mg

Oatmeal Lace Pennies

1 cup	old-fashioned rolled oats	250 mL
1 cup	granulated sugar	250 mL
3 tbsp	all-purpose flour	45 mL
¼ tsp	baking powder	1 mL
½ tsp	salt	2 mL
1	egg, beaten	1
½ cup	margarine or butter, melted	125 mL
½ tsp	vanilla	2 mL

MAKES ABOUT 66 COOKIES
Preheat oven to 350°F (180°C) • Cookie sheet lined with foil, bright side up

1. In a bowl, mix together oats, sugar, flour, baking powder and salt.
2. In another bowl, beat egg, margarine and vanilla. Add flour mixture and mix well. (If dough seems too soft, chill for 15 to 20 minutes to firm.)
3. Drop by rounded teaspoonfuls (5 mL), about 2 inches (5 cm) apart, onto prepared cookie sheet. Bake in preheated oven for 8 to 10 minutes. Cool for 2 minutes on foil, then transfer to wire racks to cool completely.

Nutritional Analysis (Per Cookie)
- Calories: 32
- Protein: 0 g
- Fat: 2 g
- Carbohydrates: 4 g
- Fiber: 0 g
- Sodium: 32 mg
- Cholesterol: 7 mg

Oatmeal Orange Coconut Cookies

¼ cup	margarine or butter	50 mL
¼ cup	brown sugar	50 mL
½ cup	granulated sugar	125 mL
1	egg	1
1 tsp	vanilla	5 mL
2 tbsp	orange juice concentrate, thawed	25 mL
½ tsp	grated orange zest	2 mL
⅔ cup	all-purpose flour	150 mL
½ tsp	baking powder	2 mL
½ tsp	baking soda	2 mL
½ tsp	cinnamon	2 mL
1 cup	corn flakes or bran flakes cereal	250 mL
⅔ cup	raisins	150 mL
½ cup	rolled oats	125 mL
¼ cup	coconut	50 mL

Make Ahead

Bake cookies up to a day ahead, keeping tightly covered in a cookie tin. Freeze cookie dough for up to 2 weeks.

MAKES 40 COOKIES

Preheat oven to 350°F (180°C) • Baking sheets sprayed with vegetable spray

1. In large bowl, cream together margarine, brown sugar and granulated sugar. Add egg, vanilla, orange juice concentrate and orange zest and mix well.

2. In another bowl, combine flour, baking powder, baking soda, cinnamon, corn flakes, raisins, rolled oats and coconut just until combined. Add to sugar mixture and mix until just combined

3. Drop by heaping teaspoons (5 mL) onto prepared baking sheets 2 inches (5 cm) apart and press down with back of fork; bake approximately 10 minutes or until browned.

Tips

- Orange juice concentrate gives a more intense flavor than orange juice. Remove some from the package, then refreeze the remainder.

- If using bran flakes cereal, do not use All-Bran or raw bran.

- Replace raisins with dried chopped dates, apricots or prunes.

Nutritional Analysis (Per Cookie)
- Calories: 51
- Protein: 1 g
- Fat: 1 g
- Carbohydrates: 9 g
- Fiber: 0 g
- Sodium: 34 mg
- Cholesterol: 5 mg

Diced Rhubarb Squares

2 cups	all-purpose flour or whole wheat flour or a combination of both	500 mL
2 tsp	baking powder	10 mL
Pinch	salt	Pinch
1 tsp	cinnamon	5 mL
1/2 tsp	nutmeg	2 mL
1/2 tsp	cloves	2 mL
1/2 cup	softened margarine or butter	125 mL
1 cup	lightly packed brown sugar	250 mL
1	egg	1
1/4 cup	milk	50 mL
1 cup	diced rhubarb	250 mL
1 cup	chopped walnuts	250 mL

MAKES ABOUT 40 COOKIES
Preheat oven to 350°F (180°C) • Greased cookie sheet

1. In a bowl, combine flour, baking powder, salt, cinnamon, nutmeg and cloves.
2. In another bowl, beat margarine and sugar until smooth and creamy. Beat in egg until well incorporated. Mix in milk. Add flour mixture and beat until smooth. Fold in rhubarb and walnuts until well combined.
3. Drop by rounded teaspoonfuls (5 mL), 2 inches (5 cm) apart, onto prepared cookie sheet. Bake in preheated oven for 18 to 20 minutes or until crisp and lightly browned. Immediately transfer to wire racks to cool.

Nutritional Analysis (Per Cookie)
- Calories: 83
- Protein: 1 g
- Fat: 4 g
- Carbohydrates: 11 g
- Fiber: 0 g
- Sodium: 48 mg
- Cholesterol: 11 mg

Whole Wheat Spice Cookies

1/4 cup	vegetable oil	50 mL
1/4 cup	molasses	50 mL
1/2 cup	granulated sugar	125 mL
1/4 cup	packed brown sugar	50 mL
2	eggs	2
1/2 cup	whole wheat flour	125 mL
1 1/2 cups	all-purpose flour	375 mL
2 tsp	baking soda	10 mL
1/4 tsp	salt	1 mL
1 tsp	ginger	5 mL
1 tsp	cinnamon	5 mL
1 tsp	cloves	5 mL

MAKES ABOUT 36 COOKIES
Preheat oven to 350°F (180°C) • Lightly greased cookie sheet

1. In a bowl, whisk oil, molasses, sugars and eggs until blended.
2. In a large bowl, mix together flours, baking soda, salt, ginger, cinnamon and cloves. Make a well in the center and add the molasses mixture, mixing until thoroughly blended.
3. Drop by teaspoonfuls (5 mL), about 2 inches (5 cm) apart, onto prepared cookie sheets. Bake in preheated oven for 8 to 10 minutes or until cookies are firm to the touch. Cool on sheets for 5 minutes, then transfer to wire racks to cool completely.

Nutritional Analysis (Per Cookie)
- Calories: 65
- Protein: 1 g
- Fat: 2 g
- Carbohydrates: 11 g
- Fiber: 0 g
- Sodium: 87 mg
- Cholesterol: 12 mg

Sesame Seed Cookies

1½ cups	whole wheat flour	375 mL
1 tsp	baking powder	5 mL
¼ tsp	salt	1 mL
¼ cup	softened margarine or butter	50 mL
¼ cup	liquid honey	50 mL
¼ cup	sesame paste (tahini)	50 mL
½ tsp	almond extract	2 mL
½ cup	sesame seeds, toasted	125 mL

MAKES ABOUT 24 COOKIES
Preheat oven to 350°F (180°C) • Lightly greased cookie sheet

1. In a bowl, mix together flour, baking powder and salt.
2. In another bowl, beat margarine, honey, sesame paste and almond extract until smooth. Add flour mixture and mix well. Stir in sesame seeds.
3. Shape dough into 1-inch (2.5-cm) balls and place about 2 inches (5 cm) apart on prepared cookie sheet. Using the tines of a fork dipped in flour, flatten, or using your hands, mold into crescent shapes. (Wet your hands first, if using to mold the dough.) Bake in preheated oven for 10 to 12 minutes or until lightly browned. Immediately transfer to wire racks to cool.

Nutritional Analysis (Per Cookie)
- Calories: 87
- Protein: 2 g
- Fat: 5 g
- Carbohydrates: 10 g
- Fiber: 2 g
- Sodium: 61 mg
- Cholesterol: 0 mg

Sesame Snap Wafers

⅔ cup	all-purpose flour	150 mL
¼ tsp	baking powder	1 mL
½ cup	margarine or butter, softened	125 mL
1 cup	packed brown sugar	250 mL
1	egg	1
1 tsp	vanilla	5 mL
1¼ cups	sesame seeds, toasted	300 mL

MAKES 72 WAFERS
Preheat oven to 350°F (180°C) • Cookie sheet, lined with parchment paper or lightly greased aluminum foil

1. Combine flour and baking powder.
2. Cream margarine, sugar, egg and vanilla. Add flour mixture. Mix until combined. Stir in seeds.
3. Drop by teaspoonfuls (5 mL) about 2 inches (5 cm) apart onto prepared cookie sheet. Bake for 6 to 9 minutes or until lightly browned. Cool for 5 minutes on sheet, then transfer to rack and cool completely.

Nutritional Analysis (Per Wafer)
- Calories: 43
- Protein: 1 g
- Fat: 3 g
- Carbohydrates: 5 g
- Fiber: 1 g
- Sodium: 20 mg
- Cholesterol: 3 mg

Vanilla Almond Snaps

¾ cup	whole blanched almonds	175 mL
¼ cup	granulated sugar	50 mL
¼ tsp	salt	1 mL
2	egg whites	2
2 tbsp	granulated sugar	25 mL
½ tsp	vanilla extract	2 mL
	Sliced almonds (optional)	

MAKES ABOUT 30 COOKIES
Preheat oven to 275°F (140°C) • Baking sheet lined with parchment paper and sprayed with baking spray

1. In a food processor, grind almonds with ¼ cup (50 mL) sugar and salt until as fine as possible. Transfer to a bowl and set aside.

2. In another bowl, beat egg whites until soft peaks form. Gradually add 2 tbsp (25 mL) sugar, beating until stiff peaks form. Fold in vanilla. Fold into ground nut mixture until blended. Drop by teaspoonfuls (5 mL) onto prepared baking sheet. If desired, sprinkle with a few sliced almonds.

3. Bake for 25 minutes or until golden.

Nutritional Analysis (Per Cookie)
- Calories: 34
- Protein: 0.9 g
- Fat: 2 g
- Carbohydrates: 3 g
- Fiber: 0.3 g
- Sodium: 19 mg
- Cholesterol: 0 mg

Oatmeal Shortbread

¾ cup	all-purpose flour	175 mL
⅔ cup	oats	150 mL
½ cup	cornstarch	125 mL
½ cup	confectioner's (icing) sugar, sifted	125 mL
¾ cup	butter, softened	175 mL

> *Shortbreads are one of the few cookies that are altered significantly when made with margarine.*

MAKES 30 COOKIES
Preheat oven to 300°F (150°C) • Cookie sheet, ungreased • Cookie cutters

1. Combine flour, oats, cornstarch and confectioner's sugar in large bowl. With large spoon, blend in butter. Work with hands until soft, smooth dough forms. Shape into ball. If necessary, refrigerate for 30 minutes or until easy to handle.

2. Roll out dough to ¼-inch (5 mm) thickness. Cut into shapes with cookie cutters. Place on cookie sheet. Decorate if desired. Bake for 15 to 25 minutes or until edges are lightly browned. (Time will depend on cookie size.) Cool for 5 minutes on sheet, then transfer to rack and cool completely. Store in tightly covered container.

Nutritional Analysis (Per Cookie)
- Calories: 76
- Protein: 1 g
- Fat: 5 g
- Carbohydrates: 8 g
- Fiber: 0 g
- Sodium: 45 mg
- Cholesterol: 12 mg

Apricot Date Biscotti

⅓ cup	margarine or butter	75 mL
¾ cup	granulated sugar	175 mL
2	eggs	2
2 tbsp	orange juice concentrate, thawed	25 mL
2 tbsp	water	25 mL
2 tsp	grated orange zest	10 mL
1 tsp	vanilla	5 mL
2⅔ cups	all-purpose flour	650 mL
2¼ tsp	baking powder	11 mL
1 tsp	cinnamon	5 mL
⅔ cup	pitted, dried and chopped dates	150 mL
⅔ cup	chopped dried apricots	150 mL

Make Ahead

Bake cookies up to 2 days ahead for best flavor, keeping tightly covered in cookie tin. Freeze cookie dough for up to 2 weeks.

MAKES 48 COOKIES

Preheat oven to 350°F (180°C) • Baking sheet sprayed with vegetable spray

1. In large bowl, cream together margarine and sugar; add eggs, orange juice concentrate, water, orange zest and vanilla and mix well.

2. In bowl, combine flour, baking powder, cinnamon, dates and apricots; add to wet ingredients and stir just until mixed. Divide dough into 3 portions; shape each portion into a 12-inch (30 cm) long log, 2 inches wide (5 cm), and put on prepared baking sheet. Bake for 20 minutes. Let cool for 10 minutes.

3. Cut logs on an angle into ½-inch (1 cm) thick slices. Put slices flat on baking sheet and bake for another 20 minutes or until lightly browned.

Tips

- Use a serrated knife to cut the logs into slices.

- Dried prunes or raisins can replace or be used in combination with the apricots and dates.

- Orange juice concentrate gives a more intense flavor than just orange juice. Use frozen concentrate, then refreeze the remainder.

Nutritional Analysis (Per Cookie)
- Calories: 62
- Protein: 1 g
- Fat: 1 g
- Carbohydrates: 11 g
- Fiber: 1 g
- Sodium: 19 mg
- Cholesterol: 9 mg

Gingerbread Biscotti

¾ cup	packed brown sugar	175 mL
¼ cup	margarine or butter	50 mL
¼ cup	molasses	50 mL
2	eggs	2
1 tsp	vanilla extract	5 mL
2⅓ cups	all-purpose flour	575 mL
2¼ tsp	baking powder	11 mL
1 tsp	ground cinnamon	5 mL
1 tsp	ground ginger	5 mL
½ tsp	ground allspice	2 mL
¼ tsp	ground nutmeg	1 mL

Make Ahead

Bake up to 1 week in advance, keeping in air-tight containers. Freeze for up to 6 weeks.

MAKES 40 TO 48 COOKIES
Preheat oven to 350°F (180°C) • Baking sheet sprayed with vegetable spray

1. In a food processor or in a bowl with an electric mixer, beat together brown sugar, margarine, molasses, eggs and vanilla until smooth. In a separate bowl, stir together flour, baking powder, cinnamon, ginger, allspice and nutmeg. Add wet ingredients to dry ingredients, mixing just until combined.

2. Divide dough in half. Form each half into a log 12 inches (30 cm) long and 2 inches (5 cm) around; transfer to prepared baking sheet. Bake 20 minutes. Cool 10 minutes.

3. Cut logs on an angle into ½-inch (1 cm) slices. Bake 20 minutes or until lightly browned.

Tips

- To add fiber, use ⅔ cup (150 mL) whole wheat flour and 1⅔ cups (400 mL) all-purpose flour.

- Increase, decrease or omit spices, according to your taste.

- For a decadent treat, melt 2 oz (50 g) semi-sweet chocolate and dip ends of cookies. Let harden.

Nutritional Analysis (Per Cookie)
- Calories: 207
- Protein: 1 g
- Fat: 1 g
- Carbohydrates: 9 g
- Fiber: 0 g
- Sodium: 27 mg
- Cholesterol: 9 mg

Pecan Biscotti

2	eggs	2
¾ cup	granulated sugar	175 mL
⅓ cup	margarine	75 mL
¼ cup	water	50 mL
2 tsp	vanilla	10 mL
1 tsp	almond extract	5 mL
2¾ cups	all-purpose flour	675 mL
½ cup	chopped pecans	125 mL
2¼ tsp	baking powder	11 mL

Make Ahead

Store in an airtight container up to 2 weeks, or freeze for up to 1 month.

MAKES 45 COOKIES
Preheat oven to 350°F (180°C) • Baking sheet sprayed with nonstick vegetable spray

1. In large bowl, blend eggs with sugar; beat in margarine, water, vanilla and almond extract until smooth.

2. Add flour, pecans and baking powder; mix until dough forms ball. Divide dough in half; shape each portion into 12-inch (30 cm) long log and place on baking sheet. Bake for 20 minutes. Let cool for 5 minutes.

3. Cut logs on angle into ½-inch (1 cm) thick slices. Place slices on sides on baking sheet; bake for 20 minutes or until lightly browned.

Nutritional Analysis (Per Cookie)
- Calories: 60
- Protein: 1 g
- Fat: 2 g
- Carbohydrates: 8 g
- Fiber: 0.5 g
- Sodium: 40 mg
- Cholesterol: 9 mg

Lemon Almond Biscotti

1¾ cups	all-purpose flour	425 mL
¾ cup	granulated sugar	175 mL
1 tbsp	baking powder	15 mL
2 tbsp	finely grated lemon zest	25 mL
¾ cup	coarsely chopped almonds	175 mL
2	eggs	2
⅓ cup	olive oil	75 mL
1 tsp	vanilla	5 mL
½ tsp	almond extract	2 mL

MAKES ABOUT 36 COOKIES
Preheat oven to 325°F (160°C) • Greased cookie sheet

1. In a bowl, mix together flour, sugar, baking powder, lemon zest and almonds. Make a well in the center.

2. In another bowl, whisk eggs, oil, vanilla and almond extract. Pour into well and mix until a soft, sticky dough forms.

3. Divide dough in half. Shape into two rolls about 10 inches (25 cm) long. Place about 2 inches (5 cm) apart on prepared cookie sheet. Bake in preheated oven for 20 minutes.

4. Cool on sheet for 5 minutes, then cut into slices ½ inch (1 cm) thick. Return to sheet and bake for 10 minutes. Turn slices over and bake for 10 minutes more. Immediately transfer to wire racks.

Nutritional Analysis (Per Cookie)
- Calories: 78
- Protein: 2 g
- Fat: 4 g
- Carbohydrates: 10 g
- Fiber: 1 g
- Sodium: 24 mg
- Cholesterol: 12 mg

Lemon and Lime Poppy Seed Biscotti

1 cup	granulated sugar	250 mL
1/4 cup	margarine or butter	50 mL
2	eggs	2
1 1/2 tsp	grated lime zest	7 mL
1 1/2 tsp	grated lemon zest	7 mL
2 tbsp	freshly squeezed lime juice	25 mL
2 tbsp	freshly squeezed lemon juice	25 mL
1 tsp	vanilla extract	5 mL
2 1/2 cups	all-purpose flour	625 mL
2 1/4 tsp	baking powder	11 mL
2 tsp	poppy seeds	10 mL

Make Ahead

Store cookies in air-tight containers for up to 1 week, or freeze in air-tight containers for up to 6 weeks.

MAKES ABOUT 40 COOKIES

Preheat oven to 350°F (180°C) • Baking sheet sprayed with vegetable spray

1. In a food processor or in a bowl with an electric mixer, beat sugar, margarine and eggs until smooth. Beat in lime zest, lemon zest, lime juice, lemon juice and vanilla.

2. In a separate bowl, stir together flour, baking powder and poppy seeds. Add wet ingredients to dry ingredients, mixing just until combined. Dough will be stiff.

3. Divide dough in half. Form each half into a log 12 inches (30 cm) long and 1 1/2 inches (4 cm) around; transfer to prepared baking sheet. Bake 20 minutes. Cool 10 minutes.

4. Cut logs on an angle into 1/2-inch (1 cm) slices. Bake 20 minutes.

Tips

- If desired, omit lime zest and juice and use double the quantity of lemon zest and juice.

- If dough is sticky when forming into logs, try wetting your fingers.

Nutritional Analysis (Per Cookie)
- Calories: 61
- Protein: 1 g
- Fat: 1 g
- Carbohydrates: 12 g
- Fiber: 0 g
- Sodium: 28 mg
- Cholesterol: 0 mg

Peanut Butter Granola Rolls

³⁄₄ cup	peanut butter	175 mL
¹⁄₄ cup	apple butter	50 mL
¹⁄₄ cup	raisins	50 mL
1¹⁄₂ cups	granola	375 mL
¹⁄₄ cup	water	50 mL
2 tbsp	wheat germ	25 mL

MAKES ABOUT 40 ROLLS

1. In a food processor, blend peanut butter, apple butter and raisins until raisins are finely chopped. Alternately add granola and water, making three additions of granola and two of water, and processing until mixture comes together.

2. Roll each 1 tbsp (15 mL) of mixture into a ball. Roll balls in wheat germ.

Tips

- Use a natural, all-peanut type of peanut butter.
- Store-bought granola can be high in fat; be sure to buy a lower-fat variety.

Nutritional Analysis (Per Roll)
- Calories: 52
- Protein: 2 g
- Fat: 3 g
- Carbohydrates: 4 g
- Fiber: 0.5 g
- Sodium: 20 mg
- Cholesterol: 0 mg

Cocoa Kisses

3	egg whites, at room temperature	3
1 cup	granulated sugar	250 mL
¹⁄₈ tsp	salt	0.5 mL
1 tsp	vanilla extract	5 mL
3 tbsp	cocoa	45 mL
¹⁄₂ cup	chopped pecans	125 mL

MAKES ABOUT 40 KISSES
Preheat oven to 250°F (120°C) • Baking sheet sprayed with baking spray

1. In a large bowl, beat egg whites until soft peaks form; gradually add sugar and salt, beating until mixture is glossy and stiff peaks form. Beat in vanilla. Sift cocoa into bowl; fold into meringue along with pecans.

2. Put mixture in a pastry bag fitted with star tip; pipe small kisses onto prepared baking sheet (alternatively, drop mixture by teaspoonfuls/5 mL onto baking sheet). Bake 1 hour or until firm and dry.

Tip

- It's easier to separate eggs when they're cold, but egg whites beat to a greater volume when at room temperature.

Nutritional Analysis (Per Kiss)
- Calories: 35
- Protein: 1 g
- Fat: 1 g
- Carbohydrates: 6 g
- Fiber: 0.3 g
- Sodium: 8 mg
- Cholesterol: 0 mg

Raspberry Cheesecake

1 cup	5% ricotta cheese	250 mL
1 cup	low-fat cottage cheese	250 mL
1/3 cup	granulated sugar or 1/4 cup (50 mL) fructose	75 mL
1/3 cup	low-fat yogurt	75 mL
2	eggs	2
1 tsp	grated lemon zest	5 mL
1/2 tsp	vanilla extract	2 mL
1 tbsp	all-purpose flour	15 mL
1 1/2 tsp	cornstarch	7 mL
1 cup	raspberries	250 mL
	Raspberry purée (optional)	

SERVES 12

Preheat oven to 350°F (180°C) • 8-inch (2 L) springform pan sprayed with baking spray

1. In a food processor, beat together ricotta cheese, cottage cheese, sugar, yogurt, eggs, lemon zest and vanilla until smooth. Beat in flour and cornstarch. Transfer to a bowl; gently fold in raspberries. Pour into prepared pan.

2. Bake 35 minutes or until a tester inserted in center comes out clean. Cool on a wire rack. Chill. Serve plain or, if desired, with raspberry purée.

Nutritional Analysis (Per Serving)
- Calories: 91
- Protein: 6 g
- Fat: 3 g
- Carbohydrates: 9 g
- Fiber: 0.5 g
- Sodium: 109 mg
- Cholesterol: 57 mg

La Costa Cheesecake with Strawberry Sauce

CHEESECAKE

2 cups	low-fat cottage cheese	500 mL
3 tbsp	fructose	45 mL
2 tbsp	lemon juice	25 mL
2 tsp	vanilla extract	10 mL
2	eggs	2
2 tbsp	low-fat milk powder	25 mL

STRAWBERRY SAUCE

2 cups	strawberries	500 mL
1	ripe banana	1
	Fresh strawberries (optional)	

SERVES 12

Preheat oven to 325°F (160°C) • 9-inch (23 cm) pie plate

1. *Make the cheesecake:* In a blender or food processor, combine cottage cheese, fructose, lemon juice, vanilla and eggs; purée until smooth. Add milk powder; blend just until mixed. Pour into pie plate. Set pie plate in larger pan; pour in enough hot water to come half way up sides. Bake 30 to 35 minutes. Remove from water bath; cool on wire rack. Chill.

2. *Make the strawberry sauce:* In a blender or food processor, purée strawberries with banana until smooth.

3. To serve, drizzle 2 tbsp (25 mL) strawberry sauce over each slice of cheesecake. Garnish with strawberries, if desired.

Nutritional Analysis (Per Serving)
- Calories: 84
- Protein: 6 g
- Fat: 2 g
- Carbohydrates: 9 g
- Fiber: 1 g
- Sodium: 168 mg
- Cholesterol: 53 mg

Individual Miniature Cheesecakes

1 cup	5% ricotta cheese	250 mL
1 cup	low-fat cottage cheese	250 mL
$\frac{1}{3}$ cup	granulated sugar	75 mL
1	medium egg	1
$\frac{1}{4}$ cup	light sour cream	50 mL
$\frac{1}{2}$ tsp	cornstarch	2 mL
$\frac{1}{8}$ tsp	vanilla extract	0.5 mL
	Fruit purée (optional)	

SERVES 10

Preheat oven to 350°F (180°C) • Line 10 muffin cups with muffin paper cups

1. In a food processor, combine ricotta cheese, cottage cheese and sugar; purée until smooth. Beat in egg. Blend in sour cream, cornstarch and vanilla until well mixed. Divide batter among muffin cups. Set muffin tin in larger pan; pour in enough hot water to come half way up sides. Bake 30 to 35 minutes or until tester inserted in center comes out clean. Remove from water bath; cool on wire rack. Chill.

2. Serve with fruit purée, if desired.

Tips

- Substitute one 8-oz (250 g) package of light cream cheese for the ricotta cheese.

- Decorate cheesecakes with berries and sliced fresh fruit; glaze with 2 tbsp (25 mL) no-sugar-added apricot spread.

Nutritional Analysis (Per Serving)
- Calories: 127
- Protein: 6 g
- Fat: 8 g
- Carbohydrates: 9 g
- Fiber: 0 g
- Sodium: 268 mg
- Cholesterol: 42 mg

Apple Strudel with Cinnamon Sauce

1¼ lbs	apples (about 4)	625 g
1 tbsp	fructose	15 mL
½ tsp	cinnamon	2 mL
¼ tsp	nutmeg	1 mL
¼ cup	raisins (optional)	50 mL
4	sheets phyllo pastry	4

CINNAMON SAUCE (OPTIONAL)

2 tsp	cornstarch or arrowroot	10 mL
1 tbsp	water	15 mL
1 cup	apple cider	250 mL
	Icing sugar	

SERVES 8

Preheat oven to 400°F (200°C) • Baking sheet

1. Peel, core and slice apples. In a bowl toss apple slices with fructose, cinnamon, nutmeg and, if desired, raisins.

2. Layer phyllo sheets one on top of the other. Put apple filling on phyllo, along short end. Roll up carefully. Tuck ends under; transfer to baking sheet. Bake 25 to 30 minutes or until golden. Meanwhile, make the sauce, if desired.

3. *Cinnamon sauce:* Dissolve cornstarch in water. In a small saucepan, bring apple cider to a boil; whisk in dissolved cornstarch. Cook, whisking, until sauce thickens.

4. Dust strudel with sifted icing sugar; serve sliced strudel with warm sauce.

Nutritional Analysis (Per Serving)
- Calories: 52
- Protein: 2 g
- Fat: 3 g
- Carbohydrates: 4 g
- Fiber: 2.3 g
- Sodium: 20 mg
- Cholesterol: 0 mg

Maple Flan with Walnuts

2	egg whites	2
1	egg	1
2½ tbsp	maple syrup	32 mL
1 tsp	vanilla extract	5 mL
1 tsp	maple extract	5 mL
1½ cups	2% milk	375 mL
	Toasted chopped nuts (optional)	
	Cinnamon Cream (optional) (see recipe, page 366)	

SERVES 6

Preheat oven to 325°F (160°C) • 4-cup (1 L) soufflé or casserole dish

1. In a bowl whisk together egg whites, whole egg, maple syrup, vanilla and maple extract until smooth. Gradually add milk, whisking constantly. Pour into soufflé dish.

2. Set dish in larger pan; pour in enough hot water to come halfway up sides. Bake for 60 minutes or until set. Remove from water bath; cool on wire rack. Chill.

3. Serve with toasted chopped nuts and/or cinnamon cream, if desired.

Nutritional Analysis (Per Serving)
- Calories: 87
- Protein: 4 g
- Fat: 3 g
- Carbohydrates: 10 g
- Fiber: 0 g
- Sodium: 65 mg
- Cholesterol: 54 mg

Pumpkin Flan

¾ cup	canned pumpkin	175 mL
2½ tbsp	fructose	32 mL
2	egg whites	2
1	egg	1
½ tsp	almond extract	2 mL
½ tsp	vanilla extract	2 mL
¼ tsp	cinnamon	1 mL
⅛ tsp	ground cloves	0.5 mL
1 cup	2% milk	250 mL

CINNAMON CREAM

1 cup	5% ricotta cheese	250 mL
4 tsp	maple syrup or honey	20 mL
¾ tsp	cinnamon	4 mL

SERVES 6

Preheat oven to 325°F (160°C) • 4-cup (1 L) soufflé or casserole dish

1. In a bowl, beat pumpkin, fructose, egg whites, whole egg, almond extract, vanilla extract, cinnamon and cloves until smooth. In a saucepan, heat milk until almost boiling; remove from heat. Whisk hot milk into pumpkin mixture. Pour into dish.
2. Set dish in larger pan; pour in enough hot water to come halfway up sides. Bake for 40 minutes or until set. Remove from water bath; cool on wire rack. Chill.
3. *Make the cinnamon cream:* In a food processor, purée ricotta, maple syrup and cinnamon until smooth. Serve with flan.

Nutritional Analysis (Per Serving)
- Calories: 111
- Protein: 6 g
- Fat: 3 g
- Carbohydrates: 13 g
- Fiber: 1.1 g
- Sodium: 75 mg
- Cholesterol: 60 mg

Frozen Jamoca Mousse

1 cup	5% ricotta cheese	250 mL
2 cups	low-fat yogurt	500 mL
½ cup	fructose	125 mL
4 tsp	cocoa	20 mL
2 tsp	instant coffee granules	10 mL
1 tsp	vanilla extract	5 mL

SERVES 12

1. In a food processor or blender, purée ricotta, yogurt, fructose, cocoa, coffee granules and vanilla until smooth.
2. In an ice cream maker, freeze according to manufacturer's directions.

Tips
- Buy extra-smooth ricotta for the smoothest mousse.
- If you don't have an ice cream maker, pour into a baking dish and freeze until solid. Break into small pieces; in a food processor, pulse on and off until smooth. Store in freezer until ready to serve.

Nutritional Analysis (Per Serving)
- Calories: 77
- Protein: 3 g
- Fat: 2 g
- Carbohydrates: 11 g
- Fiber: 0 g
- Sodium: 39 mg
- Cholesterol: 7 mg

Fresh Fruit Sorbet

2¹/₂ cups	chopped peeled soft fresh fruit (bananas, peaches, strawberries, etc.)	625 mL

SERVES 4 TO 6

1. Spread fruit on baking sheet and freeze. Purée frozen fruit in food processor and serve immediately.

Tips

- Try a combination of fresh fruits.
- Best if served immediately. If refreezing, purée again before serving.

Nutritional Analysis (Per Serving)
- Calories: 40
- Protein: 0 g
- Fat: 0 g
- Carbohydrates: 10 g
- Fiber: 1 g
- Sodium: 0 mg
- Cholesterol: 0 mg

Frozen Orange Cream

1 tbsp	grated orange zest	15 mL
1¹/₃ cups	orange juice	325 mL
²/₃ cup	skim milk	150 mL

SERVES 4

1. In a food processor or blender, purée orange zest, orange juice and milk.

2. In an ice cream maker, freeze according to manufacturer's directions.

Tips

- This makes an excellent palate cleanser between courses of a meal, as well as a refreshing dessert.
- If you don't have an ice cream maker, pour into a baking dish and freeze until solid. Break into small pieces; in a food processor, pulse on and off until smooth. Store in freezer until ready to serve.

Nutritional Analysis (Per Serving)
- Calories: 49
- Protein: 2 g
- Fat: 0.1 g
- Carbohydrates: 10 g
- Fiber: 0 g
- Sodium: 22 mg
- Cholesterol: 1 mg

Contributing Authors

Julia Aitken's Easy Entertaining Cookbook
Julia Aitken
Recipes from this book can be found on pages 24, 27, 34 (bottom), 36, 37 (top), 43, 65 (bottom), 80, 88, 100, 130, 155, 191, 232 (bottom), 258, 259, 260, 283, 284, 306 (bottom), 314 (bottom), 319 (bottom), 326 (top), 348

The New Vegetarian Gourmet
Byron Ananoglu
Recipes from this book can be found on pages 56, 59 (top), 320

125 Best Vegetarian Recipes
Byron Ayanoglu
Recipes from this book can be found on pages 28 (top), 44 (top), 57 (top), 82 (top), 89, 91 (bottom), 92 (top), 94, 105 (top), 313, 314 (top), 318, 321, 322, 324 (bottom), 325, 326 (bottom), 328 (top), 334 (top), 336, 343 (top)

Simply Mediterranean Cooking
Byron Ayanoglu and Algis Kemezys
Recipes from this book can be found on pages 82 (bottom), 103 (bottom), 104 (bottom), 106 (bottom), 108 (bottom), 109, 111, 137 (top), 145, 151, 157 (top), 158 (bottom), 164, 166 (bottom), 167 (top), 168, 173, 174, 228, 277 (bottom), 279, 289, 309 (bottom), 329

The 250 Best Cookie Recipes
Esther Brody
Recipes from this book can be found on pages 353 (bottom), 355 (top), 355 (bottom), 356 (top), 360 (bottom)

125 Best Microwave Oven Recipes
Johanna Burkhard
Recipes from this book can be found on pages 160 (top), 276 (bottom), 315, 346

300 Best Comfort Food Recipes
Johanna Burkhard
Recipes from this book can be found on pages 25 (top), 45, 49 (bottom), 53 (top), 54, 55 (bottom), 67 (top), 70, 93 (top), 133, 134 (top), 144 (top), 153, 178, 179, 193 (bottom), 234, 250, 269 (top), 271, 273, 298, 308 (bottom), 312 (top), 340 (bottom)

The Comfort Food Cookbook
Johanna Burkhard
A recipe from this book can be found on page 312

Dietitians of Canada Cook Great Food
Dietitians of Canada
Recipes from this book can be found on pages 19 (bottom), 20 (bottom), 23, 28 (bottom), 29, 32, 42 (top), 50 (top), 55 (top), 61 (top), 61 (bottom), 62 (bottom), 63 (bottom), 66 (bottom), 73 (top), 74 (top), 75 (top), 76 (top), 78 (top), 81, 84 (bottom), 86 (top), 87 (top), 90 (top), 91 (top), 92 (bottom), 96 (bottom), 97 (bottom), 99 (bottom), 102, 104 (top), 106 (top), 112, 118 (top), 123 (top), 124 (top), 127 (top), 128 (bottom), 131 (top), 131, 136 (top), 137 (bottom), 139 (top), 143 (top), 144 (bottom), 146, 147, 148, 149 (bottom), 150 (top), 154 (bottom), 156 (top), 169, 185, 189, 192 (bottom), 194 (top), 195, 197, 201, 202 (bottom), 212, 213, 223 (top), 231 (top), 239 (bottom), 240, 241 (top), 245, 246, 247 (top), 251, 253, 255, 256, 268, 270 (bottom), 278, 280, 281 (bottom), 292, 293, 296, 299, 311 (bottom), 316, 317, 327 (top), 335 (bottom), 340 (top), 342, 345 (bottom), 351

Library and Archives Canada Cataloguing in Publication

The best low-carb cookbook from Robert Rose.

ISBN 0-7788-0117-9

1. Low-carbohydrate diet--Recipes. I. Title.

RM237.73.B48 2005   641.5'6383   C2004-906428-2

Index

More Great Books from Robert Rose

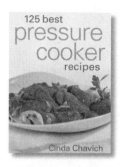

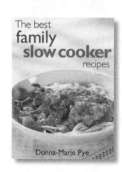

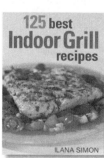

Appliance Cooking

- 125 Best Microwave Oven Recipes
  by Johanna Burkhard

- 125 Best Pressure Cooker Recipes
  by Cinda Chavich

- The 150 Best Slow Cooker Recipes
  by Judith Finlayson

- Delicious & Dependable Slow Cooker Recipes
  by Judith Finlayson

- 125 Best Vegetarian Slow Cooker Recipes
  by Judith Finlayson

- America's Best Slow Cooker Recipes
  by Donna-Marie Pye

- Canada's Best Slow Cooker Recipes
  by Donna-Marie Pye

- The Best Family Slow Cooker Recipes
  by Donna-Marie Pye

- 125 Best Indoor Grill Recipes
  by Ilana Simon

- The Best Convection Oven Cookbook
  by Linda Stephen

- 125 Best Toaster Oven Recipes
  by Linda Stephen

- 250 Best American Bread Machine Baking Recipes
  by Donna Washburn and Heather Butt

- 250 Best Canadian Bread Machine Baking Recipes
  by Donna Washburn and Heather Butt

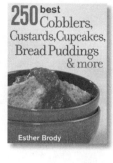

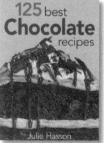

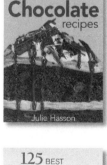

Baking

- 250 Best Cakes & Pies
  by Esther Brody

- 250 Best Cobblers, Custards, Cupcakes, Bread Puddings & More
  by Esther Brody

- 500 Best Cookies, Bars & Squares
  by Esther Brody

- 500 Best Muffin Recipes
  by Esther Brody

- 125 Best Cheesecake Recipes
  by George Geary

- 125 Best Chocolate Recipes
  by Julie Hasson

- 125 Best Chocolate Chip Recipes
  by Julie Hasson

- Cake Mix Magic
  by Jill Snider

- Cake Mix Magic 2
  by Jill Snider

Healthy Cooking

- 125 Best Vegetarian Recipes
  by Byron Ayanoglu
  with contributions from Alexis Kemezys

- The Juicing Bible
  by Pat Crocker and Susan Eagles

- The Smoothies Bible
  by Pat Crocker

- Better Baby Food
  by Daina Kalnins, RD, CNSD and Joanne Saab, RD

- Better Food for Kids
  by Daina Kalnins, RD, CNSD and Joanne Saab, RD

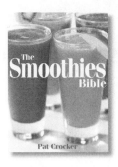

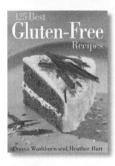

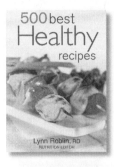

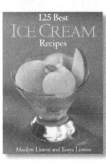

- 500 Best Healthy
  Recipes
  Edited by Lynn Roblin, RD

- 125 Best Gluten-Free
  Recipes
  *by Donna Washburn
  and Heather Butt*

- America's Everyday
  Diabetes Cookbook
  *Edited by Katherine
  E. Younker, MBA, RD*

- Canada's Everyday
  Diabetes Choice
  Recipes
  *Edited by Katherine
  E. Younker, MBA, RD*

- The Diabetes
  Choice Cookbook
  for Canadians
  *Edited by Katherine
  E. Younker, MBA, RD*

- The Best Diabetes
  Cookbook (U.S.)
  *Edited by Katherine
  E. Younker, MBA, RD*

Recent Bestsellers

- 300 Best Comfort
  Food Recipes
  by Johanna Burkhard

- The Convenience Cook
  by Judith Finlayson

- The Spice and
  Herb Bible
  by Ian Hemphill

- 125 Best Ice
  Cream Recipes
  *by Marilyn Linton
  and Tanya Linton*

- 125 Best Casseroles
  & One-Pot Meals
  by Rose Murray

- The Cook's Essential
  Kitchen Dictionary
  by Jacques Rolland

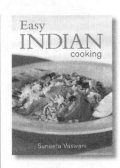

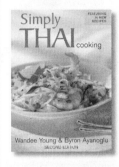

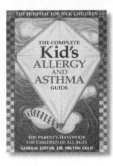

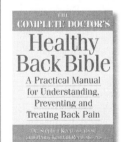

- 125 Best Ground
  Meat Recipes
  by Ilana Simon

- Easy Indian Cooking
  by Suneeta Vaswani

- Simply Thai Cooking
  *by Wandee Young
  and Byron Ayanoglu*

Health

- The Complete
  Natural Medicine
  Guide to the
  50 Most Common
  Medicinal Herbs
  *by Dr. Heather Boon,
  B.Sc.Phm., Ph.D. and
  Michael Smith, B.Pharm,
  M.R.Pharm.S., ND*

- The Complete
  Kid's Allergy and
  Asthma Guide
  Edited by Dr. Milton Gold

- The Complete Natural
  Medicine Guide to
  Breast Cancer
  by Sat Dharam Kaur, ND

- The Complete
  Doctor's Stress
  Solution
  *by Penny Kendall-Reed,
  MSc, ND and Dr. Stephen
  Reed, MD, FRCSC*

- The Complete
  Doctor's Healthy
  Back Bible
  *by Dr. Stephen Reed, MD
  and Penny Kendall-Reed,
  MSc, ND with Dr. Michael
  Ford, MD, FRCSC and
  Dr. Charles Gregory,
  MD, ChB, FRCP(C)*

- Everyday Risks
  in Pregnancy
  & Breastfeeding
  *by Dr. Gideon Koren,
  MD, FRCP(C), ND*

Also Available
from Robert Rose

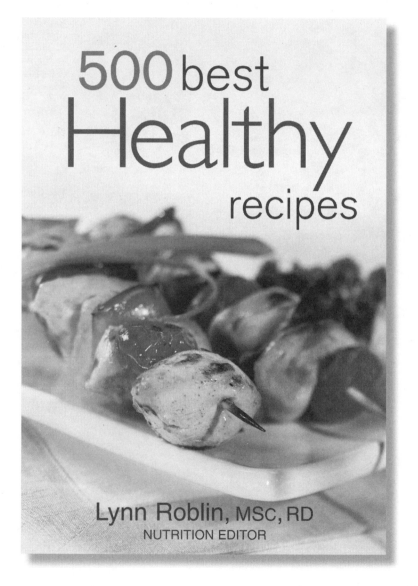

500 best
Healthy
recipes

Lynn Roblin, MSc, RD
NUTRITION EDITOR

For more great books see previous pages